MW01057035

STUDIES ON NEUROPSYCHOLOGY, DEVELOPMENT, AND COGNITION

Series Editor:

Linas Bieliauskas, Ph.D.
University of Michigan, Ann Arbor, MI, USA

To Dana, Sarah, and Megan:
For your assistance, understanding, and love. – S.B.

To my father, S.L. Drexler, my family, and friends. – M.D.

Ethical Issues in Clinical Neuropsychology

EDITED BY

SHANE S. BUSH
AND
MICHAEL L. DREXLER

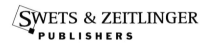
SWETS & ZEITLINGER PUBLISHERS

LISSE   ABINGDON   EXTON (PA)   TOKYO

Library of Congress Cataloging-in-Publication Data

Ethical issues in clinical neuropsychology / edited by Shane S. Bush and Michael L. Drexler.
  p. ; cm. -- (Studies on neuropsychology, development, and cognition ; v. 5)
  Includes bibliographical references and indexes.
  ISBN 9026519249
  1. Clinical neuropsychology--Moral and ethical aspects. I. Bush, Shane S., 1965- II.
Drexler, Michael L., 1954- III. Series
  [DNLM: 1 Ethics, Clinical. 2. Neuropsychology--standards. 3. Ethics, Medical, WL
103.5 E84 2002]
  RC386.6.N48 E876 2002
  174'.2--dc21

                                                                                2001057768

Cover design: Magenta Grafische Producties, Bert Haagsman
Typesetting: Grafische Vormgeving Kanters, Sliedrecht, The Netherlands
Printed by: Krips, Meppel, The Netherlands

ISBN 90 265 1924 9

Contents

From the Series Editor

With changes taking place in the American Psychological Association's *Ethical Principles*, their variability and applicability to differing areas of psychology has been drawn into focus. In particular, there are continuing discussions of the fit between these principles and the needs and practices of Clinical Neuropsychology. This volume, beautifully edited by Shane Bush and Michael Drexler, was designed to fill this void. The chapters address the special areas of attention which focus on assessment and behavioral and cognitive measurement and how those results are interpreted on the best interests of our patients. The volume also focuses on how deliberation of ethical issues applies to differing patient populations, for which neuropsychological services are provided, ranging from age groups to issues concerned with ethnic and cultural diversity and the challenges it presents. Finally, a look at ethical issues with the use of new technologies is explored along with a chapter devoted to that untoward event which we all dread, i.e. what do we do when faced with evidence of ethical violations.

The authors have pulled together current trends and concerns in ethics in a volume which is perhaps more complete than any other in psychology and which certainly is germane to Clinical Neuropsychology. This text will be of significant value for teaching to our developing students as well as extremely useful as a reference for consultation in our daily practice. I commend it to you highly and welcome this wonderful addition to our series.

Linas Bieliauskas
Ann Arbor, December, 2001

Foreword

A single volume comprising a comprehensive discussion of ethics in the burgeoning specialty of neuropsychology has long been needed and eagerly awaited. There is no question regarding the high level of interest in ethical issues among neuropsychologists. Conversation hours and discussion groups at APA and NAN conventions have always been well attended, and characterized by lively and thoughtful exchanges. A large number of excellent articles and book chapters have been published and well received. But until now there has been no single volume in which a broad and comprehensive scope of ethical questions in neuropsychology is discussed. It is gratifying to see that these editors have sought to fill that gap, calling upon leading thinkers in the area, many of whom have served with distinction on Division 40's Ethics Committee and have written compelling discussions on ethical issues in various books and journals. This is a volume that belongs on every practitioner's bookshelf.

The editors' admirable goals were achieved in varying degrees in each chapter. I was particularly pleased to see that they placed primary emphasis on the goal of increasing our sensitivity to ethical issues. Other goals, provision of guidance and extending applicability of existing ethics codes, are helpful only in the context of awareness and sensitivity to ethical concerns, which lead to thoughtful discussion and exchange of ideas. Even as we might seek clear guidance and authoritative interpretation of ethics codes we soon discover the broad range of opinions among thoughtful professionals and the value of trading thoughts and sharing experiences with our colleagues. I regard that as the primary reward of my own involvement with ethics committees: the broadening of my own outlook based upon the introduction of new ideas and new experiences. I predict that readers of this volume will find themselves disagreeing with some of the authors' statements, as I did, but I have no doubt that they will also find their horizons expanded and their judgments sharpened as a result of the ideas and experiences shared here. And I suspect that the editors, and the authors, will be pleased if they have achieved that goal.

Finally, assuming the privilege of providing an editorial opinion of my own, I would call attention to what I consider the most basic and most serious problem we face: that most ethical violations in our field are probably made by practitioners who will not read this book, who are not necessarily insensitive to the specific ethical issues discussed here, but are simply insufficiently trained to practice at a truly professional level. Lacking fundamental knowledge about the brain and its function, about psychometric qualities of tests, base rates, even the range of normal behavior, some practitioners blithely agree to provide neuropsychological consultations, unaware of their own limitations and of the serious consequences of their ignorance. Indeed, I have often felt that this is the fundamental ethical problem in our field, which can be remedied only if we effectively demand high standards of education and training for all who would practice neuropsychology. Responsible leaders have taken laudable steps in this direction, and I would urge everyone to give them our strongest support.

Bruce Becker

Preface

Neuropsychologists struggling with complex ethical issues have few published resources to turn to for guidance. In the neuropsychology literature, few specific clinical vignettes are available as examples of how to handle ethical challenges. When ethical challenges are presented in the literature, they are often without suggestions on how to resolve the challenges. As neuropsychology matures as a profession, an increased awareness of how to apply ethical guidelines to clinical interactions with specific patient populations and in specific clinical settings becomes increasingly important. This book was written to address the need for guidance regarding the application of ethical principles to clinical neuropsychology.

The idea for this book originated at the 1999 conference of the National Academy of Neuropsychology, where we were working together on the NAN Education Committee. Following discussions of ethically complex clinical cases, a search was begun for a comprehensive resource for understanding ethical issues commonly faced by neuropsychologists, as well as a guide for addressing ethical challenges. Inquiries made with the book publishers in attendance revealed a lack of such a resource. During these inquiries, an introduction was made to Jerry Sweet who had co-authored an article in press with The Clinical Neuropsychologist (Grote et al., 2000). Dr. Sweet stated that he was unaware of any book devoted to this topic and offered encouragement to embark upon such a project. Dr. Sweet provided further assistance by recommending Swets and Zeitlinger as a potential publisher, based on his positive experience of recently publishing a book with them (Sweet, 1999). Thus, Dr. Sweet played a major role in the origin of this book, and we are particular thankful to him for his encouragement and guidance throughout the process.

We also wish to express our appreciation to Linas Bieliauskas, the neuropsychology book series editor for Swets and Zeitlinger, for accepting our book into the series and providing guidance and support throughout the process. Arnout Jacobs, editor in charge of this project for Swets and Zeitlinger, was consistently supportive and responsive to our questions, and we are grateful to him for his confidence in our work. Special thanks are extended to the highly qualified and experienced authors of the book's chapters for their continued investment in this critically important but under-represented area of clinical neuropsychology.

References

Grote, C. L., Lewin, J. L., Sweet, J. J., & van Gorp, W. G. (2000). Responses to perceived unethical practices in clinical neuropsychology: Ethical and legal considerations. *The Clinical Neuropsychologist, 14* (1), 119-134.

Sweet, J. J. (Ed.) (1999). *Forensic neuropsychology: Fundamentals and practice*. Lisse: Swets & Zeitlinger Publishers.

Introduction

The American Psychological Association (APA) published the first version of *Ethical Standards of Psychologists* in 1953 in order to provide guidelines for professional conduct for psychologists (APA, 1953). Since that time, the document, commonly referred to as the Ethics Code, has undergone eight revisions. The most recent version of the APA Ethics Code, officially known as the *Ethical Principles of Psychologists and Code of Conduct*, was adopted by APA's Council of Representatives in August of 1992 and went into effect on December 1, 1992. Because the 1992 Ethics Code was designed to provide general guidelines for conducting professional behavior, it has been found difficult to apply to specific situations (Koocher & Keith-Spiegel, 1998). As a result, articles, chapters, and books have been devoted to examining ethical issues in greater detail and in specific contexts. However, relatively little information has been available to guide psychologists with ethical decision making in situations most relevant and specific to clinical neuropsychology. Throughout much of the history of neuropsychology there have been few resources available to the clinician regarding how to identify and address specific ethical issues and dilemmas. Although the Division of Neuropsychology (Division 40) of the American Psychological Association, the National Academy of Neuropsychology, and the International Neuropsychological Society were all in existence by the end of 1975 and the American Board of Clinical Neuropsychology and the American Board of Professional Neuropsychology were incorporated in 1981 and 1982, respectively, it was not until the late 1980s that articles addressing ethical issues began to appear in the neuropsychology literature with some frequency. Although a number of references involving the practice of neuropsychology have discussed relevant ethical issues (e.g., Ackerman & Banks, 1990; Banja, 1989; Bornstein, 1991; Dalby et al., 1989; Franklin et al., 1990; Kreutzer et al., 1990; Matthews et al., 1991; Meyer, 1993; Woody, 1989), the first article to examine neuropsychological assessment with respect to the current Ethics Code was published in 1995 (Binder & Thompson, 1995). A second article addressing ethical challenges in neuropsychology followed later that year (Brittain et al., 1995). In 1998 the first book chapter focusing specifically on ethical issues in neuropsychological assessment with the current ethics code was published (Anderson & Shields, 1998). However, prior to the current work, no books devoted entirely to ethical issues in clinical neuropsychology were available. Thus, this book is an attempt to integrate previous literature and to present issues of emergent importance involving the interface of ethics and neuropsychology. Consistent with the Ethics Code, the overall goal of this book is to promote the welfare and protection of the individuals and groups with whom neuropsychologists work (APA, 1992; Preamble).

The timing of this book has represented both excitement and challenge. The excitement has come from creating the first book of its kind in the maturing field of clinical neuropsychology. Whereas, the challenge has come from the need to create a work that will remain informative and relevant in the face of the anticipated publication of a new version of the Ethics Code. By focusing on the general principles and reasoning processes that underlie ethical decision making and using references to specific sections of the current Ethics Code to illustrate specific points, it is believed that the reader will be able to develop a means of conceptualizing ethical practice that allows for the integration of changes in both ethics codes and standards of practice over the years.

There are three specific goals of this book: (1) to increase sensitivity to ethical issues in clinical neuropsychology, (2) to provide guidance for negotiating difficult ethical situations in the practice of neuropsychology, and (3) to facilitate the process of evaluating the applicability of the Ethics Code to neuropsychological situations. While this book presents numerous clinical vignettes and covers a wide range of clinical situations, it cannot address all possible ethical challenges. Given the complexity and unique characteristics of many ethical problems, no ethics code or reference can provide a solution that is satisfactory to all parties or even agreed upon by all experts within the field. Furthermore, situations may arise in which two or more ethical principles or standards conflict with each other, resulting in an ethical dilemma. In other instances, clinical challenges that may at first appear to represent ethical conflicts may instead reflect professional or legal issues. This book is intended to provide direction for resolving ethical dilemmas and to provide clarification of the often related, yet distinct, ethical, professional, and legal components of neuropsychological practice. It is through the experiences and research of our experienced group of authors that we attempt to achieve our goals.

The current version of the APA ethics code is comprised of six aspirational principles and eight domains of enforceable standards. While most of the principles and standards are relevant to the practice of neuropsychology, the study by Brittain et al., (1995) revealed that the majority (56%) of the primary ethical problems reported by their sample of board certified neuropsychologists involved aspects of assessment practices. Consistent with their findings of the importance of ethical issues related to assessment, the focus of this book is on ethical standard 2 (Evaluation, Assessment, or Intervention) as it applies to neuropsychology. Since ethical challenges rarely involve just one principle or standard (Koocher & Keith-Speigel, 1998), other components of the Ethics Code are discussed when relevant. Readers seeking to understand the relationships of other principles or standards to psychology practice in greater depth are referred to more general ethics texts (e.g., Koocher & Keith-Speigel, 1998).

This book is comprised of two main sections. The first section provides an overview of ethical issues clinical neuropsychology. The second section presents ethical issues in clinical neuropsychology with specific populations and in specific settings in which neuropsychologists often work. Although neuropsychologists work in many more contexts than are covered in this book, the topics covered should provide the reader with an adequate sample of the types of ethical challenges that may be encountered and the processes through which such challenges can be resolved. There is some repetition of the Ethical Principles and Standards throughout the book, as the principles described in Part I are applied to specific clinical situations in Part II. In addition, each chapter in Part II is designed to stand on its own as a resource for a specific setting or with a particular patient population; therefore, some repetition across Part II chapters will be noted as well. However, this repetition may serve to increase the reader's familiarity with the Ethics Code and its application in clinical neuropsychology.

References

Ackerman, R. J., & Banks, M. E. (1990). Computers and ethical treatment for brain-injured patients. *Social Science Computer Review, 8 (1)*, 83-95.

American Psychological Association (1953). *Ethical standards of psychologists.* Washington, DC: Author.

American Psychological Association (1992). *Ethical principles of psychologists and code of conduct.* Washington, DC: Author.

Anderson, R. M. Jr., & Shields, H. (1998). Ethical issues in neuropsychological assessment. In R. M. Anderson, Jr., T. L. Needles, & H. V. Hall (Eds.), *Avoiding ethical misconduct in psychology specialty areas* (pp. 131-141). Springfield, IL: Charles C. Thomas Publisher.

Banja, J. D. (Ed.); (1989). Ethical and legal issues. *Journal of Head Trauma Rehabilitation, 4 (1)*; (Special issue).

Binder, L.M., & Thompson, L.L. (1995). The ethics code and neuropsychological assessment practices. *Archives of Clinical Neuropsychology, 10 (1)*, 27-46.

Bornstein, R. A. (1991). Report of the Division 40 Task Force on Education, Accreditation and Credentialing: Recommendations for education and training of nondoctoral personnel in clinical neuropsychology. *The Clinical Neuropsychologist, 5 (1)*, 20-23.

Brittain, J.L., Frances, J.P., & Barth, J.T. (1995). Ethical issues and dilemmas in neuropsychological practice reported by ABCN diplomates. *Advances in Medical Psychotherapy, 8*, 1-22.

Dalby, J. T., Arboleda-Florez, J., & Seland, T. P. (1989). Somatic delusions following left parietal lobe injury. *Neuropsychiatry, Neuropsychology, and Behavioral Neurology, 2 (4)*, 306-311.

Franklin, G. M., Nelson, L. M., Heaton, R. K., & Filley, C. M. (1990). Clinical perspectives in the identification of cognitive impairment. In S. M. Rao (Ed.), *Neurobehavioral aspects of multiple sclerosis* (pp. 161–174). New York: Oxford University Press.

Koocher, G. P., & Keith-Spiegel, P. (1998). Ethics in psychology: *Professional standards and cases*. New York: Oxford University Press.

Kreutzer, J. S., Harris-Marwitz, J., & Myers, S. L. (1990). Neuropsycholocal issues in litigation following traumatic brain injury. *Neuropsychology, 4 (4)*, 249-259.

Matthews, C.G., Harley, J.P., & Malec, J.F. (1991). Guidelines for computer-assisted neuropsychological rehabilitation and cognitive remediation. *The Clinical Neuropsychologist, 5 (1)*, 3-19.

Meyer, R. G. (1993). *Preparation for board certification and licensing examinations in psychology: The professional, legal, and ethical components.* Louisville, KY: Monkestee Press.

Woody, R. H. (1989). Public policy and legal issues for clinical child neuropsychology. In C. R. Reynolds & E. Janzen-Fletcher (Eds.), *Handbook of clinical child neuropsychology. Critical issues in neuropsychology.* New York: Plenum Press.

PART I

THE APPLICATION OF ETHICAL STANDARD 2 (EVALUATION, ASSESSMENT, OR INTERVENTION) TO CLINICAL NEURO-PSYCHOLOGY

Chapter 1

EVALUATION, DIAGNOSIS, AND INTERVENTIONS IN CLINICAL NEUROPSYCHOLOGY IN GENERAL AND WITH SPECIAL POPULATIONS: AN OVERVIEW

Jerid M. Fisher, Douglas Johnson-Greene, and Jeffery T. Barth

Introduction

The profession of clinical neuropsychology requires a considerable breadth of knowledge, encompasses a broad range of activities, and brings the neuropsychologist into contact with a diverse group of people composed of both consumers and providers of neuropsychological services. While the field of neuropsychology continues to mature, the very breadth and diversity that result in the richness of neuropsychological practice often leads to disagreements, conflicts, and uncertainties regarding optimal practice activities. Neuropsychologists, like all psychologists, have professional forums in which to discuss and debate practice parameters, have colleagues with whom to consult informally, and have a code of ethics that serves as a general guideline for what is considered to be responsible psychological practice. The ethical psychologist must, at a minimum, be competent, objective, and concerned about the best interests of his or her clients, profession, and society.

While there is considerable overlap between the ethical concerns of clinical psychologists and those in specialty areas of practice, such as neuropsychologists, the emphases often differ and unique issues arise. Nevertheless, one code of ethics governs all psychologists. In this book in general, and in this chapter specifically, many of those emphases and unique issues are examined. The current chapter examines ethical issues surrounding evaluation, diagnosis, and intervention in neuropsychology, both generally and with regard to special populations. Due to the experience of the authors of this chapter in forensic neuropsychology, an emphasis is placed on this aspect of neuropsychological practice. Because the clinical activities of many neuropsychologists are, or become, medicolegal or forensic in nature and the potential for ethical challenges in such settings is high, the emphasis on forensic neuropsychology seems warranted. However, it must be emphasized that the forensic issues in this chapter are designed to illustrate the main points of this chapter, and readers are encouraged to refer to the chapter by Sweet, Grote, and van Gorp in this text (Chapter 7) for a comprehensive examination of ethical issues in forensic neuropsychology.

This chapter begins by focusing on the need to define the relationship that the neuropsychologist will have with the examinee. Differences between the traditional treating doctor's role and the role of the forensic expert are then presented. Ethical issues pertinent to informed consent, the clinical interview, and assessment issues are then examined. The chapter concludes with an overview of ethical issues related to special populations.

Defining The Relationship

Before providing a professional service to a consumer, it is the neuropsychologist's responsibility to define, a priori, the relationship he or she is undertaking with this person or retaining party [APA Ethical Standard, 2.01(a)]. While the boundaries between clinical and forensic domains may be blurred at times, the two most common roles for a neuropsychologist are diagnostician/treater/advocate *or* impartial forensic evaluator/non-advocate. It is critical that the neuropsychologist be aware of the fundamental differences between these two roles as this understanding will inoculate him/her against common pitfalls and ethical dilemmas that can arise for colleagues who either fail to appreciate or simply choose to ignore these differences.

The Traditional Treating Doctor Role

The diagnostician/treater/advocate role, also known as a 'treating doctor', occurs when the neuropsychologist is asked to perform an evaluation or intervention with a consumer, on referral by a physician, psychologist, other provider, or in some circumstances at the consumer's direct request. The immediate requirements of this role are to provide timely assessments of the individual's neuropsychological strengths and weaknesses and to accurately communicate these findings to the referral source and the consumer.

This traditional role is defined by the need for the neuropsychologist to act principally as the consumer's advocate. Thus, the neuropsychologist should assign the highest priority to making expeditious diagnostic and treatment decisions on behalf of the consumer; in some contexts this priority supersedes (but does not preclude) the requirement to verify the accuracy of the consumer's claims about his or her past and present history. To illuminate this latter point, while it is desirable to review educational transcripts and standardized test results to confirm or disconfirm the consumer's claims about his or her intellectual accomplishments as well as to provide an estimate of base-line intelligence, the time and effort involved in securing these materials can be both lengthy and cumbersome. Delays created by this process could interfere with the principal responsibilities of the treating doctor role, to render expeditious diagnostic and treatment decisions/recommendations. Thus, the treating doctor's responsibility to act as an expedient advocate may conflict with the responsibility to gather the numerous baseline materials that are required to substantiate the history provided by the consumer. While the ability to meet the consumer's needs in a timely manner is necessary, it is advisable to make reasonable attempts to obtain relevant background information regardless of time pressures.

In outpatient settings, evaluations are often conducted at least a few days after referrals are made; in the interim, the neuropsychologist can initiate efforts to acquire the necessary records. Similarly, in the more urgent situations that often occur in inpatient settings, it may be possible for the treating neuropsychologist to obtain permission to ask family members to bring copies of records to the unit for review prior to submitting the final report. In those situations in which such information is not available, the neuropsychologist should document in the report the information that is missing and the implications that its absence has for the certainty of the conclusions. Failure to temper conclusions in the absence of relevant information could potentially result in erroneous opinions.

When undertaking the treating role, the neuropsychologist should understand that he or she is serving as the consumer's advocate. Advocacy, by definition, requires a departure from impartiality. The neuropsychologist, however, must avoid pressures that often arise when the consumer concurrently pursues litigation against one or more third parties for his or her alleged damages. Under these circumstances, the consumer's attorney may contact the treating neuropsychologist and request forensic opinions about the etiology of positive diagnostic findings or the causal relationship between an acquired injury and the need for specific treatment interventions. The treating neuropsychologist may be overtly or covertly pressured by the attorney to offer a forensic opinion or opinions but should resist succumbing to these pressures because the nature of the treating doctor role, by its very definition, fails to satisfy some basic judicial standards required to offer opinions with reasonable certainty. In addition, the APA Ethical Standard 1.17 (Multiple Relationships) advises against multiple relationships and Standard 7.03 (Forensic Activities) states: "In most circumstances, psychologists avoid performing multiple and potentially conflicting roles in forensic matters...." Similarly, the *Specialty Guidelines for Forensic Psychologists* section IV D (Relationships) states: "Forensic Psychologists recognize potential conflicts of interest in dual relationships with parties to a legal proceeding...." (American Psychology – Law Society, 1991).

The treating neuropsychologist, however, should be ever vigilant to transparent attempts by some attorneys to obtain a 'back door' neuropsychological diagnostic evaluation under the premeditated guise of having a litigant's physician initiate the referral. The most obvious red flag for a 'back door' forensic evaluation is the attorney who contacts the neuropsychologist about conducting an examination, then asserts that it would be easier as well as cost effective if the referral was made by the litigant's physician and paid for by a third party insurer. Agreeing to these circumstances, despite the strictly technical fact that the paper referral has flowed through the physician rather than directly from the attorney, arguably does not relieve the neuropsychologist from the pre-knowledge that his or her examination was conducted in contemplation of litigation (and would likely culminate in the neuropsychologist being asked at some later time to offer an opinion or opinions with a reasonable degree of certainty about the presence and cause of neuropsychological damages).

The *Specialty Guidelines for Forensic Psychologists* (1Bb) sets forth the definition of 'forensic psychology' as "...all forms of professional psychological conduct when acting, with definable foreknowledge, as a psychological expert...." If a treating neuropsychologist performs this hypothetical back door examination with definable foreknowledge of pending litigation and later offers opinions with reasonable certainty to the trier-of-fact, without following the necessary procedures and principles outlined in both the APA Ethics Code (that is, Standard 7.02, Forensic Assessments) and the *Specialty Guidelines for Forensic Psychologists,* then he or she is not immunized or excused from this significant omission error. Under these circumstances, the neuropsychologist should anticipate a cross-examination which demonstrates that he or she had 'definable foreknowledge' of the forensic context of the examination but chose to ignore important procedures that would have elevated his or her opinions to a level of certainty, useful to the trier-of-fact. Further, the neuropsychologist who agrees to conduct a back door assessment has potentially blurred the role between treating doctor and forensic expert (assuming a dual role) and should be concerned about this boundary issue. Additional omission errors may be uncovered and highlighted such as a partial or complete failure to review appropriate archival documents. This

latter responsibility is set forth in Ethical Standard 7.02(a) ("Psychologists'
forensic assessments, recommendations, and reports are based on information and techniques...sufficient to provide appropriate substantiation for their
findings") as well as VI F1 Methods and Procedures of the *Specialty Guidelines for Forensic Psychologists ("*...forensic psychologists attempt to cor-
roborate critical data that form the basis for their professional product").
Informed consent issues may also fail to be appropriately addressed under
these circumstances (see pages 8–9).

The following vignette illustrates some of the difficulties that may ensue
when a back door neuropsychological examination comes under scrutiny by a
colleague who has been hired to serve in a forensic capacity. Neuropsychologist A was retained by the defense to conduct a forensic neuropsychological
evaluation of a plaintiff who sustained a mild head injury in a motor vehicle
accident (MVA). A neuropsychological evaluation had previously been conducted by neuropsychologist B on referral by the plaintiff's primary doctor
(although evidence in the record suggested that this was actually a back door
forensic referral by the plaintiff's attorney). After reviewing neuropsychologist B's report, neuropsychologist A requested additional archival medical
records as it was clear that the plaintiff had a significant pre-MVA neurologic
history, extending to birth (peri-natal cerebral bleed and three months pre-
maturity). An array of archival file materials was requested including birth
and educational records, with the goal of obtaining objective information
about whether this early neurologic trauma resulted in demonstrable neurologic or neuropsychological injuries. The plaintiff's attorney blocked this
discovery request, accusing neuropsychologist A of engaging in a 'fishing
expedition' to 'dig up dirt' on his client, further suggesting that neuropsychologist A was serving as a hired gun for the defense. The plaintiff's attorney then secured an affidavit from neuropsychologist B, that characterized
neuropsychologist's A's record requests as "investigatory research of all possible documentation...however remote". Neuropsychologist B, instead, had
opted to rely on the self-report of the plaintiff and her mother (who was also
a party to the law suit) that there were no lasting neuropsychological or neurologic deficits as a consequence of her early birth complications/peri-natal
cerebral bleed. The court, after hearing arguments from both the plaintiff
and defense attorneys, granted neuropsychologist A's record request.

To avoid a litigation trap with its attendant ethical dilemmas, a neuropsychologist so approached should advise the litigant's attorney that if he or she
desires a comprehensive forensic workup, then the retention of the neuropsychologist and the necessary discovery of pertinent archival file materials must
come directly from the attorney. Absent this option, the neuropsychologist
should include a definitive 'disclaimer' as part of his or her final report that
clearly states that results are intended solely for the treatment and care of the
consumer; the opinions contained in the report are *not* set forth as a forensic opinion with a reasonable degree of neuropsychological certainty. This
disclaimer can also assert that additional assessment, analysis, and record

review would be necessary if forensic issues are to be addressed at a later time. By offering this disclaimer, the treating neuropsychologist effectively prevents an attempt by the litigant's attorney to extract a forensic opinion from the neuropsychologist in the setting of insufficient analysis and review.

The Forensic Expert Role

With increasing frequency, perhaps in response to a growing respect garnered by neuropsychology among attorneys as well as the litigious nature of Western society, neuropsychological professionals are being retained as experts in the context of both civil and criminal litigation. The requirements of the forensic role, however, depart significantly from the traditional treating doctor/ advocate role. In theory, the referral source in the forensic arena (typically an attorney, insurance company, etc.) desires objectivity (vs. advocacy) such that the resulting opinion or opinions of the expert neuropsychologist are credibly grounded in scientific as opposed to hearsay data. Credibility is rooted in a freedom from bias. To achieve the necessary level of objectivity that is required to truly assist the trier-of-fact, the neuropsychologist must resist pressures to serve as a biased advocate while striving to offer impartial data driven opinions. The *Specialty Guidelines for Forensic Psychologists,* in pertinent parts (Methods and Procedures), indicates that "...the forensic psychologist maintains professional integrity by examining the issue at hand from all reasonable perspectives, actively seeking information that will differentially test plausible rival hypotheses" (VIC). This latter requirement, known as 'debiasing', refers to a process in which the forensic neuropsychologist systematically applies strategies to minimize flawed judgments and reasoning. As an example, one practical debiasing strategy for understanding the cause of a low score or scores on neuropsychological testing involves listing all relevant causes for a low test score(s), then systematically eliminating those causes that are unsupported by objective data. Examples of potential causes of low neuropsychological test scores (other than an acquired brain injury) that should be considered in the debiasing process include: pre-injury educational or intellectual limitations; malingering or poor effort during formal testing; presence of a third party observer during formal testing; concurrent use of alcohol or drugs (prescription and/or illicit) that may have a potentially adverse effect on cognition; or other comorbid variables, such as sleep deprivation, pain, depression, or stress. Clearly, absent informing data about these and other potential causes of low test scores, the forensic neuropsychologist will be hampered in his or her ability to satisfactorily execute the debiasing process (as an example, if effort tests are omitted from the testing process, then vital information about this important variable has been sacrificed). It is of paramount importance, therefore, that the forensic examiner incorporate methods in his or her interview and formal evaluation to collect these critical data. These data will aid in the formulation of an informed and unbiased opinion.

In adhering to the above described debiasing process, the expert neuropsychologist is also in compliance with the *Specialty Guidelines for Forensic Psychologists,* pertinent part VII.D: "Forensic psychologists do not, by either commission or omission, participate in a misrepresentation of their evidence, nor do they participate in partisan efforts to avoid, deny, or subvert the presentation of evidence contrary to their position." In essence, the expert should ask himself or herself, 'if I was retained by the other side in this matter, would I offer the same opinion?' An affirmative answer is expected from the expert who strives to offer unbiased opinions to the trier-of-fact.

The burden of maintaining acceptable scientific standards for the field of neuropsychology falls squarely on the shoulders of the forensic practitioner. In theory, the requirement to maintain objectivity and provide qualified scientific opinions to the trier-of fact seems straightforward. However, in practice, the neuropsychologist may find himself or herself pressured (subtly or not so subtly) to deviate from this practice. As an example, some attorneys, representing either plaintiffs or defendants, may attempt to enroll the expert as a member of the "litigation team". These attempts should be recognized by the forensic neuropsychologist as either deliberate or unconscious tools of persuasion that are used by legal counsel (who, by definition, are vigorous advocates for their clients, not unbiased seekers of the truth) to bias the expert in favor of the retaining party. The forensic neuropsychologist should, of course, be familiar with and guided by Rule 702 of the Federal Rules of Evidence, which states: "If scientific, technical or other specialized knowledge will assist the trier of fact to understand the evidence or to determine a fact in issue, a witness qualified as an expert by knowledge, skill, experience, training or education, may testify thereto in the form of an opinion or otherwise."

To appreciate the pressures that are not uncommonly applied to the forensic neuropsychologist, consider a situation in which a neuropsychologist has been retained by plaintiff's counsel to evaluate his or her client with a mild head injury. The plaintiff alleges multiple acquired cognitive and emotional damages as a result of this injury. Formal testing subsequently reveals an array of low test scores. Based on a vague history provided by the plaintiff, suggestions in other file materials, and the neuropsychologist's clinical experience and knowledge of the literature, he or she strongly suspects significant pre-injury problems/limitations that could parsimoniously explain the test results. The forensic neuropsychologist believes that the plaintiff's estimated pre-injury level of functioning does not depart significantly from post-injury damage claims. In this hypothetical case, the neuropsychologist is subsequently informed by plaintiff's counsel that important pre-injury archival records, for example, educational, medical, vocational, etc., cannot be obtained. The neuropsychologist is nevertheless directed to prepare a report in support of the plaintiff's brain damage claims. Despite pressures from plaintiff's counsel to find evidence of brain damage, the forensic neuropsychologist refuses to offer an expert opinion in the absence of the necessary objective baseline of data (see Table 1).

Table 1. Important archival records to review when retained as a forensic neuropsy-
          chologist.

- Educational transcripts and standardized test results
- Cumulative school health files
- Employment and personnel records including supervisory evaluations
- Medical records
- Ambulance & police accident records (if applicable)
- Insurance appraisal and photographs of vehicles (if applicable)
- Military records
- Alcohol or other drug treatment records
- Mental health records
- Income tax returns
- Pharmacy records
- Neuropsychological reports and raw test data
- Legal documents such as the Bill of Particulars & Examinations Before Trial

---

If the neuropsychologist in this hypothetical example succumbed to these
pressures, he or she should anticipate a 'one trial learning experience' in
which he or she is confronted on cross-examination by a well prepared
defense attorney with archival file materials demonstrating a pre-injury level
of functioning in the plaintiff that did not depart significantly from his or her
post-injury level of functioning.

Ploys by the retaining party to minimize the neuropsychologist's objectivity should be vigorously detected and resisted. Since many neuropsychologists
may trace their motivation for entering this field to an abiding desire to help
and assist others, it is easy to understand why deviations from impartiality
can and do occur even among well-intentioned and well-informed practitioners. The neuropsychologist serving in a forensic capacity should constantly
monitor and assess his or her own desire for approval and ask, hypotheti-
cally, if he or she had been retained by the opposing side, would this have
resulted in a different opinion or opinions. Affirmative responses should serve
as red flags for bias. The APA Ethics Code (Standard 7.04, Truthfulness and
Candor) requires honesty and a lack of bias on behalf of the psychologist
performing assessments. While offering reliable and valid forensic opinions
may not always garner popularity from the retaining party, neuropsychologists have an affirmative responsibility to do so. Striving to be an impartial
and careful expert will shape a respected and well-deserved reputation as a
credible and unbiased reporter of data driven opinions, even if said opinions
are unpopular or contrary to what the retaining party may desire to hear.
Doing less, however, will harm both the neuropsychologist's personal reputation and ultimately undermine the trier-of-facts' more general regard for the
scientific credibility of neuropsychology. Further, it is clear that legitimate
attorneys for either plaintiffs or defendants ultimately appreciate knowing the
facts about their client or their potential exposure for damages, respectively,
well before, and not at the time of, trial.

A Division 40 newsletter describes a case (Macartney-Filgate & Snow,
2000) that illustrates many of these ethical issues. This case involved a foren-

sic neuropsychologist who was retained by the defense to evaluate a female plaintiff who sustained a mild concussion in an MVA. This plaintiff had been evaluated, on referral by her attorney, by a clinical psychologist who omitted review of pertinent archival records but subsequently opined that the plaintiff had sustained "...diffuse axonal injury resulting in permanent brain damage rendering her unemployable and posing an increased risk of early onset Alzheimer's disease." An array of 'treatments' was subsequently recommended and then provided by the same psychologist who had been retained by the plaintiff's attorney. The authors discuss the multiple ethical problems created in this vignette including "...dual and conflicting roles, rendering a diagnosis without adequate information and evaluation, practice outside the boundaries of competence, and inappropriate and potentially harmful treatment." While this case may seem, at first blush, like an aberration, in truth, it represents, unfortunately, an all too common occurrence in contemporary neuropsychology.

Considerations In The Event A Forensic Evaluation Is Not Possible

Neuropsychological consultants may be approached for retention after discovery deadlines have passed. This situation is most typically associated with a defendant's representative (lawyers or insurers) who believes that litigation will be settled prior to trial, hence money will be saved by not retaining a neuropsychological expert. When attempts at settlement fail, the neuropsychologist typically receives an eleventh-hour phone call, urgently requesting his or her expertise and opinions on a matter. In this setting, the retaining party may ask the neuropsychologist to review relevant archival file materials and evaluations by other professionals, with the goal of gaining an opinion about the injured party's cognitive and emotional injuries without benefit of an actual examination. Standard 7.02(c) of the Ethics Code cautions, however: "When, despite reasonable efforts, such an examination is not feasible, psychologists clarify the impact of their limited information on the reliability and validity of their reports and testimony, and they appropriately limit the nature and extent of their conclusions and recommendations." Similarly, the *Specialty Guidelines for Forensic Psychologists*, section VI.H states: "Forensic psychologists avoid giving oral or written evidence about the psychological characteristics of particular individuals when they have not had an opportunity to conduct an examination of the individual adequate to the scope of the statements, opinions, or conclusions to be issued. Forensic psychologists make every reasonable effort to conduct such examinations. When it is not possible or feasible to do so, they make clear the impact of such limitations on the reliability and validity of their professional products, evidence, or testimony." Thus, the forensic neuropsychologist who is asked to offer a diagnostic opinion to the trier-of-fact, without benefit of an actual examination, should proceed cautiously.

Assuming that an examination is not possible, what affirmative responsibilities does the neuropsychologist have with respect to accepting or refusing retention as an expert without benefit of an examination? Under these circumstances, the neuropsychologist should explicitly inform the retaining party that he or she is not comfortable offering a diagnosis without benefit of an examination. Many experts are also uncomfortable testifying in court absent a complete examination of the injured party, as they may lack sufficient data to constructively assist the trier-of-fact. Thus, under these circumstances, the neuropsychologist may wish to refrain from testifying about issues involving the injured party's specific diagnosis or extent of damages. These limits should be explicitly set forth with the retaining party, prior to becoming involved with the case.

In specific circumstances, it may be appropriate and beneficial for the trier-of-fact to hear testimony from an expert retained by the defense to provide a 'peer review' of the plaintiff's expert's neuropsychological evaluation. This is indicated when flawed methodologies fail to provide a minimally acceptable level of reliability/validity to support the forensic opinions proffered to the trier-of-fact by the plaintiff's expert. Testimony exposing these flaws is necessary to discourage 'junk neuropsychological science' from misleading the trier-of-fact. Furthermore, such testimony may ensure compliance with Federal Rules 702 & 703 (rules that control the admissibility of scientific evidence in federal courts). Ultimately, forensic neuropsychology will be judged by the quality of the work and the scientific credibility of testimony given at the time of trial. As a profession, we have an affirmative duty to ensure that the trier-of-fact is presented with valid and reliable data that will truly assist with the process of reaching a fair and equitable verdict.

As a general rule, the forensic neuropsychologist should strongly encourage his or her retention early in the litigation process, and discourage last minute consultation. The practice of early involvement allows sufficient time for the forensic neuropsychologist working in a civil setting to identify and acquire the necessary archival background materials (see Table 1) for an objective and comprehensive analysis of the injured person and his or her damage claims. Furthermore, this practice will also allow adequate time for the neuropsychologist to schedule and conduct the plaintiff's examination under more relaxed circumstances. Eleventh-hour examinations are stressful for all parties involved.

Informed Consent

It is the patient's right to receive full and informed consent prior to receiving any psychological services, including neuropsychological evaluations. Informed consent is ideally a shared decision-making process between a patient and their provider, or in the case of forensic neuropsychology, their evaluator. The idealistic goal of informed consent is to promote patient autonomy, a view that stands in stark contrast to the adversarial nature of forensic neuropsychology. A more myopic view shared by some neuropsychologists is that informed consent represents an obligatory practice that is fulfilled when the patient has signed on the dotted line. Indeed, the psychological community is not without neuropsychologists who abhor informed consent doctrine and procedures, perhaps because it highlights possible adverse consequences that may befall the patient, thereby diminishing their openness in the evaluation. What constitutes a reasonable separation between mindless legal requirements and patients' ethical and moral needs for information is at issue.

Historically, informed consent has been more closely associated with the practice of medicine than psychology. Indeed, legal precedents concerning informed consent have all involved patients undergoing medical procedures. Current legal standards uphold a patient's right to be given information consistent with what a 'reasonable man' would want to know prior to providing consent (Mitchell v. Robinson, 1962; Natanson v. Klein, 1960a, 1960b; Salgo v. Leland Stanford Jr. University Board of Trustees, 1957; Schloendorff v. Society of New York Hospital, 1914). The common thread implicit in all legal precedents is the ability to govern the integrity of one's body. There are no legal precedents in case law to date in any jurisdiction for providing informed consent specifically to patients seeking psychological services. However, there are federal statutory requirements for conduct of research (i.e., Guidelines of the National Committee for the Protection of Human Subjects of Biomedical and Behavioral Research), state statutes governing the practice of psychology by licensees, and ethical guidelines applicable to all psychologists who are members of the American Psychological Association (Ethical Principles of Psychologists and Code of Conduct: APA, 1992).

Despite the lack of legal precedent in this area, there is general agreement from an ethical and moral standpoint that informed consent applies to psychological treatment. There is considerably less agreement that informed consent is required for psychological assessment in general, and neuropsychological evaluations specifically (Johnson-Greene et al., 1997). The current ethical standards appear to make a distinction between assessment procedures (i.e., nature of the services) and guidelines for providing assessment results (Standard 2.09). It can be argued that the ethical guidelines pertaining to informed consent to therapy (Standard 4.02) are also applicable to assessment in that psychologists are encouraged to "obtain informed consent to therapy or *related procedures*...." One interpretation of these statements is that clients should be provided informed consent prior to initiation of assessment procedures, though this is not explicitly stated. Unfortunately, informed consent as it relates to assessment is not explicitly stated in the same manner as the guidelines that govern psychological research (Standard 6.11) and treatment (Standard 4.02). This issue has been considered closely by the American Psychological Association, and it appears that the next draft of the *Ethical Principles of Psychologists and Code of Conduct*, which has not been revised since 1992, will make explicit the need for informed consent when conducting psychological or neuropsychological assessments (APA, 2001).

Numerous articles have reviewed issues of informed consent in vulnerable populations. For example, ethical dilemmas associated with conducting research with the elderly have focused on this topic (Argarwal et al., 1996; Franzi et al., 1994; Marson et al., 1995; Wichman & Sandler, 1995). The central theme of these articles and others relates to the difficulty inherent in obtaining informed consent for research from persons who may be, by definition, not competent. One does not have to look far to see a similar irony in neuropsychology where patients are asked to provide informed consent despite being presumed to have cognitive impairments known to impede their ability to understand, conceptualize, consider, and recall important information relevant to their participation. There is a real possibility in neuropsychology that true informed consent can be obtained only from patients who turn out not to have a brain-related illness. Nonetheless, it would not be practical to do a 'mini' neuropsychological evaluation to determine if a person is competent to consent to a complete neuropsychological evaluation

The literature on informed consent and neuropsychological assessment underscores the current lack of clarity in the profession. Johnson-Greene and his colleagues (1997) outlined recommendations for the content and conveyance of informed consent, which they believe should occur prior to any neuropsychological evaluation, including medico-legal evaluations. In contrast, the only comprehensive article outlining ethical recommendations for the conduct of neuropsychological assessment practices argues against the need for informed consent. Binder and Thompson (1994) state that "the current Ethics Code, while requiring informed consent for treatment and related procedures, does not require the patient to give informed consent for assessment." Binder and Thompson (1994) go on to highlight the potential irony of situations in which some patients would "choose not to undergo a neuropsychological evaluation if they fully understood that an abnormal result could jeopardize their normal prerogatives to make important decisions." Such positions, however, may also compromise basic principles of psychology related to promotion of patient autonomy and self-determination.

Binder and Thompson's (1994) comments are not without merit. One dilemma surrounding the achievement of informed consent is that it may actually interfere with the validity of the neuropsychological evaluation. Some patients receiving neuropsychological services may be less disclosing about psychosocial variables, premorbid history, and perceived deficits, or could refuse to participate at all if they were made aware of the potential ramifications of their participation. These fears are not unfounded, as there are several potential undesirable outcomes, from the perspective of the patient, that may occur as a result of receiving these psychological services. For example, in non-medico-legal evaluations it is presumed that the information obtained is confidential. Information could, however, be disclosed against the wishes of the patient, usually as a result of legal mandate. Whether requested specifically by the patient or as a function of legal transactions, this information may affect adversely an individual's rights by denying privileges or freedoms that were previously enjoyed. Also, the ethical injunction to avoid harm (Standard 1.14) is, at times, in opposition with the ambiguities pertaining to issues of confidentiality in psychological practice in situations involving mandated disclosure (i.e., reporting of child abuse, imminent danger to self or others).

Medico-legal evaluations carry their own unique set of circumstances and disclaimers that should be clarified in advance of the evaluation (AP – Law Society, 1991). First and foremost, there is no doctor–patient relationship established in forensic proceedings. As a result, the patient has no expectation that they will be able to discuss the results of the evaluation, receive ongoing services, or have the same expectancy of confidentiality as a patient. Specifically, confidentiality is limited in cases where a person's mental state is an element of their legal proceeding. It is important to note that psychologists are not permitted to discuss aspects of a case that have not been made part of the public record. Other disclaimers that are relevant and should be discussed include clarification of the role of third parties and the adversarial nature of the proceedings.

There are no universally accepted guidelines that can be used to address clinical decisions relating to competency to consent. Indeed, the overwhelming majority of literature in this area has favored commentary and opinion over empirically validated decision models. The standard of practice at present appears to be a matter of securing consent from guardians or relatives when the patient's competency to consent is questionable. Also, the standard of competency tends to vary according to the nature and perceived invasiveness of the procedure. For example, a patient might be held to a higher standard of competence to consent to a potentially risky surgery in comparison to consent for a neuropsychological evaluation. Another maxim for consideration is the notion that patients need only provide assent and not consent for psychological services. A patient's lack of opposition to psychological services is equivalent to assent for the procedure. A standard termed *qui tacit consentiere* (i.e. silence gives assent) supports this argument and is found in English common law extending back to the 13th century.

The matter of what constitutes necessary and sufficient informed consent is an issue for debate itself. Clearly, it would not be pragmatic or desirable to provide to a patient every possible undesirable scenario, no matter how remote, that could result from a neuropsychological evaluation. Rather, it is recommended that an attempt be made to provide a reasonable explanation as to the purpose of the evaluation, the role of all parties involved, the type and nature of the procedures used, and limits of confidentiality. Such disclosure could be tailored to each specific situation depending upon the specific reason for referral for each patient. A list of suggested guidelines is presented in Table 2.

Table 2. Recommendations for providing informed consent to patients receiving psychological services.

- The patient should be provided with a basic description of the intended purpose
  of the service. Also, provide the name of the person(s) requesting the services, if
  this is someone other than the patient.
- Discuss with the patient the procedures to be used in terms that the patient can
  easily understand and, if possible, the estimated length of services. Review all
  applicable fees, financial responsibility, and scheduling issues prior to providing
  services.
- Explain the limits of confidentiality (including the possibility of record disclosure
  due to court subpoena), as well as the foreseeable uses of this information that can
  be reasonably expected given current available information about the patient and
  their reason(s) for medicolegal assessments) or anticipated or lawfully required
  breeches of confidentiality (i.e., mandatory reporting requirements) that are applicable to the patient.
- In instances where information will be placed into a medical record, provide information to the patient concerning the material to be placed in the records and where
  those records are kept.
- Every effort should be made to explain the services in terms that can be easily
  understood. In the event that a patient is unable to express an understanding of the
  services to be offered, consent is obtained, when possible, from a family member
  or legal representative. Informed consent should always be obtained from legal
  guardians prior to assessment of minors.
- Written documentation of informed consent outlining the aforementioned points
  should be obtained from the patient or legal representative prior to providing
  services.

The Clinical Interview in Traditional and Forensic Settings

Ethical Standard 2.01(b) indicates that the neuropsychologist should perform
the necessary and sufficient services to provide appropriate substantiation for
his or her findings (Standard 7.02, Forensic Assessments, is cross-referenced).
When conducting the clinical interview portion of a neuropsychological evaluation, the neuropsychologist has several distinct options. These options fall
into two categories: structured and unstructured interviews. The latter interview is more closely associated with 'bedside' or more informal examinations
of a consumer; questions are created as the interview proceeds. The scope of
questioning is entirely dictated by the interviewer's preferences, knowledge,
interests, and memory. This approach has the potential, if used repetitively
by the same examiner, to resemble a structured interview. However, the neuropsychologist is always vulnerable to bias and the vicissitudes of the moment
(such as forgetting to ask about an important area of functioning). In view
of the availability of published structured interviews, it is advised that the
neuropsychologist adopts this pre-printed format. By using a structured (written) format, the neuropsychologist ensures that he or she conducts a comprehensive interview that represents a standardized approach to data collection.
Furthermore, by relying on a structured interview format, the neuropsycholo-

Table 3. Structured interview information.

- Relevant background information such as age, birth date, marital status, living arrangements, etc.
- Chief complaints and course of each complaint
- History of injury (or illness) including loss of consciousness, presence and types of amnesia, etc.
- Educational history
- Previous assessment results; educational, psychological, neuropsychological
- Vocational history
- Medical history
- Family history
- Military history
- Mental health history
- Criminal history
- Substance use/abuse history
- Prescription regimen
- Rehabilitation history
- Typical daily routine
- Current functional abilities, such as ability to perform household chores, manage finances, prepare meals, etc.
- Ability to independently operate a motor vehicle
- Activities, hobbies, social activities. pre- and post-injury/illness

gist minimizes bias by ensuring that regardless of the setting or who the retaining party may be, virtually the same questions are asked of all interviewees.

A structured interview format is far-ranging in scope and typically inquires into an array of pre- and post-illness/injury areas (see Table 3).

Assessment Techniques: Making an Informed Selection

Current debate among neuropsychologists regarding assessment instruments, techniques, and approaches (for example: flexible vs. fixed battery approach) makes the question of what constitutes "...techniques sufficient to provide appropriate substantiation for their findings" [2.01(b)] controversial. In the interest of avoiding controversy, generic rules are discussed herein for test selection. Most importantly, regardless of the neuropsychologist's approach to assessment, the methods selected should have demonstrated reliability and validity and a good normative base for the consumer that is undergoing the evaluation (Standard 2.04(a) of the ethics code specifically states: "Psychologists who perform interventions or administer, score, interpret, or use assessment techniques are familiar with the reliability, validation, and related standardization or outcome studies of, and proper applications and uses of, the techniques they use.") A methodology to consider in test selection in a forensic context is Heilbrun's (1992) guidelines. Heilbrun's guidelines specify that a test should be commercially available and adequately documented by both a test manual (that appropriately addresses psychometric properties, administration procedures, etc.) and a publication like *Burros Mental Measurements Yearbook*. Examples of other criteria described by Heilbrun include reliability coefficients that exceed 0.80, relevance of the test to the issue, strict adherence to standard administration instructions and procedures as set forth in the test manual, and the test should be appropriate to the population as well as the purpose of the evaluation.

Assessment Techniques: Base Rates

The neuropsychologist should be familiar with the concept of base rates, particularly with relevant base rate data in relationship to tests and procedures used to formulate diagnostic opinions. Knowledge of the degree to which a condition or finding occurs among the general or normal population is essential to proper test interpretation. Standard 2.04(b) states that: "Psychologists recognize limits to the certainty with which diagnoses, judgments, or predictions can be made about individuals." As an example of the importance of knowing about base rates as they apply to statistically vs. clinically significant differences in test interpretation, consider the base rate for a difference of six scaled score points (two standard deviations) between the highest and lowest WAIS-R subtests, among the original WAIS-R standardization sample of 1880 adults. The base rate for such a difference between the highest and lowest subtest was 69%. Heaton and his colleagues (1991) administered the Halstead–Reitan Battery and the WAIS to 455 neurologically normal adults. The base rate for at least one abnormal score on this Battery was 90%. In this regard, Reitan's Impairment Index (derived from 7 HRB test variables) classifies up to two (out of seven) abnormal scores as falling in the normal range (that is, an Impairment Index of 0.0 to 0.30). Insufficient knowledge of base rates for abnormal test performance among normal individuals places a significant restriction on the neuropsychologist's ability to determine when a low test score or pattern of test scores is truly abnormal or simply a manifestation of a 'normal or expected level' of abnormality. Absence or ignorance of base-rate information may encourage the neuropsychologist to over-pathologize his or her interpretations of test results. Neuropsychologists should strive to know base rate information for abnormal test scores or test performance patterns among normal people prior to opining about abnormality on the tests they employ to evaluate neuropsychological functioning.

Assessment with Special Populations

The progress made in neuropsychological evaluation and treatment has resulted in a demand for these services across a diverse array of individuals and venues. Standard 2.04 sets forth psychologists' responsibility to "...identify situations in which particular interventions or assessment techniques or norms may not be applicable or require adjustment in administration or interpretation because of factors such as individuals' gender, age, race, ethnicity, national origin, religion, sexual orientation, disability, language, or socioeconomic status." An array of situations and variables has the potential to pose a significant threat to the use of standard normative data and require scrutiny before proceeding. There are obvious situations in which the goodness-of-fit between the consumer and assessment procedures is poor. Blatant examples include: administering the standard English version of the WAIS-R to a non-English speaker or asking a partially deaf person to take an auditory memory test in which hearing acuity is an essential prerequisite to task performance. More complex and less obvious situations that may confront the neuropsychologist might include, for example, a request to evaluate a 21-year-old consumer, born outside the United States (hence English was not his native tongue), who immigrated to this country and completed both junior and senior high school in the United States. As a bilingual speaker referred for a comprehensive forensic neuropsychological evaluation, should this evaluation be conducted in English or in this person's native language? The solution to this situation is arguably less transparent than the previously described cases.

When a neuropsychologist is asked to evaluate an individual who falls outside the normative basis for standard assessment methods, there are several alternatives to consider before accepting the referral. If the referral involves a person who speaks limited or no English, the most desirable action is to refer the consumer to a qualified colleague who can conduct an evaluation in the consumer's native language. While this is the preferable course of action, it is not always a practical alternative. Neuropsychological resources in many communities may be limited to a small number of qualified practitioners; thus, finding a goodness-of-fit between the consumer's cultural/ language background and the neuropsychologist may be a difficult, if not impossible, task. When referral to a colleague who speaks the same language (as the consumer) is precluded, what other alternatives should the neuropsychologist consider? One alternative is to simply refuse the referral, if the practitioner concludes that he or she is unable to proceed in a valid and reliable manner. A second alternative involves identifying an individual who can fluently understand and speak the consumer's language and is willing to serve as a translator. Particularly in matters of litigation, when a translator is retained, he or she should be a neutral third party without emotional or familial ties to the consumer. Furthermore, it is preferable (although not essential) that the translator possess a background in psychology or social work as well as an understanding of the consumer's cultural heritage and values. While an unbiased and competent translator may enable the neuropsychological practitioner to conduct a valid interview, formal test administration presents a far more daunting task. If the consumer has not been educated in this country and speaks a different language, then Standard 2.04(c) would clearly preclude the use of English-based test materials that rely upon a clear mastery of the English language. In this situation, the neuropsychologist who proceeds with an examination could consider administering only non-verbal tests (with the caveat that non-verbal test materials, while more resistant to language differences, may still be effected by cultural variables) or administer non-verbal tests in conjunction with selected verbal tests that have been appropriately normed in the consumer's native language. As an example, Ardila et al. in *Neuropsychological Evaluation of the Spanish Speaker* (1994) set forth test materials and appropriate norms for the evaluation of a Spanish-speaking consumer. Similar efforts have been reported by others (Campo et al., 2000; Kim & Kang, 1999; Mungas et al., 2000). While these suggestions may permit the assessment process to proceed, when the community of practitioners includes a competent neuropsychologist possessing the cultural and language heritage of the consumer, referral to this professional is preferred.

Other situations, such as the earlier example of a consumer, born outside the United States but subsequently educated in American schools from 7th–12th grades, should be approached differently than the situations just discussed with regard to non-English-speaking consumers. If English is the consumer's second language but the individual received his or her secondary education in this country and has subsequently been employed in an English speaking setting, then a strong argument can be made that English-based assessment measures are more appropriate than using tests in the consumer's native tongue.

In a recent criminal trial, the defendant was born and raised in Italy but had completed his high-school education in the United States and subsequently worked and resided in this country for more than 30 years (he spoke fluent English with an Italian accent). The neuropsychological expert for this defendant, however, faulted (in his written report) the prosecution's expert for conducting the neuropsychological evaluation in English. Examination of raw neuropsychological test data, however, revealed that the defendant actually performed better on English-speaking tests than their equivalent forms in Italian (that were administered by a translator for the defense neuropsychologist). As an example, verbal fluency (FAS word list generation) in English yielded a significantly better performance than the equivalent test in Italian. At the time of trial, the defendant's neuropsychologist was cross-examined with relevant raw test data from these examinations that demonstrated the defendant's superior abilities in English, in contrast to his performance on Italian versions of equivalent. The path to compliance with Ethical Standard 2.04(c) may be obvious in many situations but not always practical. The neuropsychological practitioner is advised to carefully weigh his or her ability to conduct a valid, reliable, and fair examination when the consumer's background deviates from the standard normative base of his or her standard approach to assessment. Whenever the consumer can be referred to a competent practitioner with a similar background, this is the most advisable course of action. As discussed, however, this may not always be possible. Under this less than optimal circumstance, an array of alternatives should be carefully considered by the neuropsychologist, from declining the referral to modifying his or her approach to assessment to allow for the most valid and reliable evaluation.

In the final analysis, common sense, concern for patient welfare, and collegial consultation should guide the practitioner's judgment and decision making when considering issues related to all of these ethical principals and guidelines.

References

Agarwall, M. R., Ferran, J., Ost, K., & Wilson, K. (1996). Ethics of informed consent in dementia research-the debate continues. *International Journal of Geriatric Psychiatry, 11*, 801-806.

American Psychological Association (1992). Ethical principles of psychologists and code of conduct. *American Psychologist, 47*, 1597-1611.

American Psychological Association (2001). Ethical principles and code of conduct draft for comment. *Monitor on Psychology, 32(2)*, 77–89.

American Psychology-Law Society and Division 41 of the APA. (1991). Specialty guidelines for forensic psychologists. *Law and Human Behavior 15*, 655-665.

Ardila, A., Rosselli, M., & Puente, A. (1994). *Neuropsychological evaluation of the Spanish speaker*. New York: Plenum Press.

Binder, L.M., & Thompson, L.L. (1994). The ethics code and neuropsychological assessment practices. *Archives of Clinical Neuropsychology, 10*, 27-46.

Campo, P., Morales, M., & Malpartida, M. (2000). Development of two Spanish versions of the verbal selective reminding test. *Journal of Clinical and Experimental Neuropsychology, 22*, 279-285.

Franzi, C., Orgren, R.A., & Rozance, C. (1994). Informed consent by proxy: A dilemma in long term care research. *Clinical Gerontologist, 15*, 23-34.

Heaton, R., Grant, I., & Mathews, C. (1991). *Comprehensive norms for an expanded Halstead–Reitan battery*. Florida: Psychological Assessment Resources.

Heilbrun, K. (1992). The role of psychological testing in forensic assessment. *Law and Human Behavior, 16*, 257-272.

Johnson-Greene, D., Hardy-Morais, C., Adams, K. M., Hardy, C., & Bergloff, P. (1997). Informed consent and neuropsychological assessment: Ethical considerations and proposed guidelines. *The Clinical Psychologist, 11*, 454-460.

Kim, J., & Kang, Y. (1999) Normative study of the Korean-California Verbal Learning Test (K-CVLT). *The Clinical Neuropsychologist, 13*, 365-369.

Macartney-Filgate, M., & Snow, W (2000). Forensic assessments and professional relations. Division 40 Newsletter 18(2), 28-31.

Marson, D.C., Cody, H.A., Ingram, K.K., & Harrell, L.E. (1995). Assessing the competency of patients with Alzheimer's disease under different legal standards. *Archives of Neurology, 52*, 949-954.

Mitchell v. Robinson, 334 S.W. 2d 11 (1960), reh'g den. 360 S.W 2d. 673 (Mo. 1962).

Mungas, D., Reed, B., Marshall, S., & Gonzalez, H. (2000). Development of psychometrically matched English and Spanish language neuropsychological tests for older persons. *Neuropsychology 14*, 209-223.

Salgo v. Leland Stanford Jr. University Board of Trustees, 154 Cal App 2d 560, 317 p2d 170 (1957).

Schloendorff v. Society of New York Hospital 211 N.Y. 125, 105NE 92 (1914).
Wichman, A., & Sandler, A. (1995). Research in subjects involving dementia and other cognitive impairments: Experience at the NIH, and some unresolved ethical considerations. *Neurology, 45*, 1777-1778

Chapter 2

COMPETENCE AND APPROPRIATE USE OF NEUROPSYCHOLOGICAL ASSESSMENTS AND INTERVENTIONS

A. John McSweeny and Richard I. Naugle

Introduction

This chapter will review and discuss three ethical dilemmas frequently encountered in the use of neuropsychological measures. The first dilemma concerns whether there is an empirical basis for the methods and interpretations made from the results of an evaluation. Second is the prevention of the misuse of test results by the neuropsychologist and by others. This second dilemma encompasses the issue of release of raw data to others. The final dilemma is related to the second and concerns the use of neuropsychological assessment techniques by unqualified persons. The first two dilemmas are covered by Standard 2.02 in the APA Ethics Code (APA, 1992), whereas the third dilemma is covered by Standard 2.06. Each standard and its implications for the behavior of neuropsychologists will be discussed in turn.

Competence and Appropriate Use of Neuropsychological Assessments and Interventions

Standard 2.02: Competence and Appropriateness of Assessments and Interventions

Standard 2.02(a)
" Psychologists who develop, administer, score, interpret, or use psychological assessment techniques, interviews, tests, or instruments do so in a manner and for purposes that are appropriate in light of the research on or evidence of the usefulness and proper application of the techniques" (APA, 1992).

Standard 2.02(a) essentially exhorts psychologists to make their practices, as much as possible, research based, and to be knowledgeable about the instruments they employ. There are several issues related to this advice including test development and test use.

Test Development

Whereas most of the standards in the Ethics Code concern professional practice, standard 2.02(a) first refers to the development of instruments. Many neuropsychologists are interested in developing new instruments or adapting existing psychological instruments for use in neuropsychological application, and it is incumbent on those who wish to do so to follow standard practice for validating and establishing the psychometric characteristics of their instruments. The process of test development and basic psychometric issues, such as the various types of validity, reliability, and normative referencing are well beyond the scope of this chapter. The current 'bible' of standards for test development is the book *Standards for Educational and Psychological Testing* (AERA, APA & NCME, 1999), which was developed as a collaborative project between the APA, the American Education Research Association (AERA), and the National Council on Measurement in Education (NCME). Clearly this is required reading for anyone who is interested in developing or adapting a test for neuropsychological applications. There are also several textbooks on psychological assessment available, such as Anastasi and Urbina (1997), that cover the issues of test development and are recommended to potential test developers or adapters.

If one is adapting a test originally developed for use with other populations for use with neurological populations one cannot assume that the psychometric characteristics reported in the test manual will generalize to the neurologically compromised. Patients with neurological disorders, because of greater variability in performance over time, may provide different test–retest reliability estimates than were obtained with normal populations, for example. Accordingly, new data with neurological populations should be collected regarding the psychometric characteristics before the test is distributed or recommended for clinical use by neuropsychologists.

In addition to establishing validity and other psychometric characteristics before 'releasing' a test for clinical use, it is important to provide sufficient information for clinicians to use it properly. This essentially refers to the development of a test manual that includes clear and unambiguous instructions for administration, scoring, and interpretation of the instrument, as well as information about proper applications and limitations. Finally, the psychometric data and related research that establish the validity for neuropsychological use should also be included. The reader is referred to *Standards for Educational and Psychological Testing* (AERA, APA & NCME, 1999) and/or textbooks on psychometric methods for more information concerning test validation and the necessary components of a test manual.

One particular practice that neuropsychologists should avoid is developing 'home-made' instruments and employing them for clinical purposes in their own practices prior to establishing their psychometric characteristics through research. Preferably such research should be based on more than one practice or institution in order to ensure the generalizability of the psychometric characteristics. Furthermore, if an experimental instrument is included in a test battery administered to a patient, the patient should be informed and consent formally to this. Indeed, most human subject review boards require that research plans for experimental assessment procedures be submitted for review and approval prior to their employment with clinical patients, even if they are not used clinically and only require a few minutes of the patient's time.

Adapting or altering an instrument developed for other purposes for neuropsychological use in one's own practice, prior to validation for such use, is also not advised. Of course, it is quite reasonable for a clinician to use instruments to assess information that is not unique to neurological patients. For example, a neuropsychologist may wish to assess occupational interests in head-injured patients in a vocational rehabilitation program.

Test Use
Section 2.02(a) also underscores the need for clinicians to be mindful of the research concerning the instruments they use in their practices. Clinicians should know for what purposes the instruments can be validly used and what the limitations of the test might be. They should be competent in the use of the tests and other instruments they employ.

Read the test manual
As interpreted by Nagy (2000), Standard 2.02(a) admonishes psychologists to "do things by the book." The best book to start with, in most cases, should be the test manual. The test manual, if properly written, contains the basic information for applications, including psychometric data, instructions for administration, proper applications and limitations, and guidelines for interpretation. It is critical that the clinicians familiarize themselves with a test's manual prior to using the test. This is also true for new versions of a test that neuropsychologist may have used in a previous edition.

We recognize that in practice some neuropsychological test instruments do not have a true manual. Rather, they are described in a research article. Neuropsychologists should be cautious about employing such instruments, especially when the data that support their use come entirely from one publication or even from a small number of publications emanating from a single laboratory.

Know the research and keep current

In addition to reviewing the test manual, it is important for clinical neuropsychologists to stay current with research on the instruments they employ. Often research that has been conducted subsequent to the release of a test manual provides information about the psychometric characteristics with new populations, such as supplementary norms. In some cases, new research allows for extended use. The research by the Mayo Clinic on extended norms for the WAIS-R and WMS-R with older Americans (Ivnik et al., 1992) provides one such example.

Seek training as appropriate

Competence requires learning, and it behooves neuropsychologists who are employing a new instrument or a new edition of an existing instrument to take advantage of Continuing Education programs that might be available. The issue of personal competence is intertwined with several or the ethical standards including 2.06 as discussed later in this chapter.

Train subordinates and others who work with you

This is essentially a corollary of the preceding point. If a neuropsychologist uses the services of a technician or psychometrist, the neuropsychologist should train that individual, or arrange to have the individual trained by others in the proper administration of the tests that the neuropsychologist uses. This issue is also directly addressed by Standard 2.06, as well as by other standards.

Stay with the intended use

This is again consistent with Nagy's (2000) admonition to "do things by the book." Neuropsychologists should avoid utilizing instruments for purposes for which they were not developed or validated. Admittedly, in some cases there is a fine line between reasonable clinical judgment and going beyond an instrument's intended use. Thus, it might be reasonable to make general statements about a head-injured patient's ability to return to work as a pilot based in part on the results of a neuropsychological evaluation, but in most cases it would not be reasonable to offer to assess pilot candidates for their potential success based on the results of typical neuropsychological tests.

Do not shorten or otherwise alter tests absent supportive research

Neuropsychologists often find themselves being pressured by managed-care organizations or hospital administrators to shorten their examinations or otherwise 'speed things up.' There may be a temptation to employ short forms of standard instruments or simply to shorten test instructions. However, unless there is clear evidence that short-forms provide equivalent data to longer versions, they should be avoided. Likewise, altering test instructions could alter a patient's performance on the test and is therefore not recommended. Nagy (2000) simply states, "do not use short cuts."

Standard 2.02(b)
"Psychologists refrain from misuse of assessment techniques, interventions, results and interpretations, and take reasonable steps to prevent others from misusing the information these techniques provide. This includes refraining releasing raw test results or raw data to persons, other to patients or clients as appropriate, who are not qualified to use such information (See also Standards 1.02, Relationships of Ethics and Law, and 1.04, Boundaries of Competence)" (APA, 1992).

Standard 2.02(b) has generated much discussion and criticism amongst neuropsychologists, both informally and in the literature. This is particularly true of neuropsychologists who perform forensic work who often find themselves presented with a subpoena from an attorney to submit all records in their possession to the attorney. "All records" would presumably include copies of test data record forms and score summary forms.

A key question about Standard 2.02(b) concerns its intent. We do not have access to the thoughts of the persons who originally drafted Standard 2.02(b), but the general intent would seem to encourage psychologists to take some responsibility for the data they collect for their evaluations, even when those data might be used by others. An obvious extension of this principle is incorporated as well, that is, taking responsibility for who has access to this information. It is this extension that has been the cause of so much controversy. Most psychologists, including neuropsychologists, are quite willing to take responsibility for their own data but have difficulty with the idea that they should take responsibility for who has access to their data, preferring to leave that responsibility to the patient or the patient's legally designated representative.

Another intent of Standard 2.02(b) appears to be the protection of the patient from the misinterpretation or other misuse of the data a psychologist collects. A frequent example that we have encountered in workshops involves the misuse of personality test data collected by a psychologist as part of a pre-employment evaluation in a corporation. In this example, the personality test answer sheet falls into the hands of a personnel officer who proceeds with recording individual responses into the employee's personnel file. This example is clear in its implications and illustrates the general wisdom of Standard 2.02(b). However, it is less clear as to how the release of neuropsychological data, with the possible exception of personality and IQ data, to non-neuropsychologists might be harmful in many cases, given that the numbers and individual responses may be meaningless to those who are not trained in neuropsychology. Furthermore, some neuropsychologists have suggested that attempting to restrict access to neuropsychological data by attorneys in the context of a legal contest places the neuropsychologists in a difficult and unnecessary legal situation and creates the impression that they have something to hide.

A second question that frequently arises in the context of discussions of Standard 2.02(b) is the definition of what constitutes 'raw test results' or 'raw data.' Do these terms refer to the sheets used to record individual responses, including those that are copyrighted, to score summary sheets, or both? For many attorneys the answer is simple: 'All of the above.'

A third question concerns who is 'qualified' to receive raw data from a neuropsychological evaluation. A few neuropsychologists have taken a very narrow view and suggested that only another clinical neuropsychologist is qualified to receive and evaluate neuropsychological data. However, given that there is no universally accepted definition of a clinical neuropsychologist at present, this places the neuropsychologist who is considering releasing the data in the awkward position of deciding whether or not the other psychologist is a 'real' clinical neuropsychologist. A somewhat less restrictive and more defensible point-of-view is that neuropsychological data may be released to another psychologist, whether or not he or she is a clinical neuropsychologist. An argument in favor of this approach is that all psychologists are bound by the same code of ethics to practice within one's bounds of competence. Accordingly, if the psychologist who receives the data is 'not qualified' by training to practice neuropsychology, he or she should adhere to the APA Ethics Code (1992) and decline to evaluate the data received. This strategy relieves the neuropsychologist with the data of evaluating the qualifications of the psychologist who is receiving the data and assumes the psychologist receiving the data will conduct a self-evaluation. This position is often seen as a reasonable compromise between being overly restrictive and overly 'loose' and is consistent with the interpretation of the code by Canter et al. (1994).

Some have noted, on the other hand, that some non-psychologists, including a few neurologists and psychiatrists, have had formal neuropsychological training, whereas most psychologists have not. These non-psychologists are usually well known to the neuropsychology community and in some cases are considered leaders in the field, including serving as editors of neuropsychological journals or publishing textbooks on clinical neuropsychology. Therefore, is it not hypocritical to refuse these non-psychologists neuropsychological data but then pass the data on to a psychologist who is probably not qualified to interpret them? The answer, although not entirely satisfactory, would seem to be that there is always an exception to every rule. Certainly there are a handful of non-psychologists who are quite qualified to interpret neuropsychological data, and it is appropriate to release neuropsychological data to them.

One apparently contradictory aspect of Standard 2.02(b) is that it allows psychologists to release data to "patients and clients as appropriate" although one would assume that in most cases these persons would not be qualified to interpret these data. However, it would seem that the intent of this provision is to recognize the overriding right of patients to have access to the data from their medical and psychological evaluations. Most jurisdictions also recognize the legal rights of patients to have access to their medical and psychological records.

Subpoenas of raw data
As noted previously, clinical neuropsychologists often find that their records, including score summaries, and even copyrighted response recording forms, can be accessed through the serving of a subpoena. However, the receipt of a subpoena does not necessarily require a neuropsychologist to automatically release the data to an attorney or another person who is unqualified to interpret them. The power and scope of a subpoena vary according to the court district, language and source. In most districts a court order signed by a judge should be considered as mandatory. Although the APA Ethics Code requires that conflicts between the Code and law be resolved "in a responsible manner" (Standard 1.02), it does not require that a neuropsychologist resist a court order.

In contrast to a court order, a subpoena signed by an attorney or a court clerk is usually negotiable. In either case, the neuropsychologist may ask that the data be supplied to another psychologist in an effort to limit the potential for abuse. Canter et al. (1994) also note that some judges will conduct an *"in camera"* (in chamber) review of data when one party has raised concerns about the release of certain evidence prior to granting release. The specific avenues available to a neuropsychologist within a specific district may be well known to more experienced forensic colleagues. Of course, it is usually prudent to seek legal advice prior to resisting a subpoena.

Routine appending of neuropsychological data summaries to reports
Some neuropsychologists routinely append a summary of neuropsychological test scores to their reports, which is a practice that has been recommended by Freides (1993) and others. The goal of appending a test-score summary is to facilitate repeated evaluations by neuropsychologists who are not in the same locale or who are at the same locale at different times. Essentially the test-score summary serves as a convenient method of communication amongst neuropsychologists. However, we have argued that routinely attaching a test score summary to reports may violate the spirit, if not the letter, of Standard 2.02(b) (Naugle & McSweeny, 1995, 1996). When a neuropsychologist *routinely* appends a test score summary, he or she is surrendering the data to who ever might receive a copy of the report either directly or indirectly. In essence, the neuropsychologist is taking *no* responsibility to ascertain the user's qualifications to interpret neuropsychological test results or to prevent

the misuse of the data once it has left his or her office. Of course, there may be many times when it makes perfect sense to attach a data summary to a report, such as when one is communicating with another neuropsychologist. In addition we believe that not providing data summaries to clinical neuropsychologists who request them with the written permission of patients is indefensible. However, we do recommend that the neuropsychologist appending the data summary should follow the logic of Standard 2.02(b) as well as the advice of most textbooks on assessment to tailor reports to the needs and expertise of the recipient. This requires that the neuropsychologist deliberately consider the issue of an appended summary on case-by-case basis rather than appending such a summary routinely.

Standard 2.06: Unqualified persons

"Psychologists do not promote the use of psychological assessment techniques by unqualified persons" (APA, 1992).

Personal Competence

As we noted previously, the issue of personal competence is intertwined with several of the ethical standards in the APA Ethics Code. The standard most directly concerned with this issue is 1.04, Boundaries of Competence. However, Standard 2.06, in addressing the issue of use of psychological assessment by unqualified persons, also implies that the psychologists who use assessment techniques should be personally competent in their use. Accordingly, we will begin this section with additional discussion of the issue of personal competence before moving on to the issue of the competence of supervisees, students, colleagues and other persons in using psychological assessment techniques.

It is commonly accepted that neuropsychologists, like other psychologists, base their scientific or professional judgments on a thorough understanding of their area of expertise. That understanding is typically obtained through years of formal coursework and extensive training under close, direct supervision by experienced and knowledgeable neuropsychologists. Once trained, neuropsychologists take steps to maintain their competence by keeping up with the scientific literature and by attending conferences and workshops to hone their understanding of various areas within neuropsychology. Only by keeping current with continuing advances in the field can one provide state of the art clinical care. The neuropsychologist whose practice relies on knowledge gained only from graduate coursework cannot improve beyond the level that he/she practiced at the time that coursework ended. The clinical skills of such an individual are doomed to atrophy and the quality of clinical service will stagnate accordingly. Recognition of the need to remain current in the advances of one's field has led most state boards to require a specified number of continuing education credit hours in order to renew one's license to practice psychology. In so doing, state boards responsible for the licensure of psychologists intend to maintain the competence of those already licensed.

It is imperative that psychologists accurately appraise their competencies and limit their professional activities to those areas in which they have sufficient education, training and experience. When faced with a referral whose needs require clinical services that the neuropsychologist cannot provide, referral to another professional is in order.

A problem exists, however, for those who practice in underserved geographic areas or provide services to underserved populations. In such situations, although the psychologist might not have obtained the necessary competence to provide the requested service, he/she may provide those services in order to ensure that the patient is not denied any intervention whatsoever. It is important, however, that the psychologist make a reasonable effort to obtain the necessary competence to provide the service in question or refer the patient to an appropriately trained provider as soon as possible.

Consider the neuropsychologist who, despite limited experience providing services to children during her training, provides services to adult patients in a rural area in the Midwest. She is miles from the nearest city and knows of no pediatric neuropsychologists within a 300-mile radius. She is referred a ten-year-old who is being considered for special education services due to learning difficulty. His parents have requested testing in order to determine what type of placement would best meet his academic needs. If the neuropsychologist were not to provide these services to the best of her ability, the student would be denied important services. Rather, it could be argued that the neuropsychologist would be best advised to consult with a colleague regarding the testing and its interpretation and provide the service.

These same issues arise when non-English speaking patients are referred for evaluation. Some have clearly stated the position that no patient should be tested in a language other than his/her own, and by a neuropsychologist who understands the subtleties of the patient's culture (Artiola i Fortuny & Mullaney, 1998). Where understanding of language, ethnicity, national origin, or socioeconomic status significantly impacts the results of one's testing, psychologists must either have or obtain the training and experience or supervision via consultation necessary to ensure that they are capable of providing such service or refer the patient to a more suitable provider. If unable to do either, testing through an interpreter may be a defensible alternative, depending upon the purpose of the testing.

Consider the case of an Arabic-speaking male who comes to the United States for a medical examination due to medically refractory seizures. He is not able to speak English, but comes for his appointments accompanied by an interpreter provided by the medical institution. His evaluation reveals that his seizures originate from the right temporal lobe and his MRI reveals a right temporal tumor. The intention of the referring epileptologist is to obtain a baseline level of ability prior to surgery, which had been scheduled to take place the following day. The neuropsychologist reluctantly agrees to the evaluation but limits the battery to those measures that are primarily visuospatial in nature and acknowledges the limitations of the results of the testing. The purpose of the testing is to establish the patient's presurgical ability on those measures as a point of comparison for his postsurgical performance. The goal, then, is not to establish his level of ability relative to a normative standard but to compare his pre- and postsurgical abilities. In this instance, the use of the interpreter to complete the testing provides the referral source with the information that is being sought, and does not impose harm on the patient by misconstruing his performance relative to an inappropriate normative standard.

In some instances, however, training and experience might not be available and referral to an appropriately trained psychologist might not be possible. To master a new technology or technique about which nobody has yet been educated and trained, the psychologist must take action to learn to the best of his or her ability the requisite skills to develop an expertise in that new area.

While the primary purpose of the standards concerning personal competence in the code is to protect patients/clients in clinical settings, it is possible to extend the principles to research as well. Consider a neuropsychologist with an interest in established neuroimaging techniques, such as MRI and PET, who might have been approached to consider developing a course of research regarding fMRI. Adherence to standards in the code concerning personal competence could be interpreted as suggesting that neuropsychologists should not avail themselves of such opportunities absent additional training. The main purpose of the code is to protect clients/patients, students, research participants, and others from harm at the hands of the practitioner who is ill equipped to provide services. But failing to develop a familiarity with fMRI might also be regarded as a disservice to patients by denying them the future benefits of that new technology. Adherence to the spirit of the code might lead the neuropsychologist to take a different tack. In emerging areas in which generally recognized standards and preparatory training do not yet exist, psychologists nevertheless should take all reasonable steps to ensure the competence of their work. Without experience in the area and no other neuropsychologists yet trained in the application of fMRI to neurologic patients, the neuropsychologist should either develop a familiarity through interactions with other specialists or through reading relevant literature. By doing so, the neuropsychologist can master new technologies for which formal training is not yet available.

Competence of Supervisees, Students, Colleagues and Others

Standard 2.06 appears to relate most directly to the situation in which a psychologist is in a supervisory role with another person. Clinical neuropsychologists frequently employ the services of a psychological technician or psychometrist who administers the majority, or in some cases all, of the tests. Neuropsychologists in academic settings or training hospitals will also recognize that 2.06 applies to students, interns, post-doctoral fellows and other trainees. Finally, many neuropsychologists will receive requests from psychology and non-psychology colleagues to borrow tests, provide them with test catalogs, or 'show me how to use this stuff.' In these situations the neuro-psychologist should consider the ultimate consequences of providing psycho-logical assessment tools to others.

Just as psychologists limit their services to those within the bounds of their competence, based on their appropriate education, training, super-vised experience, consultation, study or professional experience, they do not require, encourage or accept the work of others that exceeds their compe-tence. Toward this end, it is incumbent upon supervisors to properly train their supervisees and take steps to ascertain in an ongoing way that those supervisees execute their responsibilities in an manner that is in accordance with the Ethics Code. The portions of the Ethics Code regarding the compe-tence of individuals to conduct psychological assessments are particularly relevant to neuropsychologists by virtue of their reliance on neuropsychologi-cal test data and, frequently, the use of technicians or 'psychometrists' to collect those data. It should be noted that the administration of neuropsy-chological measures is not synonymous with 'assessment techniques.' For the purposes of this discussion, 'assessment techniques' encompasses the selec-tion, administration, and scoring of neuropsychological measures, and the integration and interpretation of the data provided by those measures in the context of the patient's academic, vocational, and medical history, including the results of relevant medical, radiological, and other tests. In the context of this conceptualization, testing is an important but small part of the evaluation process; the mastery of test administration does not enable one to conduct meaningful and useful clinical examinations of patients. Whereas it might be relatively easy to master the standardized administration of neuropsycho-logical measures and calculate the scores produced by those measures, the examination of patients requires considerably more knowledge and integra-tion of other information.

The use of bachelor's level technicians to administer and score psychologi-cal measures is commonplace and readily defensible. Using those individuals to prepare reports and assign diagnoses on the basis of those test data is not. The accurate interpretation and application of psychological measures requires training and experience that cannot be easily or quickly provided. In the case of neuropsychologists using technicians or individuals in train-ing, such as students, interns or postdoctoral fellows, the supervising neu-ropsychologist must ascertain that the supervisee has developed the requisite skills to complete the assigned responsibilities associated with his/her posi-tion. That is, psychologists who assign portions of their duties to employees, supervisees, and others or who use the services of others, including interpret-ers, must limit those assignments to tasks that the supervisee(s) can perform competently on the basis of his/her education, training, or experience, either independently or with the level of supervision being provided, and must take reasonable steps to ascertain that the individual performs those services com-petently.

Obviously, in the event that the neuropsychologist deems it appropriate to use an interpreter to administer neuropsychological measures as in the above case example, the interpreter is also considered a supervisee and must be provided with ample instruction and direction to ascertain that he or she has properly administered measures using instructions that are as close as possible to the standard instructions for each measure. The patient's responses should be carefully transcribed and subjected to scoring criteria that correspond as closely as possible to those used in the course of the routine administration of test items. It is important to note, however, that even with an interpreter experienced in the administration of neuropsychological measures, the results of testing of individuals in languages other than their primary language must be interpreted with considerable caution. Although non-English speaking patients might provide responses that can be scored, those scores cannot be assumed to carry the same meaning as those obtained from individuals who more closely match the normative group on which the standards of the test were based.

Unavoidable cultural factors affect individual's responses, and their potential influence must be recognized. The report describing the evaluation of the patient who is not English-speaking must include caveats regarding the application of tests that were developed and normed on English speaking individuals raised in the United States. Although their scores cannot be assumed to accurately characterize their performance relative to an appropriate reference group, those scores may establish their baseline performance prior to an intervention. That baseline might then be used to determine the impact of the intervention, but interpretation of those change scores is fraught with the same complications.

These notions are codified under *Standard 1.22: Delegation to and Supervision of Subordinates:*

> *"(a) Psychologists delegate to their employees, supervisees, and research assistants only those responsibilities that such persons can reasonably be expected to perform competently, on the basis of their education, training, or experience, either independently or with the level of supervision being provided.*
>
> *(b) Psychologists provide proper training and supervision to their employees or supervisees and take reasonable steps to see that such persons perform services responsibly, competently, and ethically.*
>
> *(c) If institutional policies, procedures, or practices prevent fulfillment of this obligation, psychologists attempt to modify their role or to correct the situation to the extent feasible."*

Failure to provide adequate supervision to individuals executing the various responsibilities associated with neuropsychological assessments potentially invalidates the entire examination. There are obvious risks associated with the employment of individuals with inadequate clinical skills. The risks of misdiagnosing a patient's condition are considerable. Failure to identify the etiology of neurocognitive changes is particularly damaging among individuals with progressive brain disease or expanding lesions. In the absence of correct identification and potential treatment, cognitive deterioration in those patients will certainly progress. Furthermore, if brain disease is erroneously excluded from the differential diagnosis and a functional or psychiatric disorder is assumed to be the cause of the patient's cognitive changes, the patient might receive costly psychiatric treatment from which little or no benefit will be gained.

There are additional risks to the public associated with an inadequate understanding of professional issues such as maintaining test security. Supervisees who have not been properly educated and trained are less likely to appreciate the threat posed by the indiscriminate circulation of test items or test protocols. Disclosing protocols to individuals outside of our field could lead to the widespread circulation of test stimuli. This release of materials may be an infringement of the proprietary rights of the copyright holders since a large portion of the content of the test items is included on the test protocols. Moreover, the ready availability of test items could seriously impair the validity and integrity of neuropsychological test instruments. Allowing the widespread release and potential abuse of test items and responses would potentially undermine those measures that provide much of the data upon which neuropsychologists base their professional opinions. To the extent that test items become part of the public domain, patients could be harmed. The public clearly has an interest in preserving the confidentiality and, thus, the validity of psychological and neuropsychological tests.

Consider the case of the technician who, during his training to administer neuropsychological measures, was encouraged to take testing materials home to review instructions, practice laying out test materials, and review scoring criteria. Two years later, after several of the tests had been replaced with newer versions due to wear and tear on the supplies, the technician decides to sell the original test supplies to an undergraduate student, who, in turn, reads the test manuals and practices administering the measures to his friends and neighbors in order to get some experience with neuropsychological testing prior to a course on the subject. In the event that any of those individuals who had been exposed to the test stimuli were later referred for neuropsychological examinations, they might be expected to show a 'practice effect' by virtue of their familiarity with those stimuli. To the extent that their performance on some neuropsychological measures benefited from that exposure, the interpretation of their neuropsychological profiles might be affected.

Although we have focused on supervisees in this section, many of the principles discussed also apply to the situation of under-qualified colleagues, whether they are psychologists or not. Neuropsychologists need to carefully consider requests for loans of testing materials or equipment as well as requests for instruction or assistance in obtaining or using such materials or equipment. If it is apparent that the colleague intends to engage in neuropsychological assessment without proper training, the neuropsychologist may need to say 'no' despite the risk of alienating the colleague. However, such a denial of assistance or cooperation might be accompanied with encouragement or instruction on how to obtain proper training. We should emphasize that in some cases it might be perfectly reasonable to loan colleagues materials and equipment to perform assessments that are not neuropsychological in nature. Indeed, many of the assessment tools used by neuropsychologists were developed for other purposes. The primary issue is whether colleagues intend to use the instruments for purposes for which they are not qualified.

Conclusions

Clearly, establishing the boundaries of one's competence and ascertaining the competence of one's supervisees, students and colleagues can be complicated. Few standards exist that specify the minimal competency needed to perform each assessment task; psychologists are expected to make those determinations in light of their own competencies and limitations and a thorough understanding of the demands of neuropsychological assessment techniques. As with many aspects of the ethics code, fully understanding the basis of the ethical standards regarding competence and the implications of potential breaches of the code help the neuropsychologist make informed and well-reasoned decisions about professional activities.

References

American Educational Research Association, American Psychological Association, National Council on Measurement in Education (1999). *Standards for educational and psychological testing*. Washington, DC: American Educational Research Association.

American Psychological Association (1992). Ethical principles of psychologists and code of conduct. *American Psychologist, 47*, 1597-1611.

Anastasi, A., and Urbina, S. (1997). *Psychological Testing* (7th ed.). Upper Saddle River, NJ: Prentice Hall.

Artiola i Fortuny, L., & Mullaney, H.A. (1998). Assessing patients whose language you do not know: Can the absurd be ethical? *The Clinical Neuropsychologist, 12*, 113-126.

Canter, M.B., Nagy, T.F., Jones, S.E., & Bennett, B.E. (1994). *Ethics for psychologists: A commentary on the APA Ethical Principles of Psychologists and Code of Conduct*. Washington DC: American Psychological Association.

Freides, D. (1993). Proposed standard of professional practice: Neuropsychological reports display all quantitative data. *The Clinical Neuropsychologist, 7*, 234-235.

Ivnik, R. J., Malec, J. F., Smith, G. E., Tangalos, E. G., Petersen, R. C., Kokmen, E., & Kurland, L. T. (1992). Mayo's Older Americans Normative Studies: WAIS-R, WMS-R and AVLT Norms for Ages 56 through 97. *The Clinical Neuropsychologist, 6*, Supplement, 1-104.

Nagy, T. F. (2000). *Ethics in plain English: An illustrative casebook for psychologists.* Washington, DC: American Psychological Association.

Naugle, R.I., & McSweeny, A.J. (1995). On the practice of routinely appending neuropsychological data to reports. *The Clinical Neuropsychologist, 9,* 245-247.

Naugle, R.I., & McSweeny, A.J. (1996). More thoughts on the practice of routinely appending raw data to reports: Response to Freides and Matarazzo. *The Clinical Neuropsychologist, 10,* 313-314.

Chapter 3

ETHICAL ISSUES IN TEST CONSTRUCTION, SELECTION, AND SECURITY

Robert M. Anderson, Jr. & Ann M. Palozzi

Introduction

This chapter will discuss the ethics of test construction, test selection, and test security. At first glance, it might seem unnecessary to have a chapter on these topics. We have the ethical principles, and the standards are reasonably specific in spelling out the do's and don'ts for psychologists (American Psychological Association [APA], 1992). Why then do we need chapters like this one and books about ethical issues in clinical neuropsychology?

The answer to this question is complex and provides a framework for our analysis in this chapter. First of all, ethical considerations are often complex, as complex as human life, and contain elements not specifically delineated in a set of ethical standards. Secondly, additional complexity is introduced in specialized areas of clinical psychology, such as clinical neuropsychology where inferences to and from brain function and behavior are added to the psychologist's area of expertise (Anderson, 1994; Anderson & Shields, 1998). Thirdly, ethical situations often involve conflicts: (1) conflicts between the interests of different parties to which one has an ethical-professional duty, (2) conflicts between ethical principles, (3) conflicts between the principles and one's personal morality (Schumacher, 1998), and (4) conflicts between the principles and the law. Lastly, the ethical principles themselves may be subject to ethical criticism. They may be examined for consistency in application and scrutinized from the perspective of more fundamental values, values from which the principles derive their credibility. As practicing psychologist we rarely take ethical issues to this level; however, for the ethical well-being of clinical neuropsychology, it is helpful to occasionally transcend our professional self-interest and look at the issues from a more inclusive perspective.

Ethical problems arise for people, professionals and clients, in specific situations. For this reason we will use fictional but realistic vignettes to examine ethical issues that may arise regarding test construction, test selection, and test security. In analyzing each example, we will take a bottom-up approach. We will look first at the vignettes on the most concrete level. We will attempt to answer the question, 'Given the complexity and conflicts in the described situation, what is the appropriate application of the ethical principles?' We will also attempt to address any ethical issues specific to clinical neuropsychology. We will then take our analysis to a meta-level and critique the ethical principles themselves. Unless otherwise indicated, references to Ethical Standards refer to the 1992 APA Ethics Code.

Test Construction

Vignette 1

Dr. King uses a flexible battery approach to neuropsychological testing. To fill a gap in the set of tests that he relies on when constructing batteries, he designs a test that he believes can assess verbal and conceptual flexibility. Surprise Story (SS) consists of a short story for which the patient must write five different endings: humorous, sad, logical, aggressive, and joyful. The SS is quantitatively scored for level of flexible thinking, composition, writing mechanics, and fluency. Dr. King first piloted his test on his ten male staff members in his clinic. He then administered it to 40 Caucasian male mild head injury outpatients at the King Institute of Psychology. He markets his test via flyers sent to psychologists in his state. The flyers read as follows: Surprise Story — Use this brief new test to measure cognitive flexibility, the ability to shift set, and the capacity to solve novel problems in children and adults with cortical impairments. Surprise Story is comprised of an unfinished story. The endings, provided by the patient, are scored quantitatively. Normative data are available from individuals both with and without brain injury.

Relevant Ethical Standards

2.02(a) Psychologists who develop, administer, score, interpret, or use psychological assessment techniques, interviews, tests, or instruments do so in a manner and for purposes that are appropriate in light of the research on or evidence of the usefulness and proper application of the techniques.

2.03 Psychologists who develop and conduct research with tests and other assessment techniques use specific procedures and current professional knowledge for test design, standardization, validation, reduction or elimination of bias, and recommendations for use.

Discussion

In developing and marketing his test, did Dr. King meet these two standards? To determine this, one could consult the *Standards for Educational and Psychological Testing* (American Educational Research Association, 1999) for a more detailed description of the professional expectations for psychological test development. One could also consult texts on test construction by experts in the field regarding current expectations for adequate test development. In Dr. King's case, a student who had taken an undergraduate course in tests and measurement could probably see that the development of the Surprise Test was inadequate. The normative sample is not representative, there is no reliability data, and the test has not been formally validated.

Other issues arise regarding the subjects that he used for piloting the test. Since his employees and patients were used as subjects, there may have been an element of coercion in their participation. Questions to be considered include the following: Did Dr. King protect these individuals from potential adverse consequences of declining or withdrawing from participation [Standard 6.11(c)]? Did Dr. King bill for the administration of a test that was in the research and development stage?

Due to the extremely inadequate development of the test, Dr. King's claims about the test in the flyers may be seen as false and unwarranted. He may have violated Standard 3.03(a), *Avoidance of False or Deceptive Statements*.

The Dr. King vignette is clear-cut and can be addressed through straightforward application of Ethical Standards 2.02(a) and 2.03. The following example is more complex and subtle and demonstrates that a knee-jerk application of these Standards is not always appropriate.

Vignette 2

Dr. Loose has developed a method for describing and analyzing test behavior for a well-accepted and standardized test marketed by a major test publisher. The method contains some test items, scales, and testing procedures that were not part of the original standardized test. Normative data, reliability, and validity are minimal or, for some scales, entirely lacking. Claims are made that the method can assist in the diagnosis of cognitive deficits and brain dysfunction. The test publisher publishes the method, and it is marketed as an adjunctive qualitative procedure useful for diagnosing cognitive impairments and brain dysfunction. Dr. Tight lodges an ethics complaint with the APA Ethics Committee alleging violations by Dr. Loose of Standards 2.02 and 2.03.

Discussion

In this vignette it is not clear that there has been a violation of these Standards. The method is presented not as a means by which the psychologist can collect and analyze quantitative data but as a procedure by which meaningful qualitative data can be collected. Since some validity studies have been completed and experts have found the procedure to be useful, it is probably appropriate to conclude that the procedure has some usefulness or validity. Dr. Tight might argue that conclusions about cognitive impairments and brain dysfunction should not be made on the basis of normless, qualitative data. In doing so, Dr. Tight would open up the philosophical-scientific debate between advocates of qualitative approaches and supporters of purely quantitative approaches to test data interpretation in clinical neuropsychology. He would find, however, that many of the most prominent clinical neuropsychologists support a qualitative approach (Kaplan, 1988; Lezak, 1995; Walsh, 1991), at least as an adjunct to quantitative approaches. Even strong supporters of quantitative approaches, such as Golden et al. (1985), provide extensive descriptions of the qualitative use of data from the Luria Nebraska Neuropsychological Battery. Given the controversy and divided opinion in the field, Dr. Tight would be likely to have great difficulty advancing her allegations further.

Test Selection

Vignette 3

An eight-year-old Hawaiian-Chinese boy, Pono, who has documented absence seizures, was referred to Dr. Dudly for a neuropsychological evaluation to determine the nature and extent of his educational difficulties. Previous WISC-III testing conducted by school personnel revealed a Full Scale I.Q. of 55. Based on this one test, he was classified as a Special Education Student and diagnosed as having moderate mental retardation. Pono's parents objected to this diagnosis. They reported that his primary language is Hawaiian, that he only had a vocabulary of 50 to 100 English words, and that he cannot fully comprehend directions provided in English. Without interviewing Bono, his parents, or school personnel, Dr. Dudley decided to measure Pono's cognitive ability with the Leiter International Performance Scale and the Bender Visual Motor Gestalt Test.

Relevant Ethical Standards

2.04(a) Psychologists who perform interventions or administer, score, interpret, or use assessment techniques are familiar with the reliability, validation, and related standardization or outcome studies of, and proper application and uses of, the techniques they use.
2.04(b) Psychologists recognize limits to the certainty with which diagnoses, judgments, or predictions can be made about individuals.
2.04(c) Psychologists attempt to identify situations in which particular interventions or assessment techniques or norms may not be applicable or may require adjustment in administration or interpretation because of factors such as individual's gender, age, race, ethnicity, national origin, religion, sexual orientation, disability, language, or socioeconomic status.

2.07(a) Psychologists do not base their assessment or intervention decisions or recommendations on data or test results that are outdated for the current purpose.

2.07(b) Similarly, psychologists do not base such decisions or recommendations on tests and measures that are obsolete and not useful for the current purpose.

Discussion

Dr. Dudley appears to be conforming to 2.07(a) in that she is not simply accepting the old test results as definitive of Pono's intellectual capacity. She is also attempting to comply with 2.04(c) by using tests that require little language competence and may, therefore, provide a better measurement of Pono's intelligence than the WISC-III. The Leiter can be administered using gestures and are solely manual manipulations. Unfortunately, the Leiter that she is using has norms that are more than 30 years old and would likely provide an inaccurate measure of intelligence. In addition, many areas of cognitive, motor, and sensory functioning would not be assessed with this set of tests. The addition of the Bender Gestalt Test would add a constructional component, but this combination of measures would appear to be far from adequate.

Dr. Dudly, lacking fluency in the Hawaiian language, would probably not be the ideal neuropsychologist for this assessment. However, even with a Hawaiian-fluent examiner, there would be numerous methodological hurdles to be overcome in such an assessment (Fletcher-Janzen et al., 2000).

Test Security

Vignette 4

Rudy is a 17-year-old boy who suffered viral meningitis during his junior year of high school. Prior to this infection, he maintained a 3.7 GPA. The infection resulted in impairments with speech, auditory information processing, concentration, sequencing, cognitive flexibility, and auditory and visual memory. Rudy spent six months in the Higgins Rehabilitation Hospital. He was evaluated by his school's neuropsychological consultant, Dr. Wise, prior to his return to school. Dr. Wise noted that Rudy's scores were in the superior range on the Rey Auditory Verbal Learning Test (Spreen & Strauss, 1998) and on the Benton Visual Retention Test-Revised (Sivan, 1992). When discussing the results with Rudy and his parents, Dr. Wise noted the scores and the wide discrepancy between scores on similar tests. At this juncture, Rudy stated that he 'practiced' those tests with his speech therapist (Mr. Lang) and at home every day for the past month.

Relevant Ethical Standards

2.10 Maintaining Test Security. Psychologists make reasonable efforts to maintain the integrity and security of tests and other assessment

techniques consistent with law and other contractual obligations, and in a manner that permits compliance with the requirements of this Ethics Code.
2.06 Unqualified Persons. Psychologists do not promote the use of psychological assessment techniques by unqualified persons.

Discussion

First of all, this vignette underscores the importance of asking patients whether they have had prior experience with the tests being administered in a neuropsychological battery. Even if Dr. Wise responded to this information in a minimal way by dropping these tests from his battery and not contacting the speech therapist, he probably would not be seen as promoting the use of psychological assessment techniques by unqualified persons. Nevertheless, he would probably be well advised to contact Dr. Lang and inform him, in a diplomatic way, that the Benton Visual Retention Test-Revised is classified as a level C product by The Psychological Corporation (2001) and requires specialized training (Wong, 1998). Mr. Lang could also be informed about how his misuse of the test resulted in invalid results for the that measure on the neuropsychological evaluation and about how breaching test security is a violation of the purchaser's agreement with The Psychological Corporation.

Since Mr. Lang is not a psychologist, the APA Ethics Code does not govern his behavior. If Mr. Lang does not seem to appreciate the harm resulting from his actions, Dr. Wise might consider reporting him to the local speech therapy licensing board or to the American Speech and Hearing Association. Mr. Lang might be seen to be in violation of the American Speech and Hearing Association's code of Ethics (1994).

Vignette 5

Dr. Friendly is a clinical neuropsychologist with a thriving private practice specializing in assessment of, and therapy with, traumatically brain-injured individuals. She receives a subpoena requesting the release of any and all records of her patient, Mr. Hurt, to an attorney, Mr. Sue. Apparently, Mr. Hurt has filed a lawsuit, and Mr. Sue is the defendant's attorney. After receiving written consent from her patient, Dr. Friendly provides the attorney with a report and a statement that raw data and test protocols have not been included because to do so would require that she violate the Ethics Code. Dr. Friendly then receives a call from Mr. Sue who demands that she turn over all of the data to him immediately. She sites the Ethics Code and suggests that she could turn all of the data over to a qualified psychologist of his choosing. He responds that he is not ready to retain an expert yet and that she must turn over all of her data to him. He threatens that if she doesn't do as he asks, he will be forced to obtain a court order, and she will have to pay the cost of his doing so.

Relevant Ethical Standards

2.10 Maintaining Test Security, as stated above.

2.02(b) Psychologists refrain from the misuse of assessment techniques, interventions, results, and interpretations and take reasonable steps to prevent others from misusing the information these techniques provide. This includes refraining from releasing raw test results or raw data to persons, other than to patients or clients as appropriate, who are not qualified to use such information.

1.02. If psychologists' ethical responsibilities conflict with the law, psychologists make known their commitment to the Ethics Code and take steps to resolve the conflict in a responsible manner.

Discussion

Dr. Friendly appears to be doing her best to maintain test security. However, she is in danger of capitulating due to the significant pressure that she is experiencing from the attorney. She could benefit from some specific guidelines for how she should proceed at this point. Fortunately, an algorithm has been proposed by the National Academy of Neuropsychology (2000b, 2000c) for responding to subpoena's for records.

Although Ethical Standard 2.02(b) is commonly accepted without question by psychologists, it is possible to see that there are some problems with the standard if we take our analysis to a higher critical level. Certainly there are compelling reasons for maintaining test security (APA, 1999). If information about a secure test is made public and made known to an individual who is to be assessed with the test, that individual may produce an inaccurate score. Inferences may be made on the basis of that score which could result in harm. There have been clear cases in which information about tests has been used by attorneys to coach clients and thereby subvert the assessment process (Youngjohn, 1995). If information about a secure test is made public, it will damage the usefulness of the test. If the test is not useful, it will not be purchased, and publishers will not be able to recover the money spent in test development and make a profit. If developing and marketing tests is no longer profitable, publishers will cease publishing tests, and tests would not be available. This would be a great loss for the public and for the profession of clinical neuropsychology.

On the other hand, an extremely rigid policy on test security could be harmful to some patients (Anderson & Shields, 1998). For example, a patient may wish to know more about the tests she has been administered than is provided in the feedback they receive from the neuropsychologist. According to Principle D, "Psychologists accord appropriate respect to the fundamental rights, dignity, and worth of all people. They respect the rights of individuals to privacy, confidentiality, *self-determination*, and *autonomy*, mindful that legal and other obligations may lead to inconsistency and conflict with the exercise of these rights" (italics added). It would seem that we, as a profession, are lacking in respect for the autonomy and self-determination of our clients when we deny them knowledge of procedures and instruments by which they are assessed. This secrecy does not have an analog in most professions. An attorney's client can, in principle, have access to all of the legal information available to the attorney. There are not secret sections of law libraries.

Another more controversial issue that arises out of the above vignette is the appropriateness of including raw test data in neuropsychological reports. The strictest interpretation of Standard 2.02(b) is that absolutely no raw data should be present in a report. According to this interpretation, it would be unethical to include a grip strength measurement in a neuropsychological report. But such practice would seem to be overly restrictive. Raw data, such as grip strength scores, can be easily comprehended by most healthcare professionals, and its inclusion in reports can actually help referral sources obtain a clearer understanding of the patient's capabilities. If test security is not violated, there would seem to be little reason not to include raw data in situations in which the data increases the recipient's knowledge. Such information would seem to be much less susceptible to misinterpretation than phrases such as "moderately impaired executive functioning," which are so vague as to be almost meaningless. If a primary purpose of Standard 2.02(b) is to encourage psychologists to prevent the misinterpretation and misuse of psychological evaluations, then this exception to the raw data rule would seem appropriate.

A much more extreme departure from Standard 2.02(b) has been proposed. Freides (1993) has suggested that all quantitative data be routinely appended to neuropsychological reports. According to Freides, this would make reports more efficient because data would not be located in the body of the report. If would make reports less biased because all of the data would be present in the appendix. Data would be available for comparison when retesting is performed. This proposal has been energetically debated (Freides, 1995; Matarazzo, 1995; Naugle & McSweeny, 1995). The primary problem with Freides' proposal is that it would provide referral sources and patients with a set of raw data with no clear explanatory context. This would be likely to lead to misinterpretation and misuse of results, exactly what 2.02(b) was formulated to prevent. To meet Freides' goal of facilitating comparisons across evaluations, subsequent evaluators need only to contact the previous neuropsychologist and request the original data.

Vignette 6

Dr. Smart, who has limited forensic experience, is hired by an attorney, Mr. Gladiator, to perform a thorough neuropsychological evaluation of his client, Ms. Hurt. Dr. Smart is to document any cognitive deficits that are due to brain trauma caused by a motor vehicle accident and to provide an opinion regarding Ms. Hurt's prognosis. Dr. Smart receives a call from Ms. Jugular, the attorney hired by the defendant's insurance company, who demands that she be present during the evaluation. Dr. Smart expresses concerns about test security and threats to the validity of the evaluation. Ms. Jugular is unmoved. Dr. Smart then communicates these concerns to Mr. Gladiator. Rather than supporting Dr. Smart, Mr. Gladiator insists that he be present also. In the face of this pressure from both attorneys, Dr. Smart reluctantly agrees to the presence of the attorneys.

Discussion

In agreeing to third-party observation without further protest, Dr. Smart may be violating several ethical and professional standards. First of all, test security would be violated by having an unqualified third-party observer present. Secondly, according to the National Academy of Neuropsychology (2000a), the presence of a third-party observer during the administration of formal test procedures creates the potential for distraction or interruptions and may, therefore, compromise the validity of the examination. Also, since neuropsychological tests are normed under conditions in which no third-party observer is present, the presence of a third-party observer introduces an extraneous variable into the testing situation which may make established norms inapplicable and preclude valid inferences from the test data. Therefore, the National Academy of Neuropsychology (2000a) concludes that "neuropsychologists should strive to minimize all influences that may compromise accuracy of assessment and should make every effort to exclude observers from the evaluation" (p. 380). Dr. Smart might have dealt with this situation in a more effective manner if she had obtained a mentor to guide her through her initial forensic cases (Tsushima & Anderson, 1996).

Having stated our profession's official position on third party observers, let us now take our analysis up one level and subject this position to criticism. The first problems for the official position is that there is very little research on the effect of third-party observers on neuropsychological evaluations (Lynch, 1997). The effect size and circumstances under which there is a greater effect are virtually unknown. This fact is especially troubling when the NAN Statement distinguishes between potential third-party observers that should be forbidden to observe neuropsychological evaluations — court reporters, attorneys, and attorney representatives — versus third-party observers who may observe – students, other professionals in psychology, and parents. It is argued the "trainees have sufficient instruction and supervision in standardized measurement and clinical procedures, such that their presence would not interfere with the assessment process" (National Academy of Neuropsychology, 2000a; p. 380). No evidence or study is cited in support of this statement. If we are to have an official statement that is based on evidence and not merely professional opinion, we should provide empirical support for statements such as this one.

A policy statement for the American Academy of Clinical Neuropsychology made the distinction between involved observers and uninvolved observers (Hamsher et al., 1999). An involved third party is someone who has some investment in the outcome of the examination, such as an attorney, whereas an uninvolved third party, such as a student, has no stake in the outcome.

In a recent survey of NAN members that resulted in 817 respondents, 70% indicated that they would consider it acceptable to have either a neuropsychologist or a trained technician observe examinations (Sewick et al., 1999). That is, of the responding NAN membership, 70% agreed that observation by a trained third party poses no threat to test security, standardization concerns, or ethical behavior of neuropsychologists. Thus, issues of observer training, observer involvement, and examination context have all been considered relevant in discussions of the appropriateness of third-party presence during neuropsychological evaluations.

Videotaping and audiotaping have also been discussed as less intrusive means of monitoring the examination process. However, these procedures may also impact the evaluation process in unknown, and potentially harmful, ways.

Conclusion

In this chapter the ethics of test construction, test selection, and test security were reviewed. Many of the issues involved are at the core of ethical debate in neuropsychology, and the field does not appear to be approaching consensus at this time. As more and more neuropsychologists continue to turn to the forensic arena for referral sources in this time of diminishing income from managed care, the ability to anticipate, identify, and successfully negotiate ethical challenges will become increasingly important. By reviewing these professional issues, the relevant sections of the Ethics Code, and their clinical application, it is hoped that the reader has gained an increased appreciation of factors contributing to ethical neuropsychological practice.

References

American Educational Research Association, American Psychological Association, National Council on Measurement in Education (1999). *Standards for educational and psychological testing*. Washington, D.C.: American Educational Research Association.

American Psychological Association (1992). Ethical principles of psychologists and code of conduct. *American Psychologist, 47*, 1597-1611.

American Psychological Association (1999). Test security: Protecting the integrity of tests. *American Psychologist, 54*, 1078.

American Speech and Hearing Association (1994). Code of ethics. Available at: http://professional.asha.org/library/code of ethics.htm.

Anderson, R.M. (1994). *Practitioner's guide to clinical neuropsychology*. New York: Plenum Press.

Anderson, R.M., & Shields, H. (1998). Ethical issues in neuropsychological assessment. In R.M. Anderson, Jr., T.L. Needles, & H.V. Hall (Eds.), *Avoiding ethical misconduct in psychology specialty areas*. Springfield, IL: Charles C. Thomas Publisher, Ltd.

Fletcher-Janzen, E., Strickland, T.L., & Reynolds, C.R. (Eds.) (2000). *Handbook of cross-cultural neuropsychology*. New York: Kluver/Plenum.

Freides, D. (1993). Proposed standard of professional practice: Neuropsychological reports display all quantitative data. *The Clinical Neuropsychologist, 7*, 234-235.

Freides, D. (1995). Interpretations are more benign than data. *The Clinical Neuropsychologist, 9*, 248.

Golden, C.J., Purisch, A.D., & Hammeke, T.A. (1985). *Luria-Nebraska Neuropsychological Battery: Forms I and II Manual*. Los Angeles: Western Psychological Services.

Hamsher, K., Baron, I.S., & Lee, G.P. (1999). *Third party observers: Policy Statement for the American Academy of Clinical Neuropsychology*.

Kaplan, E. (1988). A process approach to neuropsychological assessment. In T. Boll & B.K. Bryant (Eds.), *Clinical neuropsychology and brain function: Research, measurement, and practice* (pp. 129-167). Washington, DC: American Psychological Association.

Lezak, M.D. (1995). *Neuropsychological assessment* (3rd ed.). New York: Oxford University Press.

Lynch, J. (1997). The effect of observer's presence on neuropsychological test performance: A test of social facilitation phenomenon. *Dissertation Abstracts International: Section B: The Sciences and Engineering, 57(11-B)*: 7230.

Matarazzo, R.G. (1995). Psychological report standards in neuropsychology. *The Clinical Neuropsychologist, 9*, 248-250.

National Academy of Neuropsychology (2000a). Presence of third party observers during neuropsychological testing: Official statement of the National Academy of Neuropsychology. *Archives of Clinical Neuropsychology, 15*, 379-380.

National Academy of Neuropsychology (2000b). Test security: Official statement of the National Academy of Neuropsychology. *Archives of Clinical Neuropsychology, 15*, 383-386.

National Academy of Neuropsychology (2000c). Test security: Official statement of the National Academy of Neuropsychology. *National Academy of Neuropsychology Bulletin, 15*, 5-7.

Naugle, R., & McSweeny, J. (1995). On the practice of routinely appending neuropsychological data to reports. *The Clinical Neuropsychologist, 9*, 245-247.

Schumacher, J.A. (1998). Philosophy, ethical theory, and the APA Ethical Principles. In R.M. Anderson, Jr., T.L. Needles, & H.V. Hall (Eds.), *Avoiding ethical misconduct in psychology specialty areas* (pp. 7-25). Springfield, IL: Charles C. Thomas Publisher, Ltd.

Sewick, B.G., Blase, J.J., & Besecker, T. (1999). Third party observers in neuropsychological testing: A 1999 survey of NAN members [abstract]. *Archives of Clinical Neuropsychology, 14*, 753-754.

Sivan, A.B. (1992). *Benton Visual Retention Test* (5th ed.). San Antonio, TX: The Psychological Corporation.

Spreen, O., & Strauss, E. (1998). *A compendium of neuropsychological tests: Administration, norms, and commentary*. New York: Oxford University Press.

The Psychological Corporation (2001). *The catalog for neuropsychological assessment and intervention resources* [Catalog]. San Antonio, TX: Author.

Tsushima, W.T., & Anderson, R.M. (1996). *Mastering expert testimony: A courtroom handbook for mental health practitioners*. Mahwah, NJ: Lawrence Erlbaum Associates.

Walsh, K.W. (1991). *Understanding brain damage: A primer of neuropsychological evaluation* (2nd ed.). Edinburgh: Churchill Livingston.

Wong, T.M. (1998). Ethical issues in the evaluation and treatment of brain injury. In R.M. Anderson, Jr., T.L. Needles, & H.V. Hall (Eds.), *Avoiding ethical misconduct in psychology specialty areas* (pp. 187-200). Springfield, IL: Charles C. Thomas Publisher, Ltd.

Youngjohn, J.R. (1995). Confirmed attorney coaching prior to neuropsychological examination. *Psychological Assessment, 2,* 279-283.

Chapter 4

ETHICAL ISSUES IN INTERPRETING AND EXPLAINING NEUROPSYCHOLOGICAL ASSESSMENT RESULTS

Laetitia L. Thompson

Introduction

Given the emphasis on assessment in neuropsychology and the fact that most clinical neuropsychologist practitioners devote considerable time to performing, interpreting, and explaining neuropsychological test results to patients, ethical issues in this area deserve serious consideration and discussion. As noted by Koocher and Keith-Spiegel (1998), "One cannot underestimate the political and social significance psychological testing has come to have in America, and the converse impact of public attitudes to the field of psychometrics" (p.145). Messick (1999) asserted that not only should tests be evaluated in terms of their measurement properties, testing applications should be evaluated in terms of their potential social consequences. This latter task involves evaluating the present and future consequences of interpretation and use and brings ethics as well as science to the forefront of discussion.

In this chapter, the focus will be on Sections 2.05, *Interpreting Assessment Results* and 2.09, *Explaining Assessment Results* of the American Psychological Association's (APA) Ethical Principles of Psychologists and Code of Conduct (referred to as the Ethics Code; American Psychological Association, 1992). Obviously, many other sections of the Ethics Code apply in interpreting and explaining assessment results; these will be identified and discussed as appropriate. Another excellent source of information and guidance regarding interpretation and explanation of assessment results is the recently published *Standards for Educational and Psychological Testing* (American Educational Research Association, American Psychological Association, National Council on Measurement in Education, 1999).

It is important and instructive to keep in mind that the ethical 'rules' of test interpretation and explanation ultimately tie back to the Ethical Principles, which are portrayed as 'aspirational goals' rather than enforceable rules for conduct. The six Principles form the basis for all of the Standards in the Ethics Code, provide the underlying rationale for making ethical decisions, and assist in complex or conflictual cases where the appropriate course(s) of action is (are) ambiguous.

The Ethics Code principle of *Competence* (Principle A) reminds us that we only interpret those neuropsychological tests for which we are qualified to do so by education, training, and/or experience. Further, it is incumbent upon neuropsychologists performing assessments to know relevant scientific and professional information related to the tests and procedures they use. It is also imperative to recognize that attaining competence in neuropsychological assessment does not imply a static concept; therefore maintaining competence involves ongoing education and continual updating of knowledge and procedures.

Principle B, *Integrity,* emphasizes the need to be honest, fair, and respectful of others. This involves considering all of the data in neuropsychological assessments, even data that seem discrepant or unsupportive of the primary hypothesis. Moreover, integrity means involving the patient from the outset in explaining the purpose of the evaluation, how assessment results will be communicated, and what the psychologist's role is.

Principle C refers to *Professional and Scientific Responsibility*. In neuropsychological assessment, several aspects apply. The principle refers to "clarifying professional roles and obligation." This overlaps with Integrity in apprising the patient as fully as possible of the assessment situation and the possible consequences of the results. Principle C also refers to adapting methods to the needs of different populations. In neuropsychological assessment, this involves considering demographic and cultural factors in interpreting test results. This principle would also apply to interpreting the test results of individuals with peripheral impairments (blindness, paralysis, etc.) that necessitate modifying testing procedures and then dealing with interpretation of non-standard testing. Finally, Principle C refers to taking appropriate responsibility by obtaining consultation with colleagues, when needed.

Principle D: *Respect for People's Rights and Dignity* is extremely important in neuropsychological interpretation and in the explanation of the interpretation to patients. This principle emphasizes respect for privacy and confidentiality of the information as well as an understanding of individual differences and a respect for diversity.

Principle E pertains to *Concern for Others' Welfare*. This is fundamental to all clinical work with patients, and the terms *beneficence* and *non-maleficence* most succinctly describe this principle. In both interpreting and explaining assessment results to patients, psychologists consider the welfare of the patient and, above all, attempt to do no harm.

Principle F: *Social Responsibility* relates to neuropsychological assessment primarily in two ways. Psychologists attempt to prevent the misuse of neuropsychological assessment results, and psychologists are encouraged to contribute a portion of their time for little or no personal advantage. In a neuropsychology assessment practice, this might involve seeing patients with limited financial resources.

The remainder of the chapter focuses on the more concrete, specific, and enforceable ethical standards through discussion and presentation of scenarios that may commonly arise in neuropsychological practice. The above principles serve as important guideposts in situations that are complex, murky, and/or ambiguous. When I am tempted to get 'stuck' in thinking too concretely or rigidly about an ethical standard, I find it useful to reflect back on the six aspirational principles to refocus on the underlying philosophical reasons for ethical reasoning and behavior.

Section 2.05, Interpreting Assessment Results

Section 2.05 of the Ethics Code states:

> "*When interpreting assessment results, including automated interpretations, psychologists take into account the various test factors and characteristics of the person being assessed that might affect psychologists' judgments or reduce the accuracy of their interpretations. They indicate any significant reservations they have about the accuracy or limitations of their interpretations.*"

In his excellent book on the APA Ethics Code for psychologists, *Ethics in plain English*, Nagy (2000) translated Section 2.05 as follows:

> "In assessing others, always remember to consider both (a) the characteristics of the person and (b) the test factors themselves that might affect your judgment or reduce the usefulness of the results. Also be sure to disclose any reservations you may have, out loud or in writing, when giving your results or creating a report" (p. 67).

For the purpose of discussing the ethics of interpretation in neuropsychological assessment in this chapter, Section 2.05 is subdivided into four major areas. In addition to test factors, patient characteristics, and reservations about interpretation alluded to by Nagy, the use of automated interpretations also will be discussed.

Test Factors in Interpretation

Although given brief attention in the Ethics code, this provision covers a range of significant issues in neuropsychological assessment. This section implies that neuropsychologists not only use tests that have acceptable psychometric properties in general (Section 1.04, *Boundaries of Competence*), but that neuropsychologists know and use information about the tests that are applicable in the individual evaluation context (see also Section 2.02, *Competent and Appropriate Use of Assessment and Intervention*). To the extent that there are test factors that might affect the accuracy/utility of the interpretation, it is incumbent upon the neuropsychologist to consider those test factors carefully. A number of these issues are cogently presented in Koocher and Keith-Spiegel (1998) in their discussion of ethical issues in the broader realm of psychological assessment. Accurate and meaningful interpretation of scores requires an understanding of the psychometric properties of the test including the standard error of measurement, test–retest reliability, criterion-related and construct validity, and what represents reliable change over time. For example, interpretation relies upon knowledge of the normative data that are available and how closely the normative sample resembles the patient being assessed (Mitrushina et al., 1999). Consideration of the appropriateness of the norms needs to address whether there is potential cultural or language bias, what the age and ethnic background of the normative group are, and whether norms were derived from small or idiosyncratic samples of subjects (Section 1.06 of the Ethics Code, *Basis for Scientific and Professional Judgment,* is also relevant to consider in this regard).

Neuropsychologists need to consider whether the test was, in fact, administered in the standardized manner, or, in the case of some tests or procedures, which one of several standardized administration and scoring procedures was followed. If several different administration procedures are described in the published literature, the administration and scoring procedures used in the clinical context must match the administration procedures used for the group upon which the normative data were collected in order for the interpretation to be valid.

The Ethics Code emphasizes that the neuropsychologist must practice only within areas of competence (see Ethics Code Standards 1.04, *Boundaries of Competence,* and 2.04, *Competent and Appropriate Use of Assessment and Intervention*). Competence is not a static phenomenon; as new research is published, neuropsychologists must incorporate new findings into neuropsychological test interpretation in order to maintain expertise (see Standard 1.05). In neuropsychological assessment, it is especially important for clinicians to attend to publication of new normative data for tests that they use and to understand the normative data and how the norms apply to individual practice.

The existence of high-quality tests and a set of standards or principles for test publishers, distributors, and consumers does not guarantee that tests will be administered and interpreted properly (Aiken, 1991). Neuropsychologists engaging in assessment must understand how using a high-quality, standardized test applies to the individual case in terms of interpreting results ethically.

Vignette 1: The Importance of Psychometrics

Dr. L evaluated a patient with a traumatic brain injury on two occasions, the first time one year after the injury and the second time 20 months after the injury. In the second report, Dr. L interpreted the first IQ scores from the Wechsler Adult Intelligence Scale – Third edition (WAIS-III; The Psychological Corporation, 1997) as reflecting a depression in the patient's intelligence caused by the brain injury and the second set of IQ scores from the WAIS-III as reflecting recovery and bringing the patient closer to her premorbid level of intellectual functioning. In this interpretation, Dr. L did not review the test–retest reliability data for the WAIS-III, nor did he consider data about 'practice effects' for the test. He also failed to review other information from the patient's history that was relevant to estimating her premorbid intellectual functioning. Failure to consider test factors important for interpretation may have resulted in an incorrect interpretation of the results. Conclusions such as this have implications for decisions about treatment and recommendations about returning to premorbid tasks and activities. Dr. L needs to review the psychometric data for the test and to familiarize himself with the emerging research on how to assess change in a reliable and valid manner.

Vignette 2: Incorporating New Norms into Test Interpretation

Dr. N saw Ms. Q, a 67-year-old teacher because of concerns about possible early dementia. Dr. N administered the California Verbal Learning Test (CVLT; Delis et al., 1987) as part of the evaluation and interpreted the results as within normal limits, per the published, age-corrected normative data for the test. Ms. Q had a few other test results that were outside of the normal range, but they did not clearly indicate problems at a level commensurate with early dementia. Dr. N wrote a report, fully explaining the findings and communicated them to the patient and her neurologist. Approximately one year later, Ms. Q returned to Dr. N for a reevaluation because she was still concerned about her functioning. Dr. N retested Ms. Q. When he interpreted the CVLT, he used newly published norms that not only corrected for age but also education, gender, and ethnicity. The new norms placed several of Ms Q's CVLT scores in the impaired range. When Dr. N compared her performances across the two occasions, it appeared that Ms. Q performed more poorly in the second evaluation. If the new norms had been available when he interpreted her first test results, however, several scores would have been in the mildly impaired range and the apparent decline was attenuated. Dr. N debated about how to portray these findings in his report. He was reluctant to revise his previous interpretation, but he did not want to mislead anyone. After considering the situation carefully, Dr. N disclosed in the new report that new, more precise norms had become available during the test–retest interval. He then interpreted both of the patient's sets of test results using the new norms and clarified that what initially appeared to be dramatic decline in her performance was actually only a mild decline (see also Section 1.06, *Basis for Scientific and Professional Judgments*, which is relevant for this vignette).

Vignette 3: Interpretation of Non-Standard or Problematic Testing
Dr. K used the MicroCog Assessment of Cognitive Functioning (Powell et al., 1993) to screen patients. When she obtained a new computer to use for this purpose, her assistant loaded the software and told Dr. K that the test was working properly. This same assistant also typically administered the test to patients. In discussing some problematic results with a patient, the patient complained to Dr. K that the glare from the computer screen had interfered with his seeing the stimuli well, and he also complained that the auditory stimuli were barely audible (Dr. K became a little concerned about the patient's hearing although it seemed fine during the interview and normal conversation). The patient reported that because of these problems with the test, his cognitive ability had not been validly assessed. Dr. K assured the patient that she would check on the test and report back to him her conclusions. Much to her surprise, at certain times of the day there was significant glare and the auditory stimuli were rather faint. She was quite distressed and notified the patient that he was correct and that she would administer another screening evaluation to him without cost. Dr. K also reviewed all of the protocols of patients who had taken the test since the new computer was installed and notified patients whose results were below normal that there had been 'technical difficulties.' She indicated that she would be happy to do further evaluation to be sure that the conclusions were valid. Finally, she resolved to maintain a closer watch over such matters to ensure that this type of problem did not happen again (Section 1.22, *Delegation to and Supervision of Subordinates*, also is relevant to this vignette).

Patient Characteristics Affecting Interpretation

In recent years, much attention has been devoted to understanding the effects of chronological age and educational achievement level on adult neuropsychological test performance. The realization that both of these factors explain considerable variance in test scores has resulted in the development of more precise normative data that take such variables into consideration (e.g., Heaton et al., 1991). Even more recently, interest has developed in exploring the relationship between expected neuropsychological test performance and patient characteristics such as gender, ethnicity/race, and language proficiency/fluency. Studies have shown significant effects of these variables, but norms for specific gender groups, ethnic groups or bilingual individuals are still rare. As research assessing the effects of such patient variables becomes available, it should be incorporated into neuropsychological interpretation.

Other patient characteristics such as the motivation and effort of the patient in the testing and the patient's premorbid level of functioning are essential variables to consider in interpreting neuropsychological test results. While Grote et al. (2000) indicated that assessment of motivation is especially important if litigation or disability is involved, adequacy of effort is crucial to all valid neuropsychological testing. Therefore, a careful evaluation of the patient's approach and effort is always necessary. Similarly, in order to interpret neuropsychological test results accurately, the clinician must estimate premorbid level of functioning by using available information and the research literature. Grote et al. (2000) cite the failure to consider these types of issues as potentially violating this section of the Ethics Code.

Vignette 4: Effects of Ethnicity and Language on Interpretation
Dr. A saw Mr. B for a neuropsychological evaluation because of a history of head trauma. Mr. B was a 63-year-old Hispanic male with ten years of education. He spoke English fluently, although his family of origin had mostly communicated in Spanish and he was bilingual. Dr. A administered his usual battery of tests and carefully interpreted the results according to the normative data. He realized, however, that most of the test norms that he used were for more highly educated subjects from English monolingual families. He used his clinical judgement to correct for the lower educational achievement and possible language issue, and issued his report. He thought that Mr. B had some impairments as a result of the head injury, and he did not want to 'water down' his report by hedging his conclusions too much, so he did not qualify his conclusions in the written report. While Dr. A's efforts to present his patient's results with conviction may be laudable, this case appears to involve a number of patient characteristics (education, ethnic background) that affected test interpretation. Dr. A needed to discuss these issues in the report, justifying his conclusions on the basis of data about the patient or the tests. He also needed to note any reservations he had or limitations in his interpretation because of these factors (see next subsection, Limitations of Interpretation).

Vignette 5: Effort and Motivation as Patient Characteristics
Dr. G evaluated a patient, Ms. H, at the request of her neurologist. The patient had been in a motor vehicle accident about a year before and was diagnosed with a concussion. She had persisting pain and cognitive complaints, so the neurologist thought a neuropsychological evaluation would be helpful in delineating problem areas and their etiologies. At the initial interview with Dr. G, the patient seemed pleasant and friendly and as though she would be easy to test. A psychometrist who had been testing for Dr. G for approximately two months was assigned to do the formal testing. The psychometrist rated the patient as very cooperative and hardworking in the assessment. Dr. G's inter-

pretation of the test results revealed mild to moderate deficits, which Dr. G attributed to the accident. He communicated this to the patient and her neurologist, with recommendations regarding compensating for her deficits and possible rehabilitation strategies. About one year later, Dr. G was approached by the patient's attorney to testify in an upcoming personal injury lawsuit. Dr. G did testify and, on the stand, was confronted with evidence from other evaluations of symptom exaggeration and questionable effort. Dr. G's interpretation was weakened by his failure to formally assess the patient's motivation and effort during the neuropsychological evaluation and by his relying on the opinion of a novice psychometrist. Through this case, Dr. G was reminded that even though he might delegate testing to another person, he remained responsible for ensuring the quality of the testing and the interpretation of the results. He resolved to supervise psychometrists more closely, especially new, inexperienced examiners. This situation is a complicated one, involving not only Section 2.05, but also Sections 1.22, *Delegation to and Supervision of Subordinates*, and 7.01, *Professionalism in Forensic Activities*.

Vignette 6: Ethnicity and Language as Patient Characteristics

Dr. E was asked to perform a neuropsychological evaluation on a male patient because of questions of cognitive impairment secondary to toxic exposure on the job. The patient was a 47-year-old Hispanic male, born and raised in a rural community in which the residents spoke primarily Spanish. He learned to speak English in school and went through the 12th grade. For the past 18 years, he had worked at an industrial plant, doing cleaning and janitorial work. He began to complain of headaches and trouble remembering and was being evaluated for possible long-term, low-level exposure to cleaning agents containing volatile solvents. As an adult, he spoke both English and Spanish regularly and considered himself to be fluent in both languages. Dr. E worked in a large metropolitan area. She had considerable experience in evaluating toxic exposure cases and considered herself knowledgeable and competent in the area. She was a monolingual English speaker, however, and did not consider herself to be an expert in bilingual or bicultural aspects of neuropsychology. Dr. E did not know of any neuropsychologists in the community who were expert in both areas, so she agreed to take the case, with the agreement that she would need to consult with a colleague about the effects of language and cultural issues on the interpretation. She decided that in this way, she could evaluate the patient competently and ethically (see also Sections 1.08, *Human Differences*; 2.04, *Competent and Appropriate Use of Assessment and* Intervention; and 5.06, Consultations).

Limitations of Interpretation

It is essential that psychologists acknowledge limitations about the accuracy or precision of test interpretation. As seen in several of the vignettes above, occasions arise frequently in neuropsychological assessment where limitations in knowledge or problems with procedures create situations in which the test(s) is (are) 'interpretable' only with qualifications and reservation. Also, as recognized by Binder and Thompson (1995), neuropsychologists need to recognize the "limits of certainty with which diagnosis, judgments, predictions can be made about individuals [as opposed to groups of patients]" (p.33). Less is known about individual prediction in most cases than group membership. Furthermore, in spite of relatively little empirical data about the ecological validity of neuropsychological tests for everyday behavior, neuropsychologists are frequently asked to draw conclusions about a patient's competency, employability, ability to benefit from treatment, etc. It is appropriate to do so as long as one relies on scientific data to base conclusions or, when the data are scarce, predictions and recommendations are made with appropriate caution and reservation.

Vignette 7: Non-Standard Administration and Absence of Education Corrected Norms

Dr. C saw Ms. D for a neuropsychological evaluation because the patient had complaints of increasing memory loss, and her neurologist had not found any etiology thus far. Ms. D was a 48-year-old female with advanced degrees and a high level position at a private research facility. Dr. C had just purchased the Wechsler Memory Scale-III (WMS-III; The Psychological Corporation, 1997) and had been doing some reading about the test, but she had never used it with a patient. Because of the breadth and depth of memory functions tested with the WMS-III, Dr. C thought that Ms. D would be an appropriate patient to take the test. After giving and scoring the test, Dr. C became aware of two factors that might affect interpretation. The first involved test administration factors; she realized that she had inadvertently changed the instructions for two subtests, thereby administering the subtests in a slightly non-standard manner. The second factor that might affect interpretation concerned specific patient characteristics rather than the test itself. Ms. D had masters' degrees in physics and chemistry, and Dr. C was uncertain how to 'adjust' expected memory performance on the basis of this high educational level. After much agonizing, Dr. C decided she needed to consult with a colleague who had more experience with the WMS-III. She did so, and they discussed the consultant's clinical experience with level of performance in highly educated individuals. Dr. C then wrote the report, acknowledging the limitations in interpretation because of non-standard administration, and she provided a lengthy discussion of the patient's performance relative to the normative group and how this might not be totally appropriate. She acknowledged the lack of education-corrected norms for the WMS-III, but cited literature from other tests indicating that more highly educated groups generally performed better on certain types of memory testing.

Vignette 8: Reservations about Validity of the Data

Dr. E saw Mr. F for a neuropsychological evaluation to help differentiate between dementia and depression. Per her usual protocol, she had Mr. F complete the MMPI-2 (Butcher et al., 1989) and Beck Depression Inventory (BDI; Beck et al., 1996) as well as neuropsychological tests. Mr. F completed the MMPI-2 and BDI independently, and he did not report any difficulty. Unknown to the neuropsychologist was the fact that Mr. F, although a high school graduate, had had life-long problems with reading. Because the evaluation focused on the issue of diagnosing dementia, she did not include any academic testing in the protocol. By failing to consider the reading level requirements of the tests, Dr. E was unable to incorporate that test feature into her interpretation. While reading through medical records, Dr. E came across some information about the literacy issue. Even though the test profile was not obviously invalid, she realized that it was possible that Mr. F did not understand some of the MMPI-2 items because of his limited reading skills. Dr. E was unable to schedule the patient for a return appointment before writing the report, but she was careful to state in the report the problems with the psychological testing that had been done. She reported that Mr. F had not reported significant depression either on the MMPI-2 or the BDI, but this may have been because of a lack of understanding of the items.

This vignette relates to both administration and interpretation issues. It was important that Dr. E report her reservations about the validity of the psychological tests. If she had written her report before learning about the reading problem, it would have been her responsibility to amend her report with the appropriate qualifications. It was also her responsibility to follow up in order to obtain additional data about the patient's emotional status, whether through psychological testing or interview (See also Standard 1.14, *Avoiding Harm*).

Vignette 9: Making Predictions without Specific Norms or Data

Dr. I was asked to see Dr. J, a 67-year old pediatrician, because of complaints to the State Medical Board of Examiners about the doctor's judgment and treatment decisions in a couple of different cases. Dr. I administered a comprehensive battery of tests to Dr. J, who was cooperative although somewhat irritated by being asked to undergo a cognitive evaluation. Dr. J's test results were within normal limits for his age, but Dr. I did not think that Dr. J's level of performance necessarily indicated that he was cognitively capable of practicing medicine. Dr. I compared Dr. J's results with a young adult normative group, reasoning that this would be a better indication of how Dr. J was functioning relative to other physicians. Compared to the young normative sample, many of Dr. J's results were in the impaired range, especially measures of information processing speed and spatial analysis. Dr. I concluded that Dr. J should not be practicing medicine. Dr. J was quite angry about the findings and challenged the neuropsychologist's conclusions on the basis that Dr. I had no normative information from physicians and no information that competently practicing physicians in their 60s were not showing the same age-related changes as Dr. J was. Dr. I was still concerned about Dr. J's level of functioning, but did write an addendum to his report, indicating that no physician specific norms were available. He modified his conclusions by noting that his interpretation was limited by the absence of physician norms and drew more circumspect conclusions about considering the physician's practice performance in light of the neuropsychological findings of age-related decline.

Use of Automated Interpretations

The first computer-based test interpretation programs were developed in the early 1960s, many for interpreting the MMPI (Aiken, 1991). The availability of computerized test interpretations has grown in the past several years along with the growth of computer technology and ease of use. Still, the most widely used computerized test interpretation programs in neuropsychological assessment pertain to the MMPI-2 (Garb, 2000). Computer-based test interpretation for neuropsychological tests or test batteries has been much slower to develop. Russell (1995) reviewed the research literature on automated programs developed to detect and/or lateralize brain dysfunction using the Halstead–Reitan Battery. Based on his review, Russell concluded that such programs were generally not as accurate as expert clinical judgment, but one of them (Neuropsychological Key Approach) reached adequate levels of accuracy. Russell concluded that more work on such programs might lead to increased accuracy, as computer programs are 'correctable' when new data become available. One of the most important points of the review was that, like any test or summary score, each program must be validated before being used clinically. In that regard, surprisingly little research has been devoted to computer-based test interpretation in neuropsychology.

Computerized interpretation programs may be appealing to busy clinicians because of their 'face' validity, ease of use, and efficiency. As Turkington (1984) pointed out, because test interpretations come from a computer, they may give a false impression of infallibility. However, when using automated interpretation programs, it is important to remember that the responsibility for the accuracy of the interpretation remains with the psychologist conducting the assessment. It is his/her responsibility to determine the validity of any automated program and to assess the utility of the program with the individual in question. Because automated programs come nicely packaged and presented, it may be tempting to assume that validity has been established. Early in the development of such programs, the validity of such programs was challenged (Adams & Heaton, 1985; Matarazzo, 1986). Even as recently as 1998, however, most automated assessment programs had not been shown to be valid (Garb, 1998). This suggests caution in embracing automated interpretation programs and suggests the need for the same critical scrutiny that one would give to any new (neuro)psychological test.

Automated programs *can* rely on statistical prediction rules, resulting in actuarial judgments and predictions. Grove et al. (2000) recently published a meta-analysis of 136 studies that compared actuarial (also called mechanical) prediction with clinical prediction. Studies included were those that predicted human behavior, assessed psychological states and traits, or made psychological or medical diagnoses. The meta-analysis included a few studies involving neuropsychological assessment and prediction, but the authors did not restrict the meta-analysis to such studies. Overall the actuarial programs were about 10% better at predicting than were the clinicians. Further, the clinician predicted more accurately than the mechanical method in only a small number of studies. However, as noted above, few of the studies pertained specifically to neuropsychological assessment. A perusal of hit rates among those studies that employed neuropsychological diagnosis or classification as the goal revealed that the clinical and mechanical methods were essentially the same. This meta-analysis illustrates that with rigorous methods, it may be possible to develop accurate and useful automated prediction programs in neuropsychology, but at present the science is in its infancy.

Advantages of computer based test interpretation include the fact that the same input data will always produce the same output (reliability) and both scoring and interpretation can typically be performed very quickly (efficiency). Disadvantages include the fact that computerized test interpretation programs seldom consider all of the salient variables affecting interpretation even when the basic program has been validated. Also, because of the apparent ease of use, such programs may appear attractive to individuals who do not have the necessary training and expertise to use them wisely (See Standards 1.04, *Boundaries of Competence,* and 2.02, *Competent and Appropriate Use of Assessment and Intervention*). A recent survey of psychologists suggests that, at the present stage of development, most view computer-based test interpretation programs as providing a supportive role along with more traditional methods of interpretation, and most of the psychologists responding to the survey thought it unethical to rely on computer interpretation as the primary resource for case formulation (McMinn et al., 1999).

Vignette 10: Reliance on Computer-based Interpretation

Dr. Z was asked by a managed care company to include a particular 'malingering' test that he had never used before. Dr. Z had heard of the test but had not studied it. He agreed to purchase and include the test in the evaluation. When the test arrived, it came with an automated interpretation program that conveniently printed at the end of the test administration. Dr. Z administered the test, but never found the time to thoroughly read the manual or any other materials about the test. He found the computer interpretation to be clear so included segments of it in his written report.

Dr. Z succumbed to the temptation to 'shortcut' the research that must be done when thinking about using a new neuropsychological procedure. The ease and convenience of the computerized program made this omission easy, but Dr. Z was obligated to find the time to research the test before using it clinically. Without doing that, he could not know whether the test was validated for the questions asked in this particular evaluation, and he could not know whether the normative sample was appropriate for use with this patient (see also Standards 1.04, *Boundaries of Competence*, 2.02, *Competent and Appropriate Use of Assessment and Intervention*, and 1.06, *Basis for Scientific and Professional Judgments*).

Vignette 11: Computer Interpretation and Patient Characteristics

Dr. Y included the MMPI-2 in a neuropsychological evaluation with an African American woman who had completed 13 years of formal education. Dr. Y had grown accustomed to using computerized interpretive reports for the MMPI-2. She had found the reports to be quite accurate and useful, and generally relied on them a great deal. In the evaluation of this woman, she utilized the computer interpretation. After writing the report, she met with the patient and the patient's therapist to communicate the results of the evaluation. At that time, she realized that the automated interpretation did not consider ethnicity, race, or cultural factors. Dr. Y was aware of research indicating that African Americans as a group tended to score higher on certain MMPI-2 clinical scales, and as she discussed the results, she realized that this information should have been incorporated into her interpretation. She discussed this with the patient and her therapist and provided a brief addendum to her report, modifying her previous interpretation. Dr. Y viewed this situation as a useful 'wake-up call' regarding her almost automatic use of the computer-generated interpretive report.

Section 2.09, Explaining Assessment Results

Section 2.09 of the Ethics Code, *Explaining Test Results*, states: *consent*

> *"Unless the nature of the relationship is clearly explained to the person being assessed in advance and precludes provision of an explanation of results (such as in some organizational consulting, pre-employment or security screenings, and forensic evaluations), psychologists ensure that an explanation of the results is provided using language that is reasonably understandable to the person assessed or to another legally authorized person on behalf of the client. Regardless of whether the scoring and interpretation are done by the psychologist, by assistants, or by automated or other outside services, psychologists take reasonable steps to ensure that appropriate explanations of results are given."*

In his casebook, Nagy (2000) translated this section for psychologists in general as:

> "Explain the results of your formal assessments in simple English — not 'psychologese' — to the person you are evaluating unless, of course, you are prohibited from discussing test results by virtue of your role or the setting (e.g., personnel screening, mental competency examinations). In those cases, be sure to tell test takers in advance that you will not be giving them any results or interpretations" (p.74).

Historically, explaining/communicating test results has received much less attention than the administration and interpretation components of the process (Pope, 1992). It is somewhat disturbing to note that patients who have been evaluated often report that they were not informed about their test results (Gass & Brown, 1992). Although Anastasi (1982) indicated that psychologists had given much thought to the communication of test results in a meaningful and useful way, her statement refers mainly to communicating results to third parties. She addresses feedback to patients as follows: "Last but by no means least is the *problem* [italics added] of communicating test results to the examinees themselves, ..." (p. 55). From an ethical perspective, it is imperative to reframe this 'problem' as an integral and important part of the evaluation. Unfortunately, in the neuropsychological literature, little attention has been given to this. An important article, therefore, is a guide provided by Gass and Brown (1992) regarding feedback of neuropsychological test results. They discuss the process and provide a step-by-step approach to providing feedback that includes the neuropsychologist reviewing the purpose of the testing, defining the tests, explaining behavior and results in various cognitive domains, describing consequent strengths and weaknesses, addressing diagnostic and prognostic issues, and making recommendations. The reader is referred to this article for a number of helpful suggestions in how to convey test results to patients and others.

This article is a useful addition to the literature, because many other authors have assumed that if a competent psychologist knows how to interpret neuropsychological data, he or she will automatically know how to communicate the results to the examinee (or appropriate others) in a competent and ethical manner. This section of the Ethics Code suggests that the communication of assessment results is a skill requiring competency and sensitivity that may be different from the skill of interpretation, per se.

Pope (1992) emphasized that feedback should be thoughtful as well as dynamic and interactive. It is important to check on what the patient hears and understands during the feedback process as well as to ascertain the patient's reaction to the results. Information should be presented in understandable language, but this does not mean that the results should be diluted or simplified to the point of distortion. If the results are somewhat contradictory or ambiguous, this needs to be conveyed to the patient. How the results are presented can have a significant influence on how the patient will receive the information. In spite of pressure from managed care and limited reimbursement at times, this aspect of the evaluation should be done with the same level of conscientiousness and care as the basic interpretation. Neuropsychologists should be sensitive to the impact that the evaluation results may have on the patient. Patients may invest the neuropsychologist with a certain sense of infallibility (Pope, 1992), so the neuropsychologist should discuss the results and their impact with an appropriate degree of circumspection.

Another issue is whether test scores should be included in the written report of neuropsychological testing (and whether scores should be discussed with the patient). Freides (1993) proposed that test scores be included in the written report, perhaps in an Appendix. He proposed that such a procedure would increase efficiency in the report, ensure the integrity of the data in that no data would be omitted, and provide opportunity for more direct comparison in the event of retesting. Naugle and McSweeny (1995) responded to the proposal by pointing out some potential disadvantages. They included the test scores under the umbrella of raw data and suggested that it may be unethical to release raw data because it may lead to misuse of the scores. They also noted that the inclusion of test scores might be regarded as an intrusion on the patient's privacy. Freides (1995) then responded by reiterating his point that including test scores encouraged interpretation of all the data, not just data that 'fit' with the author's hypotheses, and he questioned the assertion that the test data might be more harmful than verbal judgments about the meaning of the data. Matarazzo (1995) echoed Freide's opinion that reporting scores is no more an invasion of privacy than is a narrative interpretation of the data. She also expressed the opinion that the persons most likely to want and use the scores would be other psychologists who would appreciate the immediate availability of the information. There does not appear to be a uniform standard or policy at this time, and opinions continue to differ regarding the ethics of providing this type of quantitative information to patients and others. It is unlikely that a provision of scores without a narrative interpretation of their meaning would ever be regarded as ethical.

For the purposes of further discussion, vignettes that highlight common ethical issues in explaining assessment results will be presented under the following three subheadings: (1) Feedback to the patient; (2) feedback to others with the consent of the patient or feedback to those who have legal authority over the patient; and (3) situations in which feedback is prohibited.

Feedback to the Patient

Most psychologists agree that patients have the right of access to information about themselves, or in the case of children, that parents have access to assessment information about their minor children (Koocher & Keith-Spiegel, 1998). Furthermore, Koocher and Keith-Spiegel (1998) recommend that psychologists assume that any patient may ask to see his/her records and that those who persist are likely to be able to obtain copies, whether the psychologist thinks that this is a good idea or not. Therefore, it probably is prudent to write neuropsychological reports, keeping in mind that the patient may get the report. When the patient does access the report, the psychologist "should be willing to share the material, along with an explanation of terms and answers to other questions that the client may have" (Koocher & Keith-Spiegel, 1998, p. 128). This passive style of providing feedback (waiting for the patient to demand it) may not be the ethical approach, however. Standard 2.09 implies that understandable information about the evaluations should be provided willingly and proactively.

Vignette 12: Feedback with a Memory-impaired Patient
At the encouragement of his primary care physician (PCP) "to be sure that everything was all right", Mr. U went to Dr. T for a neuropsychological evaluation. Mr. U was a 78-year-old man whose children had contacted the PCP because of an apparent decline in Mr. U's memory and cognition. Mr. U lived independently in a townhouse, he was widowed, and he had two grown children, one of whom lived in the area. Mr. U had been a high-level executive in business prior to his retirement at age 65. He had periodic assistance in maintaining his home (lawn care and house cleaning) but continued to drive, travel, and manage his finances. He prided himself on his independence. He took an active part in the evaluation and expressed a strong interest in returning to discuss the results with Dr. T. The neuropsychologist and Mr. U discussed that it would be helpful to bring his son, with whom he was close, to the feedback session. Mr. U's evaluation revealed significant memory deficits in the context of relatively normal functioning in other areas.

Mr. U arrived for his feedback session alone. When asked about his son's attendance, he initially seemed surprised and then said that his son was not able to make the appointment. Dr. T offered to reschedule the feedback at a time when Mr. U's son could attend, but the patient wished to proceed. In discussing the results, Mr. U was polite and courteous, but seemed to minimize the importance of what Dr. T was saying about his memory. He did not want Dr. T to contact any one else about the results, because he thought he was functioning well and was concerned that others might try to restrict his freedom. Although Dr. T thought that Mr. U understood the feedback, she was concerned about his ability to remember and use the information. She provided him with a copy of the report and encouraged him to provide it to his doctor so that it could become part of the medical record. Although Dr. T was concerned about Mr. U's memory deficit, it did not appear that Dr. U was in immediate danger to himself or others and it appeared that he was competent and understood the results. As a result, Dr. T did not feel that she should violate confidentiality and contact

Mr. U's doctor against his wishes (see Ethics Code Principle D: *Respect for People's Rights and Dignity*).

Vignette 13: Neuropsychological Feedback to a Depressed Patient
Ms. W was having significant problems following a motor vehicle accident about four months previously that had caused a mild concussion and cervical strain. Initially, she had been in considerable pain, but that had subsided considerably. Now her complaints centered around feeling overwhelmed, distractible, inattentive, and forgetful. She found her job to be very stressful, and she found herself withdrawing from social and recreational activities. Her attorney suggested that she contact her neurologist, which she did, and he referred her for a neuropsychological evaluation to obtain information about her mental functioning and why she was having so much trouble. Dr. V performed the evaluation. Ms. W wished to obtain the results directly, and she requested that the report also be sent to her neurologist and her attorney. Dr. V found Ms. W to be clinically depressed, and on neurocognitive testing, she showed mild problems with sustained attention and new learning. Dr. V could not determine whether these deficits were related to the concussion, to the patient's depression, or to a combination of the two. Dr. V was concerned about how Ms W would receive the results. When he met with Ms. W, he tried to explain things carefully because he did not want to exacerbate her depression, and he was concerned that she was likely to interpret the results in an overly pessimistic way. He was sensitive to the issue of avoiding harm to the patient in considering her emotional reaction to the findings from the evaluation. He spent extra time with her, focusing on both the areas of difficulty and the cognitive strengths. He also emphasized that he thought that treatment for her depression would be very helpful and made specific recommendations for how she might proceed to initiate treatment. Ms. W seemed worried, but she agreed to contact potential therapists for treatment. Two weeks later, with permission from the patient, the new therapist contacted Dr. V because Ms. W was distraught about her brain injury. Her attorney had emphasized to her that she was 'brain-damaged' and that Dr. V probably had tried to soften the news to her about this. Dr. V was distressed by this turn of events. He attempted to schedule a session with both the patient and her attorney, but the attorney was never available. He did meet with Ms. W and her therapist to reiterate his findings and conclusions, and he telephoned Ms. W's neurologist to emphasize his concern that an overemphasis on the 'brain injury' would be counterproductive to Ms. W's treatment and recovery from her depression.

Feedback to Others

In some cases, parties other than the examinee may have the legal right to the evaluation results, such as in the cases of minor children or adults who have guardians. In these cases, it is ethically important to consider this at the outset of the evaluation and to clarify the roles and responsibilities of each person before the evaluation takes place (see also Sections 1.21, *Third Party Requests for Services* and 5.01, *Discussing Limits of Confidentiality*).

Vignette 14: Feedback to Adolescent Patient and Family

Dr. P was asked to evaluate a 16-year-old boy, R, at the request of his parents because his grades were declining, and the parents were concerned about an undiagnosed learning disability. Recognizing that multiple issues may be contributing to a decline in grades in a 16-year-old, Dr. P administered a battery of tests that not only evaluated academic skills and related cognitive abilities, but also assessed depression. As part of the history taking, Dr. P interviewed R and his parents separately regarding a variety of issues, including use of illicit drugs. Dr. P viewed all of this as essential in conducting a comprehensive and clinically meaningful evaluation. After the evaluation, he arranged a time to meet with R and his parents to discuss the results. At the beginning of this meeting, as he began to discuss the evaluation, R appeared uncomfortable and blurted out that he did not want some of the information provided to his parents. His parents looked alarmed and accused him of having 'secrets'. They insisted that Dr. P reveal everything to them because they were R's parents after all and they were paying for the evaluation. Dr. P felt 'stuck' and realized that he should have informed both R and his parents at the outset about his policies of who would have access to what information. Dr. P requested a few moments to meet with R alone, to which his parents reluctantly agreed. Dr. P then apprised R of the information he planned to go over in the meeting. R did not have any objection to that information; he was concerned about his parents learning of his drug experimentation. Dr. P did not think that this was salient information for the evaluation, but given R's protest in front of his parents, he and R discussed how to provide the information to his parents. The four of them then met, Dr. P provided the evaluation feedback, and R disclosed (minimally) his concerns. The parents expressed concern, but also relief, that the information was not worse. Dr. P was relieved that the outcome was positive, but resolved to provide patients at the outset more detailed information about confidentiality and who would have access to what information.

Vignette 15: Feedback in a Rehabilitation Setting

Dr. L worked in an outpatient rehabilitation setting. Treatment was based on an interdisciplinary model in which it was considered important to share information about the patient with both involved family members and with rehabilitation staff. Dr. L was always careful to inform patients of this at the outset of any neuropsychological evaluation. He provided both written and verbal information that the results of the evaluation would be discussed with the patient and family, and that the results would be provided to the rest of the treatment team to help with planning of treatment and monitoring of progress. Because many of the patients presented with memory impairment, Dr. L repeated this information several times during the evaluation, and reminded the patient of it at the beginning of any family or treatment team discussion. His proactive stance helped patients to feel comfortable with this approach and to appreciate the benefit from information being provided to those involved with the treatment program. He also provided feedback to patients in brief installments and typically reviewed the findings in treatment as appropriate. This helped cognitively impaired patients gradually incorporate the information about areas of strength and deficit.

Situations that Prohibit Feedback

In neuropsychological assessment, one of the most common situations in which feedback is prohibited is an evaluation conducted for legal purposes. Neuropsychological assessment is common in personal injury cases, and in the case of 'independent evaluations' feedback to the examinee is prohibited. It is important to remember that the examinee is not the client or patient. Rather, the third party seeking the evaluation is the client. This may be confusing for the examinee (and for the naïve neuropsychologist), and it should always be discussed at the beginning of the evaluation. For the discussion here, the salient information to be conveyed to the examinee is that the psychologist performing the evaluation is not permitted to give the results to the examinee (either in written or oral form).

Vignette 16: Independent Neuropsychological Evaluations
An employer requested that Dr. N perform an independent neuropsychological evaluation on an individual involved in a worker's compensation claim. The claim concerned a traumatic brain injury suffered on the job, when Mr. O was hit in the head by a falling beam at a construction site. Dr. N spent several hours testing and interviewing Mr. O. They developed a good rapport. Mr. O felt comfortable with Dr. N and revealed some personal data that he had been reluctant to discuss with others. Dr. N explained to Mr. O that the evaluation was being done because of the job-related injury but did not explicitly explain that there was no doctor-patient relationship and that he could not meet with Mr. O to discuss the test results. At the end of the evaluation, Mr. O asked Dr. N when they would be meeting again and how Dr. N would be able to help him. When Dr. N then explained that he would not be meeting with Mr. O because of the nature of the exam, Mr. O became angry and tearful and claimed that Dr. N had tricked him. Although late in the process, Dr. N spent some time explaining the limits of his role to Mr. O and he apologized for not being clearer at the outset. While Dr. N did not feel that he could appropriately make treatment suggestions, he did say to Mr. O that he might contact his neurologist for suggestions, should he wish to pursue follow up treatment (other

standards of the Ethics Code relevant to this situation include 1.21, *Third Party Requests for Services*; 7.01, *Professionalism in Forensic Activities*; and 7.02, *Forensic Assessments*).

Related Issue of Whether to Seek Informed Consent

A related issue that affects feedback of results (as well as a number of other aspects of neuropsychological assessment) concerns informed consent for assessment. The 1992 APA Ethics Code requires informed consent for therapy and for research but not for assessment. A number of authors writing about assessment, however, argue for informed consent prior to evaluation (Aiken, 1991; Koocher & Keith-Spiegel, 1990; Nuttall et al., 1999). In neuropsychological assessment, it appears likely that some patients do not understand (or remember) the purpose of the evaluation, how the results will be used, and who will have access to the results, in spite of the neuropsychologist's efforts to explain simply and sometimes repeatedly.

As noted by Binder and Thompson (1995), "It is a sad irony that some patients referred for evaluation of their competency to manage their own funds or make decisions regarding their own health and welfare would choose *not* [emphasis added] to undergo a neuropsychological examination if they fully understood that an abnormal result could jeopardize their normal prerogatives to make important decisions" (p.39).

It is not clear how these situations should be handled, but these are the types of situations where it is important to consider carefully who is the patient, how the results of the evaluation will be used, and who will have access to the information. After the neuropsychologist reaches clarity regarding these issues, the neuropsychologist has the responsibility to convey the information to the examinee as clearly as possible (using language the examinee can understand) and as often as necessary. This may still fall short of obtaining informed consent, but appears to generally follow the guidelines in the current Ethics Code.

Conclusions

These vignettes have been provided to highlight common evaluation situations and the ethical issues they raise. It is important to remember that ethical issues are an integral part of clinical practice, not a crisis that arises when one misbehaves. As such, ethics permeates all of our actions as professionals.

There will always be ethical issues in neuropsychological assessment interpretation and feedback. This does not mean that only one method or approach of handling situations is appropriate or 'ethical'. Nor does it mean that a good neuropsychologist never feels the tension and pressure that some ambiguous or conflictual situations present.

This chapter has attempted to present both successful and problematic scenarios, as each of us will encounter both in clinical practice. When problematic situations arise in the scenarios, discussion is provided for actions that might be taken to minimize harm or, if possible, to remedy the situation. The scenarios are not meant to describe the best or the preferred way to handle difficult situations. Rather, the vignettes raise issues, present one course of action and, hopefully, generate thoughts and ideas for how to approach situations that arise in individual clinical practice.

References

Adams, K.M., & Heaton, R.K. (1985). Automated interpretation of neuropsychological test data. *Journal of Consulting and Clinical Psychology, 53*, 790-802.

Aiken, L.R. (1991). *Psychological testing and assessment* (7th ed.). Boston: Allyn and Bacon.

American Educational Research Association, American Psychological Association, National Council on Measurement in Education (1999). *Standards for educational and psychological testing.* Washington, DC: American Educational Research Association.

American Psychological Association (1992). Ethical principles of psychologists and code of conduct. *American Psychologist, 47*, 1597-1611.

Anastasi, A. (1982). *Psychological testing* (5th ed.). New York: Macmillan Publishing Co., Inc.

Beck, A.T., Steer, R.A., & Brown, G.K. (1996). *Beck Depression Inventory manual* (2nd ed.). San Antonio: Psychological Corporation.

Binder, L.M., & Thompson, L.L. (1995). The Ethics Code and neuropsychological assessment practices. *Archives of Clinical Neuropsychology, 10*, 27-46.

Butcher, J.N., Dahlstrom, W.G., Graham, J.R., Tellegen, A., & Kaemmer, B. (1989). *Minnesota Multiphasic Personality Inventory – 2.* Minneapolis, MN: NCS Assessments.

Delis, D.C., Kramer, J.H., Kaplan, E., & Ober, B.A. (1987). *California Verbal Learning Test.* San Antonio, TX: The Psychological Corporation.

Freides, D. (1993). Proposed standard of professional practice: Neuropsychological reports display all quantitative data. *The Clinical Neuropsychologist, 7*, 234-235.

Freides, D. (1995). Interpretations are more benign than data? *The Clinical Neuropsychologist, 9*, 248.

Garb, H.N. (1998). *Studying the clinician: Judgment research and psychological assessment.* Washington, DC: American Psychological Association.

Garb, H.N. (2000). Computers will become increasingly important for psychological assessment: Not that there's anything wrong with that! *Psychological Assessment, 12*, 31-39.

Gass, C.S., & Brown, M.C. (1992). Neuropsychological test feedback to patients with brain dysfunction. *Psychological Assessment, 4*, 272-277.

Grote, C.L., Lewin, J.L., Sweet, J.J., & van Gorp, W.G. (2000). Responses to perceived unethical practices in clinical neuropsychology: Ethical and legal considerations. *The Clinical Neuropsychologist, 14*, 119-134.

Grove, W.M., Zald, D.H., Lebow, B.S., Snitz, B.E., & Nelson, C. (2000). Clinical versus mechanical prediction: A meta-analysis. *Psychological Assessment, 12*, 19-30.

Heaton, R.K., Grant, I., & Matthews, C.G. (1991). *Comprehensive norms for an expanded Halstead-Reitan Battery: Demographic corrections, research findings, and clinical applications.* Odessa, FL: Psychological Assessment Resources.

Koocher, G.P., & Keith-Spiegel, P.C. (1990). *Children, ethics, and the law: Professional issues and cases.* Lincoln, NE: University of Nebraska Press.

Koocher, G.P., & Keith-Spiegel, P. (1998). *Ethics in psychology: Professional standards and cases* (2nd ed.). New York: Oxford University Press.

Matarazzo, J.D. (1986). Computerized clinical psychological test interpretations: Unvalidated plus all mean and no sigma. *American Psychologist, 41,* 14-24.

Matarazzo, R.G. (1995). Psychological report standards in neuropsychology. *The Clinical Neuropsychologist, 9,* 249-250.

McMinn, M.R., Ellens, B.M., & Soref, E. (1999). Ethical perspectives and practice behaviors involving computer-based test interpretation. *Assessment, 6,* 71-77.

Messick, S. (1999). Test validity and the ethics of assessment. In D.N.Bersoff (Ed.), *Ethical conflicts in psychology* (2nd ed.) (pp. 285-286). Washington, DC: American Psychological Association.

Mitrushina, M.N., Boone, K.B., & D'Elia, L.F. (1999). *Handbook of normative data for neuropsychological assessment.* New York: Oxford University Press.

Nagy, T. F. (2000). *Ethics in plain English: An illustrative casebook for psychologists.* Washington, DC: American Psychological Association.

Naugle, R.I., & McSweeny, A.J. (1995). On the practice of routinely appending neuropsychological data to reports. *The Clinical Neuropsychologist, 9,* 245-247.

Nuttal, E.V., Romero, I., & Kalesnik, J. (1999). *Assessing and screening preschoolers: Psychological and educational dimensions* (2nd ed.). Boston: Allyn and Bacon.

Pope, K.S. (1992). Responsibilities in providing psychological test feedback to clients. *Psychological Assessment, 4,* 268-271.

Powell, D.H., Kaplan, E.F., Whitla, D., Weintraub, S., Catlin, R., & Funkenstein, H.H. (1993). *MicroCog Assessment of Cognitive Functioning manual.* San Antonio: Psychological Corporation.

Russell, E.W. (1995). The accuracy of automated and clinical detection of brain damage and lateralization in neuropsychology. *Neuropsychology Review, 5,* 1-68.

The Psychological Corporation (1997). *WAIS-III, WMS-III Technical Manual.* San Antonio: Author.

Turkington, C. (1984). The growing use and abuse of computer testing. *APA Monitor, 7,* 26.

PART II

ETHICAL ISSUES IN NEURO-PSYCHOLOGY WITH SPECIAL POPULATIONS

Chapter 5

ETHICAL ISSUES IN PEDIATRIC NEUROPSYCHOLOGY

Eileen B. Fennell

Introduction

Beginning in the 1990s, there has been an increase in the number of publications addressing issues in the practice of clinical neuropsychology. Topics addressed in these publications have included the presence of third party observers in clinical neuropsychological evaluations (e.g., McSweeny et al., 1998), the release of raw test data to the courts (e.g., Lees-Haley & Courtney 2000), the use of test technicians in clinical practice (e.g., NAN Policy and Planning Committee, 2000a), ethical issues in forensic neuropsychological consultation (Guilmette & Hagan, 1997), and clinicians' responses to perceived unethical practices in clinical neuropsychology (e.g., Grote et al., 2000). Despite this expanding body of opinion, relatively little information has been provided on these issues as they may arise in the practice of pediatric neuropsychology. While it is assumed that the *Ethical Principles of Psychologists and Code of Conduct* (American Psychological Association, 1992) apply to all practitioners (see Chapter 1, this volume), as well as the standards regarding test construction and application (see Chapters 2 and 3, this volume), discussion of the application of these principles and standards to neuropsychological practices involving children and their families is still needed.

In this chapter, issues in three main arenas of practice will be addressed: (1) hospital based practice issues; (2) forensic evaluations; and (3) evaluations for school specialty services. A general discussion of issues specific to testing and education and training in pediatric neuropsychology follows. The chapter concludes with some general guidelines for practice with children and adolescents.

Pediatric Neuropsychology in a Health-Care Setting

Woody (1997) recently cautioned that the growing recognition of the specialty of child (pediatric) neuropsychology has increased the potential for legal liability by virtue of the specialty being part of the health care industry. He argues that there are four reasons why the specialty of child neuropsychology is at greater risk for legal action, such as a malpractice claim, than is likely in a general child clinical practice: (1) there is an absence of a unifying standard of training in clinical child neuropsychology; (2) the increased identity as a health care provider in a medical context increases the risk for legal action; (3) the principle of vicarious liability can apply to any member of a health care team, including the neuropsychologist, despite any direct claim of fault against the neuropsychologist; and, (4) neuropsychology, by virtue of its focus on brain-related issues, has the potential to increase the basis of legal action claims (p.719).

Consultation Requests and Consent to Treatment

Several situations arise in which a pediatric neuropsychologist may be asked to provide consultation to a child who is hospitalized. A common request is for the minor patient to be assessed for the presence of brain dysfunction. This request can arise because the child's primary illness directly involves neurological dysfunction, as in the case of a child being treated for a head injury or CNS infection or when dysfunction is a secondary effect of illness or its treatment (e.g. the leukemias). Parents may consent to the consultation request but many times may be unaware that a request for neuropsychological services has been initiated by an attending physician. In either case, it is the neuropsychologist's ethical responsibility to fully inform the parents of the request for and purpose of the assessment, of potential limitations in assessment imposed by the child's condition, and of potential implications of the findings regarding treatment. Legally, parents have the right to consent to treatment, while minors do not. Assent to treatment which involves soliciting the agreement to treatment by a child aged eight years or older is now a standard practice in research IRB protocols and is also employed by many practitioners for non-experimental treatment protocols (Rae et al., 1995). Determining voluntary assent must take into account the child's capacity to understand the purpose of any treatment, including an assessment, its benefits and risks, and the likely outcomes of undergoing or withholding treatment. This task can, in fact, be quite difficult to achieve because it involves evaluating the child's stage of development of cognitive abilities and emotional status (Rae et al., 1995). As such, a solid background in cognitive development, children's conceptualizations of illness, and psychological complications of medical illness are essential to the appropriate assessment of the child's capacity.

Confidentiality and Record Keeping

A second issue that can arise in hospital settings relates to confidentiality of records. Record keeping in a hospital setting may involve both a written consultation note and on-going notes of contact with a patient or with the child's family. While the APA (1992) Ethics Code states that the psychologist will maintain appropriate confidentiality in handling of patient records (Standards 1.24 and 2.10), as a member of a health-care team, the consulting neuropsychologist may be required by hospital policy to place the report of an evaluation or contact notes directly into the child's medical record. Access to the medical record is open to all health care providers for the child; therefore, it is imperative that the neuropsychologist considers the limited control over who may be reading their reports or notes. While release of medical records to a third party such as an insurance carrier, parent, or attorney requires a written authorized release, it is helpful to require that the release specify psychological reports or treatment notes to obtain these records. Even with a legal request for release of records, the neuropsychologist should follow general APA guidelines regarding release of records and the protection of the client (see Chapter 2, this volume).

Abbreviated Test Batteries and Standards of Care

A final issue that may arise in a hospital setting relates to the use of an abbreviated testing protocol when examining a child. The fundamental issue here is whether the abbreviated battery can reliably provide valid indicators of the neuropsychological status of a child who may be physically unable to undergo a comprehensive exam due to limitations imposed by the illness and its treatment. Outcome predictions based upon comprehensive batteries obtained in outpatient settings may not be applicable to the hospitalized child. There is the potential that the question of medicolegal/psycholegal appropriate standard of care could be raised under such circumstances (Woody, 1997). For this reason, it is ethically necessary that the neuropsychologist's report clearly identify: (1) the reasons for using an abbreviated testing battery; (2) the limitations of data derived from the abbreviated battery; and (3) the relevance of the findings to the current status of the child. Predictions regarding the relationships of the current findings to future outcomes should be carefully and cautiously offered, acknowledging clearly the limitations of the current test results to predictions of longer-term outcomes.

One special instance in the use of abbreviated batteries can be undergoing an experimental treatment protocol that includes routine neuropsychological assessments. Clinical trials for children's cancer treatments, HIV treatment, and organ transplantation often contain abbreviated testing batteries. While it is the case that the parents (and the child) may have signed an Informed Consent to participate in the treatment, the parents (and child) still retain the right not to participate in this aspect of the protocol. Whether failure to comply with the neuropsychological testing requirements of the protocol will result in their withdrawal from the study should be clearly indicated on the Informed Consent for treatment. Even with a signed consent, it is still ethically necessary that the neuropsychologist explain the same limitations of an abbreviated battery as described above in the case of a non-experimental treatment. Use of abbreviated test batteries in an outpatient setting carries the same ethical obligations by the pediatric neuropsychologist. Limitations of the diagnostic and or predictive validity of an abbreviated battery should be considered and noted in the report, although research on this issue in the pediatric age group is currently lacking (Fennell, 1999). Use of an abbreviated battery, based upon reimbursement limitations by an insurance carrier rather than appropriateness to the diagnostic question, raises concerns regarding appropriate standards of care for the practitioner (Woody, 1997) and may raise liability questions for such practice decisions. Documentation of the reasons for the use of a screening battery along with the appropriate limitations of the testing results as these relate to diagnostic and treatment recommendations should be included in any neuropsychological report written under these restrictions. If the abbreviated battery is the result of difficulties in obtaining child or parental completion of an examination, these difficulties should be noted along with the constraints placed by the shortened battery on comparability to normative data available on the tests utilized in assessment.

Pediatric Neuropsychology in a Forensic Setting

Broadly defined, forensic practice may take place in the context of criminal or civil proceedings. In criminal law, the individual is charged with the commission of an act which violates a state or federal statute and which is punishable by imprisonment or a fine (Melton et al., 1997). In contrast, a civil proceeding involves a dispute between two or more private individuals (a 'plaintiff' and a 'defendant'). Pediatric neuropsychologists may be asked to provide consultation or evaluation services in either system of law.

Criminal Process Consultations

The two most likely ways in which a pediatric neuropsychologist may be involved in a criminal proceeding are (1) as a defense expert, testifying as to the competence of a juvenile charged with a crime or (2) as a prosecution expert testifying as to the neuropsychological effects on a victim of a crime committed by an adult or juvenile (e.g., child abuse). What defines a neuropsychologist as expert in court proceedings? Most, but not all, state courts have adopted the so-called Federal Rules of Evidence regarding opinions and expert testimony (Melton et al., 1997). Rule 702 of the Federal Rules of Evidence states that: "If scientific, technological, or other specialized knowledge will assist the trier of fact to understand the evidence or determine a fact at issue, a witness qualified as an expert by knowledge, skill, experience, and training or education, may testify thereto in the form of an opinion or otherwise" (Melton evaluation, p. 16). Thus, most neuropsychologists who are asked to testify as experts in criminal (or civil) proceedings will be examined regarding education, training, and experience relevant to the opinions to be offered in the case. Once admitted as an expert, the neuropsychologist may provide testimony in a juvenile court hearing regarding the juvenile's competency to proceed to trial or competency with regard to appreciation of and/or ability to inhibit/prevent the commission of the alleged criminal acts. Recently, juveniles may now be charged as adults for certain types of major, usually violent, crimes, such as murder.

A pediatric neuropsychologist may become involved in assessing a juvenile when the question of competence arises as a consequence of a pre-existing brain injury (e.g. traumatic brain injury) or medical condition (e.g., epilepsy). Occasionally, a question regarding competency can arise when injury occurs between the time of commission of the criminal act and the criminal proceedings. I was once asked to testify prior to sentencing about a teenager who had sustained a severe brain injury in a motor vehicle accident after having committed a crime of breaking and entering and theft. The question raised was whether the juvenile's changed mental status should/would affect the proposed punishment (incarceration in a juvenile facility). As a consequence of the severe brain injury, the juvenile had no memory of the crimes with which he was charged nor could he assist his attorney in his defense as to the facts of the crime. Because of a prior juvenile record, the defendant served a 'modified' sentence in a state forensic residential school. In a second example, I was asked by an attorney to assess a juvenile with complex partial seizures who had been charged with indecent exposure. As part of the automatisms of his epilepsy, the juvenile had unzipped his pants in a public setting (a grocery store). In this instance, the primary expertise was that of the treating neurologist who testified to the child's type of epilepsy and the automatisms he had witnessed while treating the child. My role was limited to describing the neuropsychological profile of the child in support of his neurological status, as well as in evaluating him for the presence of psychological factors in the patient and the family that might indicate a basis for 'sexually deviant behavior'. The charges against the juvenile were eventually dismissed.

A second situation in which pediatric neuropsychological expertise might be sought is in determining the effects of brain trauma on a child victim. In these instances, I have most often been asked to evaluate the status of a child by the state agency for Child Protective Services. To a large degree, this type of assessment is quite similar to an assessment that might be requested by a referring physician in that the tests and procedures employed in the comprehensive test battery would be the same. Where the procedures may differ in a parental abuse case is in the availability of parent report data on the child's development prior to the injury, as well as in the limitations of data about the child's current behavior due to placement in foster care or other childcare arrangements. Sometimes, the agency requesting the evaluation may request an opinion regarding the future placement of the child victim. It is important that the pediatric neuropsychologist be aware of the limitations of their evaluation data in addressing this question. Neuropsychological tests are not designed to provide direct information about child residential care or therapeutic placement per se. While more traditional psychological testing may provide some data on the child's emotional state, determination of child placement is a complex process requiring multidimensional assessment and custody expertise. If the pediatric neuropsychologist typically would not be involved in ascertaining appropriate child placement decisions, ethics require that this limitation in expertise needs to be clearly stated to the referring agency. Referral to another individual with such expertise is an appropriate professional response (Koocher & Keith-Spiegel, 1990).

Civil Process Consultations
Probably the two most common situations in civil trials that involve a pediatric neuropsychologist's expertise are civil suits involving personal injury and malpractice suits. A third, more recent arena of practice relates to claims of failure to comply with Federal Regulations regarding special services to the handicapped in school settings and Social Security Disability determination for a handicapped child.

Personal injury claims filed on behalf of a child by parents that involve claims of brain damage are apparently becoming increasingly common (Woody, 1997). The pediatric neuropsychologist may become involved in such claims either on behalf of the injured party's attorney (plaintiff) or on behalf of the defendant's attorney who may represent an individual or a business such as an insurance carrier. States vary in the limitations of liability in the requirement for court-ordered mediation. The practicing pediatric neuropsychologist should become familiar with the state statutes that apply regarding these issues as well as court-ordered rules regarding the presence of third party observers, videotaping of the examination, test data release, and required distances to travel to an examination (McSweeney et al., 1998; Barth, 2000; NAN Policy and Planning Committee, 2000b; Shapiro, 2000). In order to comply with ethical practice guidelines by the individual's state Psychology Board of Professional Regulation, the neuropsychologist may request that raw test data only be released to a qualified licensed psychologist and that such data, along with videotapes, be sealed by the court upon conclusion of the trial. Ethical practice requires the pediatric neuropsychologist to conduct not only a comprehensive assessment of the child alleged to have sustained a brain injury but also that there be a comprehensive review of the child's developmental and medical history, school records prior and subsequent to the alleged injury, and treatment records, including any diagnostic laboratory studies (e.g., EEG), imaging studies (e.g., CT, MRI) and any prior psychological and/or neuropsychological assessments. The pediatric neuropsychologist should integrate this information with what is known about the effects of the alleged brain injury, what research studies suggest about likely outcomes (short and long term) of mild, moderate, or severe injury, and the role of family factors in recovery from a brain insult (Yeates et al., 1997).

Similar practice issues may emerge when the pediatric neuropsychologist is asked to evaluate a child for injuries or harm sustained as a consequence of alleged malpractice by a treating professional, most often a physician. Whether being asked to evaluate the child as a defense or plaintiff's expert, the same comprehensive approach to the evaluation should be followed. Limitations in the data should be addressed where these arise. A further concern relates to the limitations of the pediatric neuropsychologist when asked to testify regarding so-called "Life Plans" for habitation and rehabilitation necessary as a consequence of the injuries sustained. Relatively few pediatric neuropsychologists have received specialty training in determining educational interventions and the work/employability economic estimates, which are often elements of a Life Plan. Similarly, some jurisdictions request that a formal determination of disability be assessed by an evaluator. If the pediatric neuropsychologist has not been formally trained or certified in these areas, rendering opinions on such issues may be beyond the scope of that practitioner's expertise. Because forensic consultation often involves a so-called 'battle of experts' (Glass, 1991) the expert may feel pressured to render opinions on information about which the pediatric neuropsychologist has limited experience or expertise. The ethical practitioner should advise the attorney of these limits to avoid being asked to comment on these issues in deposition or in trial testimony. Wherever possible, referral to an appropriately certified professional should be provided in these situations (Standards 1.04 and 1.06).

With the passage of PL94-142 (Education for all Handicapped Children Act) in 1975 and the revision of the act in PL101-476 (Individual with Disabilities Act – IDEA) in 1990, children with various disabilities are required by Public Law to be provided with free and appropriate public education (Latham & Latham, 1998). Pediatric neuropsychologists may be asked to examine a child to determine whether that child is eligible for special educational services under the specific state's requirements of eligibility. Requests for the evaluation may be initiated by the child's parent, by the child's school, and, occasionally, by state-funded programs for the education of handicapped children. Specialized educational and rehabilitation services are specified by an individualized education program (IEP) which must (by Federal regulation) be provided to a child who meets state guidelines for services. Typically, reports of a pediatric neuropsychological evaluation undertaken to provide information regarding a child's eligibility for services should include an introduction explaining the purpose of the examination, a 'fact' section that includes the history, interview information and testing results, and a final opinion section stating whether the child meets eligibility criteria (Latham & Latham, 1998). These elements are necessary in order to meet three criteria: (1) legal impairment; (2) impact of impairment on the child's functioning in the school setting (major life activity); and (3) recommended accommodations for the impairment. Lorber and York (1999) present a detailed review of the different criteria for eligibility under PL101-476 for a variety of developmental conditions, including autism, sensory impairments, emotional disorders, mental retardation, multiple disabilities, specific learning disabilities, and other health impairments. Children who do not meet criteria under PL101-146 may still be eligible for accommodations under section 504 of the Rehabilitation Act. This information should be included in a pediatric neuropsychologist's report where necessary and recommended accommodations are outlined.

Pediatric neuropsychologists may also be asked to evaluate a child for Social Security Disability under the Social Security Act. In order to be deemed eligible for SSI benefits, a child must be found to have a qualifying disability, and the family must lack the income and resources to manage the medical and rehabilitative services necessary to treat or manage the qualifying conditions (Latham & Latham, 1998). There has been considerable controversy regarding the inclusion of children with ADHD under these guidelines, in part because of varying state interpretations of a child's eligibility. The controversy involves, in part, whether such children meet the SSI criteria of substantial limitation in major life activities, as well as the economic concern over the increasing numbers of children who were qualified for SSI financial support. In my experience, careful documentation of specific impediments in life functioning and adjustment is necessary in neuropsychological reports being utilized for SSI eligibility. As a result, documentation beyond neuropsychological test results and diagnosis may be needed. For example, documentation of behavioral disorders, emotional disorder, and familial impact should be included. The pediatric neuropsychologist should include specific measures of these problems and document how these measures reliably indicate the impact of the child's ADHD diagnosis on 'major life functioning.' However, in my experience, neuropsychological assessments conducted in another context, for example, in response to a pediatric neurosurgeon's request for an evaluation of a child's cognitive functioning following surgery for a cerebellar astrocytoma, may be solicited by a state's Social Security office, accompanied by a signed parental release. In these circumstances, all of the information required for eligibility may not be included in the report. This is often the case when the neuropsychologist has had only a single consultative contact with the child. In addition to copies of the report, the state may send a detailed request for information regarding the child's condition that the pediatric neuropsychologist may simply not have. In these instances, a cover letter explaining the context and limits of the original consultation should accompany the report in order not to adversely affect the child's disability determination (Standard 2.09).

Other Ethical Issues in Pediatric Neuropsychology

There are several issues related to the general practice of pediatric neuropsychology which touch upon adherence to the General Ethical Principles of

Psychologists and Code of Conduct (APA, 1992). These include: (1) limited age-based norms on standardized tests; (2) limited data on neuropsychological profiles for many pediatric disorders; and (3) training and educational criteria for practice of the specialty of pediatric neuropsychology.

As a recent review has noted (Fennell, 1999), the validity of neuropsychological testing in general, and pediatric/child neuropsychological testing in particular, rests upon the availability of well-normed, age-appropriate measures of memory, visuospatial, language, motor, and executive functioning. Although recent compendiums of test norms have included some child-oriented tests (Spreen & Strauss, 1998), there is still a need for a compilation of test data on many widely used child instruments. A particular issue, familiar to pediatric neuropsychologists, is the age-gap in referenced norms for ages 15 to 21 years. As a result, there are no norms on many instruments for the adolescent years despite the fact that pediatric neuropsychologists are well aware of age effects on the development of various cognitive abilities (Fennell, 1999). If the pediatric neuropsychologist employs an instrument with minimal norms, there is an ethical obligation to document the potential impact of these limited norms on a reasonable interpretation of the data and on conclusions about the presence or absence of brain dysfunction (Standards 2.05 and 2.09).

A second issue relates to the need for information about the brain behavior effects of many childhood disorders (Fennell, 1999). Recent publications have begun to provide data on neuropsychological effects of a variety of primary childhood CNS disorders, for example, brain tumors or stroke disorders, of secondary CNS effects of primary medical diseases such as renal and cardiac disease, and on the CNS effects of treatment for medical disorders such as acute leukemias (Baron et al., 1995; Yeates et al., 2000). Assuming that knowledge about a disorder should guide, in part, interpretation of neuropsychological test data (Fennell & Bauer, 1997), the lack of sufficient information about a childhood disorder may limit the practitioner's ability to integrate the specific findings from an exam with the medical diagnosis (see Chapter 4 this volume) in order to derive meaningful recommendations for future care and/or special needs that the child may have. Reliance upon global measures of intellectual functioning such as intelligence testing, achievement, and/or memory batteries may be insufficient to describe the specific effects on brain functioning of a childhood disorder. The ethical neuropsychologist should formally acknowledge any limitations in the application of such global measures when asked to describe disorder-specific consequences of a neurological or medical condition affecting a child or adolescent.

A final issue relates to education and training in pediatric neuropsychology. At the present time, two major credentialing boards, the American Board of Professional Psychology (ABPP) and the American Board of Professional Neuropsychology (ABPN), provide certification of training for the practice of clinical neuropsychology per se. Neither Board offers sub-specialty certification in Pediatric/Child Neuropsychology. Increasing membership in the

Pediatric Neuropsychology Interest Group (PNIG), which meets at the annual meetings of the National Academy of Neuropsychology and the International Neuropsychological Society, documents the number of practitioners who indicate that they have a primary or exclusive focus on clinical and research activities in pediatric neuropsychology. Yet, as of now, no sub-specialty certification of education and training in pediatric neuropsychology is available.

The problem of credentialing for a specialty practice is not new to psychology in light of the lack of universally accepted criteria for training and expertise in neuropsychology (Woody, 1997). Because pediatric neuropsychologists must approach assessment from a normal and abnormal development context and because specific information regarding child neurology (Menkes, 2000) is a necessary part of understanding the effects of acquired or congenital neurological abnormalities on the developing CNS, as a rule, pediatric neuropsychologists eschew the use and interpretation of child assessment instruments by those who have not had specific training in pediatric neuropsychology. Further, because the pediatric neuropsychologist examines the child in the context of a family, including parents and siblings, pediatric neuropsychologists must also obtain general training in child clinical and/or pediatric psychology (Roberts, 1995). Unfortunately, a practicing pediatric neuropsychologist often encounters reports written by individuals whose training at the internship and/or postdoctoral level has been exclusively directed at adult disorders and whose practice is primarily directed at the adult population. Such reports often lead to descriptive interpretations of test scores (as abnormal) or quantitative interpretations (as above or below group means) or are unable to go beyond an acceptance of the face validity of the scores. Ethical principles (see Chapter 2, this volume) require that the psychologist practice in his/her area of competence by education, training, and experience (Standards 1.04 and 1.05). Those whose practice is primarily in the area of pediatric neuropsychology would argue that specific expertise is needed in the area of childhood disorders that goes beyond simply administering and interpreting widely available childhood tests and assessment instruments.

Closing Comments
Koocher and Keith-Speigel (1990, p. 67) offer a number of helpful guidelines for clinical practice with children and families, which are equally helpful in the ethical practice of pediatric neuropsychology. Regarding child assessment, the authors offer the following practice guidelines (slightly modified by the present author):

(1) When developing, administering, or interpreting psychological assessment tools, assure that the APA Standards for Educational and Psychological Testing are met;

(2) Report conclusions based on test results accurately and in a manner appropriate for the intended audience;

(3) Avoid making decisions that are based on test data that are inconsistent with the normative or intended use of the test instrument;
(4) Do not use test instruments that you have not been trained to administer or interpret;
(5) Do not assess a child or adolescent without parental consent.

Regarding issues of confidentiality and competence in working with children, Koocher and Keith Spiegel (1990, p. 87-88) also offer some of the following general guidelines for clinical practice (again, slightly modified by the present author):
(1) Carefully consider the differences in confidentiality requirements in working with children and adolescents as compared to adults;
(2) Practitioners must be aware of the state legal requirements and limitations placed on their professional relationships with child clients, including such matters as reporting child abuse, duty-to-protect rules, and family members access to child records;
(3) Careful consideration of the consequences of release of confidential materials to third parties (insurance carriers, schools) with information provided on a 'need-to-know' basis.

As Woody (1997) notes, all neuropsychological services should be based on education, research, and training, which is consistent with standards for being both a generalist and a specialist (p. 723). He asserts that there is a bright future for pediatric neuropsychology as long as the following issues are addressed by both the practitioner and the field in general: (1) identification of the limitations in assessment strategies; (2) the need for modifications in guiding theory and practice through research; (3) the need for advanced training in this practice area beyond doctoral degree programs; and (4) the need for prudence and caution by the termed 'psychological' issues in child clinical neuropsychology. He has surely identified issues of ethical relevance to all whose practice involves neuropsychological assessment of children and adolescents.

References

American Psychological Association (1992). *Ethical principles of psychologists and code of conduct*. Washington, DC: American Psychological Association.
Baron, I.S., Fennell, E.B., & Voeller, K.K.J. (1995). *Pediatric neuropsychology in a medical setting*. New York: Oxford University Press.
Barth, J.T. (2000). Commentary on "Disclosure of tests and raw test data to the courts" by Paul Lees-Haley and John Courtney. *Neuropsychology Review, 10*, 179-180.
Fennell, E.B. (1999). Issues in neuropsychological assessment of children and adolescents. In R. Vanderploeg (Ed.), *A clinician's guide to neuropsychological practice* (2nd ed.), (pp. 357-382). Hillsdale, NJ: Earlbaum Associates.

Fennell, E.B., & Bauer, R.M. (1997). Models of inference in evaluating brain–behavior relationships in children. In C.R. Reynolds & E. Fletcher-Ganzen (Eds.), *Handbook of child clinical neuorpsychology* (2nd ed.) (pp. 204-215). New York: Plenum Press.

Glass, L.S. (1991). The legal base in forensic neuropsychology. In H.O. Doerr & A.S. Carlin (Eds.), *Forensic neuropsychology: Legal and scientific bases* (pp. 3-16). New York: The Guilford Press.

Grote, C.L., Lewin, J.L., Sweet, J.J., & van Gorp, W.G. (2000). Responses to perceived unethical practices in clinical neuropsychology: Ethical and legal considerations. *The Clinical Neuropsychologist, 14*, 119-134.

Guilmette, T.J., & Hagan, L.D. (1997). Ethical considerations in forensic neuropsychological consultation. *The Clinical Neuropsychologist, 11*, 287-290.

Koocher, G.P., & Keith-Spiegel, P.C. (1990). *Children, ethics, and the law.* Lincoln, Nebraska: The University of Nebraska Press.

Latham, P.S., & Latham, P.H. (1998). Selected legal issues. In C.E. Coffey & R.A. Brumback (Eds.), *Textbook of child neuropsychiatry* (pp. 1491-1506). Washington, DC: American Psychiatric Association.

Lees-Haley, P.R., & Courtney, J.C. (2000). Disclosure of tests and raw test data to the courts: A need for reform. *Neuropsychology Review, 10*, 169-175.

Lorber, R., & York, H. (1999). Special pediatric issues: Neuropsychological applications and consultations in schools. In J.J. Sweet (Ed.), *Forensic neuropsychology: Fundamentals and practices* (pp. 369-418). Lisse: Swets & Zeitlinger Publishers.

McSweeny, A.J., Becker, B.C., Naugle, R.I., Snow, W.G., Binder, L.M., & Thompson, L.L. (1998). Ethical issues related to presence of third party observers in clinical neuropsychological evaluations. *The Clinical Neuropsychologist, 12*, 552-560.

Melton, G.P., Petrila, J., Poythress, N.G., & Slobogin, C. (1997). *Psychological evaluation for the courts* (2nd ed.). New York: The Guilford Press.

Menkes, J.A. (2000). *Child neurology* (6th ed.). Philadelphia: Lippincott, William, & Wilkins.

NAN Policy and Planning Committee (2000a). The use of neuropsychology test technicians in clinical practice: Official statement of the National Academy of Neuropsychology. *Archives of Clinical Neuropsychology, 15*, 381-382.

NAN Policy and Planning Committee (2000b). Presence of third party observers during neuropsychological testing: Official statement of the National Academy of Neuropsychology. *Archives of Clinical Neuropsychology, 15*, 379-380.

Rae, W.A., Worchel, F.F., & Brunnquell, D. (1995). Ethical and legal issues in pediatric psychology. In M.C. Roberts (Ed.), *Handbook of pediatric psychology* (2nd ed.) (pp. 19-36). New York: The Guilford Press.

Roberts, M.C. (1995). *Handbook of pediatric psychology* (2nd ed.). New York: The Guilford Press.

Shapiro, D.L. (2000). Commentary: Disclosure of tests and raw data to the courts. *Neuropsychology Review, 10*, 175-176.

Spreen, O., & Strauss, E. (1998). *A compendium of neuropsychological tests* (2nd ed.). New York: Oxford University Press.

Woody, R.H. (1997). Psychological issues for clinical child neuropsychology. In C.R. Reynolds & E. Fletcher-Janzen (Eds.), *Handbook of clinical child neuropsychology* (2nd ed.) (pp. 712-725). New York: Plenum Press.

Yeates, K.O., Ris, M.D., & Taylor, H.G. (2000). *Pediatric Neuropsychology.* New York: The Guilford Press.

Yeates, K.O., Taylor, H.G., Drotar, D., Wade, S.L., Klein, S., Stancin, T., & Schatschneider, C. (1997). Pre-injury family environment as a determinant of recovery from traumatic brain injuries in school-age children. *Journal of the International Neuropsychological Society, 3*, 617-630.

Chapter 6

ETHICAL ISSUES IN THE PRACTICE OF GERIATRIC NEUROPSYCHOLOGY

Joel E. Morgan

Introduction

The practice of geriatric clinical neuropsychology is no different from any other sub-specialty of neuropsychology in terms of the ethical responsibilities expected of its practitioners. Indeed, the APA Ethical Principles of Psychologists and Code of Conduct (1992) (hereinafter referred to as the Ethics Code) requires that all psychologists adhere to its principles and standards. In fact, the Ethics Code specifically calls attention to working with "special populations." 'Special populations' refer to groups of individuals whose demographics fall outside the norm. Individuals over the age of 65 constitute a special population in the practice of clinical neuropsychology. While many groups of individuals fall outside the expected normative ranges for education, primary language, race, national origin, ethnic affiliation, and so forth, it is the demographic of *age* that stands apart because the relationship between age and neuropsychological performance is both robust and well documented (Heaton et al., 1991). One could not, therefore, ethically practice *pediatric neuropsychology* without specific training in, and knowledge of, the unique characteristics of the brain–behavior relationships of children and adolescents. The same reasoning must be applied to senior citizens who may manifest a host of physical, cognitive, emotional, and demographic differences that set them apart, as a group, from the norm. In this regard, the ethical practice of geriatric neuropsychology must take cognizance of these differences. In addition to the Ethics Code in general, neuropsychological practice with geriatric patients specifically raises ethical issues involving competence of the practitioner (Standards 1.0x, 2.0x), assessment issues (Standard 2.0x), and confidentiality (Standard 5.0x). In addition, the proposed revision of the Ethics Code would require that informed consent take place prior to performing assessment services (Proposed Standards 3.10, 9.03) (APA, 2001). This change, if enacted, would raise specific issues for many geriatric assessments.

This chapter will focus on these aspects of the practice of geriatric clinical neuropsychology that have particular relevance to the Ethics Code and possible future revisions affecting practice. After a review of the most common ethical issues that may arise in geriatric practice, a case vignette approach will be utilized to illustrate common situations with the elderly. Case analysis and discussion will follow. It is hoped that this chapter will heighten the awareness and sensitivity of the clinical neuropsychologist to the special nature of working with geriatric clients and prepare the clinician for potential ethical situations and dilemmas that may arise in their geriatric practice. The avoidance of a pitfall is far easier than digging one's way out of the 'pit,' so to speak.

Geriatrics and Ethics: What are the issues?

Principle A of the Ethics Code concerns *Competence*. Most clinical neuropsychologists want to be, and certainly believe that they are, competent. But are special competencies required to work ethically with geriatric clients above and beyond those for general competence? What factors constitute a concern for special competencies? Standard 1.04 (Boundaries of Competence) calls for a psychologist to, "...provide services, teach, and conduct research only within the boundaries of their competence, based on education, training, supervised experience, or appropriate professional experience..." (a). Standard 1.04 (b) further stipulates that psychologists provide services in new areas only after appropriate training (paraphrasing), and (c) psychologists take reasonable steps to ensure the competence of their work in new or emerging areas where standards for preparatory training do not yet exist. It should certainly be obvious that for neuropsychologists who have not specifically worked with the elderly, their lack of experience with this population may render their work with geriatrics as *less than competent*. Take for example a young neuropsychologist recently completing training in a primarily pediatric/adolescent setting. Although some adults were seen during the training program, he or she really worked with many more children than adults and had only two previous geriatric cases. Familiarity with medical/physiological issues of aging and geriatric norms gleaned from a reference text is crucial to competent work. But such preparation alone may be insufficient in achieving a level of competency in geriatric neuropsychology that is compatible with independent practice and Ethics Code standards. Rather, having seen many geriatrics under the supervision of an experienced, senior neuropsychologist is crucial. In so doing, the nature of geriatric presentations, the kinds and degrees of disorders, and the myriad nature of establishing a professional relationship, eliciting full cooperation, and maintaining rapport with the elderly client can be *practiced clinically*. It is incumbent upon the professional who has a minimum of experience in direct patient care of the elderly to get supervision by an experienced colleague before engaging in independent professional work. It should go without saying that the reverse is certainly true (i.e., that pediatric neuropsychology should not be practiced by the professional with limited experience in the field), but this chapter concerns the elderly.

The reader may wonder why such experience is crucial? It is because the elderly have a unique set of factors that make them different from younger adults, and certainly from children. Among these factors are the effects of aging on sensory, motor, and cognitive functions[1]; medical disorders in the elderly[1]; the prevalence of depression and other emotional changes among the elderly[1]; educational, background, ethnic, and other demographic factors[2]; as well as others.

The effects of aging on sensory, motor and cognitive processes

Picture the following scenario: You have a new referral of an 81-year-old widow whose family has contacted you for an evaluation because they are worried about her 'memory'. After all of the appropriate questions, arrangements, and so forth have been made, the day arrives for the patient's appointment. The elderly lady is escorted to your office by her son and daughter-in-law. The patient is using a walker to assist her ambulation. You immediately notice her hands holding the bar of the walker: they are twisted, swollen and knurled with apparent arthritis. The patient's daughter-in-law says that, "...mom is hard of hearing so you must please speak up..." In conversation, you are further told that, "...mom has cataracts...and still sees but not perfectly..." To complicate matters more, they tell you that mom's memory seemed fine until recently when the death of her lifelong friend and neighbor occurred, "...she says she's not depressed about it.... but she just hasn't been the same.... what do you think doctor?" What *do* you think? What are the relevant issues?

The reader should not think for one moment that the above scenario is an exaggeration or an unusual experience. Rather, it is practically an everyday occurrence in the practice of geriatric clinical neuropsychology. The issues raised in the above scenario include: sensory processes (audition and vision), motor functioning (arthritis of the hands), and possible emotional factors (loss, depression). Do any of these factors have a potential effect on neuropsychological testing? Clearly the answer is 'yes.'

Accommodating to the patient's needs

It is well known that reduced sensory and motor functioning accompany aging (Tuokko & Hadjistavropoulos, 1998). Practitioners who wish to

---

[1] Factors that may affect performance.
[2] Factors that may affect data interpratation.

administer tests which were originally normed on younger, healthier adults may have to adjust administration procedures in order to accommodate the needs of geriatric patients with sensory and/or motor decline. The neuropsychologist should be aware that such procedural accommodations may violate standardized administration procedures, thus rendering results of dubious merit and utility, or invalidating them altogether. As a rule of thumb, the neuropsychologist should therefore always strive to use tests that were specifically developed for and normed on geriatric patients, where available (e.g., Dementia Rating Scale; Mattis, 1988). In the above brief vignette, for example, the patient's arthritis may be so severe that any tests of motor, praxis, construction, psychomotor, or manipulative abilities may not be able to be completed. Likewise, her visual acuity may be so poor as to make any testing in the visual modality impossible. The neuropsychologist may wonder about the feasibility of leaving vast areas of neurocognitive functioning untested, but this is precisely what one does in cases of complete and partial sensory or motor loss (e.g., hemiplegia, hemiparesis). The experienced neuropsychologist will attempt to glean as much useful and valid information from the patient as is possible, given the patient's limitations. It should be stressed, however, that appropriate norms should be used for age, education, gender, and where available, ethnic background, geographical region, and language. Finding appropriate norms for testing procedures that were performed under significant conditions of accommodation, however, may be very problematic. Standard 2.02(a)[3] addresses the appropriate use of assessment techniques and notes the importance of research-based evidence for such techniques. Neuropsychologists who accommodate to geriatric patients' needs must therefore do so in light of this standard. Where tests must be used which were not standardized and normed on the elderly, accommodations for administration procedures may be used only if the neuropsychologist explicitly states so in the evaluative report and expressly notes that such results must be interpreted with appropriate, conservative caution. Where significant reservation exits about such results, (i.e., has accommodation been so great so as to stretch the essential intent of the test and render the results dubious?) the neuropsychologist should state so, or perhaps not administer such tests at all, since validity is at issue. In all cases, that which is most important is fairness to the patient and an honest attempt to portray the patient's true abilities compared against his or her demographic peers.

Standard 2.04 requires the psychologist to be familiar with reliability, validation, standardization and outcome studies in the proper application of tests (a), to recognize the limits of certainty of their judgments (b), and to attempt to identify situations in which techniques and norms may not be applicable or require adjustment in administration because of demographic

---

[3] See also Standard 2.02(b) "Psychologists refrain from misuse of assessment techniques..."

factors (c). While on the surface this standard would 'permit' the neuropsychologist to accommodate to the patient's needs and abilities as required,
how does one really know that this departure from administration standards
yields results with any real validity? Here is where training and experience
become most important.

'Covert Agendas' in testing the elderly

Imagine this scenario: You are contacted by a woman who asks for a neuropsychological evaluation for her father. "He has Alzheimer's Disease,
doctor...the attorney requires a report from you before we can proceed..."
You think, "the *attorney? Proceed?*" You then find out that the elderly gentleman lives alone and is a retired, successful businessman with considerable financial assets. "Who diagnosed him as having Alzheimer's Disease",
you query. "Well, that's why we need your report – the family doctor said
we needed to see a neuropsychologist...and our attorney can't initiate the
paperwork until we do so..."

This scenario, like the last, is unfortunately quite common in the practice
of geriatric neuropsychology. It should at least raise some suspicion in the
practitioner. Perhaps the entire thing is quite legitimate; maybe the gentleman is demented and incompetent. But what if not? Maybe he is only mildly
demented, then what? How should the ethical neuropsychologist proceed?
In either case, it is incumbent on the qualified and ethical neuropsychologist
to understand these issues from the beginning, proceed with competence and
care, and always have the *patient's* interests at heart.

Informed consent for assessment

Standard 3.10(a) of the proposed revision to the Ethics Code would require
that psychologists obtain informed consent to, "...conduct research, provide
assessment, psychotherapy, or counseling...using language that is reasonably
understandable to that person...informed consent ordinarily requires that
the person has the capacity to consent, has been provided information that
might affect his/her willingness to participate, and is aware of the voluntary
nature of participation and has freely and without undue influence expressed
consent..."

Imagine attempting to gain informed consent in the above scenario: "Mr.
Jones, please sign here indicating that you agree to take these tests which
would ultimately result in your being declared incompetent to participate in
your own care, make decisions, and handle any of your financial affairs. Oh,
your family will end up with all your assets. Yes, thank you very much..."
It will likely not be that easy. Indeed, in cases of suspected diminished intellectual capacity and reduced ability to comprehend the ultimate possible consequences of neuropsychological testing, what is the ethical and appropriate
thing for the neuropsychologist to do? Likewise, in cases such as the above
scenario where it may be that family members have an apparent unexpressed
agenda to gain substantial financial resources, and where the patient does

not appear to warrant such decision from a neuropsychological perspective, what is the appropriate course of action?

Providing feedback and the limits of confidentiality

In geriatric practice, as in all clinical practice, it is incumbent upon the psychologist to provide appropriate feedback to the patient, medico-legal and forensic assessments aside (Standard 2.09). In the case of the geriatric patient, an explanation of results is no less important than with other adults. With geriatric patients, feedback to family and other professionals is common, and a release of information from the client may be required to do so, depending on the situation. The neuropsychologist may also be called upon to provide emotional support to the client and/or the family, depending on the results.

Clearly, issues of confidentiality regarding assessment results are common in geriatric practice. Imagine for a moment the case of the geriatric patient who is demented but who refuses to let his family know. This could be a potentially dangerous situation for the client, as you may have determined that he needs to be supervised. Where, then, are the boundaries of confidentiality drawn?

Case Vignettes, Analysis, and Ethical Resolution

In this section we will look at more detailed vignettes that may present multiple ethical issues imbedded in a single case. The reader is encouraged to examine each case carefully and determine the ethical issues, decide on potential resolutions, and determine how to avoid such situations, where appropriate, in the future.

Case Study 1

Imagine the following scenario: You assess a 76 year-old, single male, Mr. A. You note that he lives alone, drove himself to the evaluation alone, and apparently takes care of his own needs. He tells you his only living relative is a niece who lives out of state. You do the evaluation. You cannot believe the results.... but you are quite certain that he tried his best on all of the tests. He has a Master's Degree in Accounting and worked for over 45 years as a corporate CPA, rising to the rank of Assistant Vice President for Finance. You obtain a Wechsler Adult Intelligence Scale-Revised (WAIS-R) Full Scale IQ of 88, with slightly better verbal than performance scores. He earns a T-Score of 27 on the California Verbal Learning Test (CVLT), Wechsler Memory Scale-Revised (WMS-R) Verbal Memory Index of 77, Visual Memory Index of 58. He took 300 seconds on Trail Making Part B before you cut it off, after 6 errors, and less than halfway done. His score on the Mattis Dementia Rating Scale (DRS) was 98. He completed only one category on the Wisconsin Card Sorting Test (WCST) and made over 30 perseverations. His copy of the Rey figure was unintelligible. He only knew 38 items on the Boston Naming Test

(BNT) and he made numerous semantic paraphasic errors and circumlocutions (e.g., for bench: "a place to sit in the park...made of wood..."). Animal Naming score was 12; FAS was 19.

You had little doubt that this gentleman had a dementia syndrome and with no cardiovascular history, otherwise normal labs, and "...mild to moderate atrophy and ventricular dilatation..." on his MRI, it was consistent with Probable DAT. Now, how was this man driving, living alone, and attending to his needs?

You find out more: You ask him how he spends his time, how he takes his meals, etc. "Oh", he says, "Margaret helps me." After a rather circumstantial story with much perseveration, you glean that 'Margaret' is someone he picked up in a bar. He takes his 'dinner' at this bar, and dines on the free hors d'oeuvres. He proudly tells you, "...she used to be a prostitute, you know."

At any rate, you find out that he lent her some money over the past six months: $55,000.00 to be exact. You are practically choking now: "Mr. A., why did you lend her so much money?", you ask, practically sick by now. "She needs it — sick mother, you know." Is there no decency?

What are the issues in this case? What should the neuropsychologist do?

Case study 1: analysis and ethical resolution

It should be emphasized that although it seems somewhat dramatically portrayed, this is an actual case from the author's clinical practice. In fact, Mr. A. had "lent" (i.e., given) 'Margaret' a total of $77,550.00 over the past 11 months, confirmed by his niece somewhat later after she got involved. Margaret was indeed a prostitute, among other occupations. The ethical issues in this case are: (1) providing appropriate feedback to Mr. A. Indeed, Mr. A. was told that he had a serious problem with his memory and judgment and that this was likely to be a dementia. Mr. A. was told that he must no longer drive an automobile and was encouraged to voluntarily give it up. "But then how will I take Margaret to the bank to withdraw money for her?", he wanted to know. His niece had to be told — Mr. A. was literally throwing away vast sums of money, as his judgment was so impaired. In the end, Mr. A. had to move into an assisted living facility and his niece became his power-of-attorney. He never quite seemed to understand that Margaret was not looking out for his best interests.

What are the ethical issues in Case 1?

Competence — (1.04 Boundaries of Competence; 2.01 Evaluation, Diagnosis, and Intervention in a Professional Context; 2.02 Competence and Appropriate Use of Assessments and Interventions; 2.05 Interpreting Assessment Results).

One would certainly have to have basic neuropsychological competence in the assessment of dementia and related disorders in the elderly in order to have correctly assessed Mr. A and to have drawn the conclusions that his judgment was impaired with regard to his finances, that he was not properly caring for himself, and that he was potentially dangerous to himself or others because he continued to drive an automobile. It should also be understood that the correct clinical conclusions concerning the patient required knowledge of appropriate assessment techniques, most compatible norms, and sufficient knowledge of dementia and related disorders.

Providing Feedback — (2.09 Explaining Assessment Results).
Like it or not, Mr. A. had to be told that he was cognitively impaired, and that he had to stop driving, and not waste further funds on his 'friend' Margaret. Mr. A. balked at the whole thing and was at first not a willing subscriber to this input. The resolution of this dilemma raised the other important ethical issue in this case, confidentiality.

Confidentiality — (5.05 Disclosures (a) "Psychologists disclose confidential information without the consent of the individual. ...where permitted by law for a valid purpose such as ...(3) *to protect the patient, client, or others from harm*").
Mr. A. did not accept the recommendations of the neuropsychologist, and his niece had to be enlisted to help. She obviously had to be told what was going on, such as his diagnosis, the fact that he was still driving (he had had a number of accidents by now), and what poor financial judgment he was manifesting. A breech of confidentiality and of professional privilege was necessary to protect both the patient and others. Mr. A. had become prey to a woman who exploited his cognitive deficits and poor social judgment. Margaret had taken over $77,000 from Mr. A. and, although she argued that he gave it to her willingly and freely of his own choice, the presence of his dementia, likely to be DAT, made her argument irrelevant. It was also discovered by Mr. A.'s niece that he had also become prey to some telemarketers and had given his credit card number out. Serious financial difficulties for the family were the result, a sad situation since Mr. A. was going to require his assets for placement in a nursing home. Mr. A. also never voluntarily relinquished his driver's license, and the state Department of Vehicles had to be contacted. In all, the ethical neuropsychologist in this case will be competent, use assessment techniques correctly, provide appropriate feedback, and disclose pertinent case information to appropriate family and government officials in order to protect the patient, his resources, and the public.

Case Study 2
The situation: Dr. Smith is a neuropsychologist at a large, urban Midwest medical center. He is called one day by a hospital surgeon to evaluate Mrs. R. for, "...competency to refuse medical treatment..." Mrs. R. was in the hospital with gangrene of her right foot and ankle. She had a long history of poorly controlled diabetes and spotty medical care over the more recent past. The surgeon informs Dr. Smith that, "...if we don't remove her foot she will

die..." But the situation was problematic for the physicians because Mrs. R. apparently was refusing to have the surgery, "...I'm too old and sick...just leave me alone", she told the surgeon. The surgeon felt that she was not mentally competent to make decisions on her own behalf, that she did not understand the seriousness of her condition, and that she had impaired judgment — "...otherwise, surely she would have given her consent for the life-saving surgery. I don't think she understands that she will die unless she has this done. She is otherwise reasonably healthy and could have more time." The hospital social service worker had been called and could not locate any family to provide informed consent. Hence, a call was placed to Dr. Smith, the neuropsychologist.

Mrs. R. was a widowed woman in her late 70s who had been living on her own. She was living on a small pension, having worked for 40 years as a bookkeeper for a local business. To her neighbors, she had been managing apparently well for many years, but more recently hadn't been seen by her neighbors in some time. Mrs. R. had no children and although she spoke of some distant relatives "upstate', no one knew for sure about the existence of these relatives, and none of her neighbors had ever seen them. The social worker reported that her apartment was reasonably neat and, although not spotlessly clean, was acceptable. Her neighbors indicated that Mrs. R. was a pleasant woman who minded her own business. They used to see her come and go with groceries but hadn't seen her in a while. They wondered if she had taken sick, and knew she had 'sugar.' She ended up in the hospital after her neighbor from the adjacent apartment became concerned that she hadn't seen her and knocked on the door. The neighbor found her with a 'black foot,' unable to move. She immediately called an ambulance.

At the hospital, Mrs. Smith was told about her diagnosis by the surgeon and his associates. They were very concerned because her condition was critical, and they were afraid of the further spread of gangrene. "She said she didn't want it — she must not understand. She must have Alzheimer's...", the surgeon told Smith; "...just tell us that she's incompetent so that we can do the surgery and save her life, Dr. Smith."

At first Mrs. R. was not amenable to Dr. Smith's assessment, but after several visits over a day and a half, he was able to elicit her cooperation. She agreed to take "these silly tests..." Mrs. R. completed High School in a city in the Midwest and had two years of college. Smith's results are as follows: Mattis Dementia Rating Scale — 139; WAIS-R FSIQ — 103; WMS-R General Memory Index — 98; California Verbal Learning Test — Trials 1–5 — T = 43, Recognition — 14 hits, 2 false positives, Perseverations = 1, Intrusions = 4; Boston Naming Test 56/60; Animal Naming 29; CFL — 49; Trail Making A — 47"; Trail Making B — 96" (no errors); Halstead Category Test — 41 errors; Rey figure copy 33/36; Rey figure immediate 26/36; Rey figure delayed 24/36; Beck Depression Inventory — 46.

Is Smith's battery appropriate? What is the apparent conclusion? What is now the appropriate course of action for Smith in consideration of his professional ethical responsibilities? Take note about the increasing pressure from the Department of Surgery and the hospital administration. The reader is asked how he or she would now proceed?

Case 2 analysis and ethical resolution

On the basis of his neuropsychological assessment and interview, Dr. Smith concluded that Mrs. R. was indeed competent to provide informed consent for her medical care and that if she decided she was not going to have the surgery, it was not because she did not understand the consequences, or because of reduced cognitive capacity. She had no evidence of dementia or other severe cognitive disorder, but the BDI was consistent with a moderately severe depression. Mrs. R. denied that she had suicidal thought but simply stated, "...I'm just too old...I have no one...let it be..." A psychiatric consult was called for, and the psychiatrist, agreeing with Dr. Smith's clinical assessment, prescribed Prozac. Meanwhile, the surgeon was worried, as Mrs. R.'s condition was deteriorating, and they were afraid of "blood poison — a life-threatening condition." At this point, Mrs. R. was still refusing surgery. The social worker informed that there was no family, and the 'upstate' relatives did not seem to exist. The surgeon would ask a Judge to intervene and get a court order, but Smith argued that Mrs. R. was fully cognizant and that there were no legal grounds to force her to have the operation. The psychiatrist informed that it would probably be at least two weeks for the medication to have any demonstrable effect. Smith decided to attempt to engage the patient in psychotherapy with more frequent visits. He determined that the lady was fearful of having to live without her foot, "...how will I get around...what will become of me...I'm all alone..." In a real life 'Deus ex machina', Smith finally convinced Mrs. R. to have the surgery. "O.K., O.K.", she said, "I suppose you're right."

Indeed, Mrs. Smith was competent to make decisions on her own behalf. She was neither demented nor mentally ill to the extent that would warrant a declaration of being mentally incompetent. She could give informed consent. However, Smith correctly determined that the patient's depression was probably related to her decision. The only recourse was to attempt counseling, which was successful.

What are the ethical issues in Case 2?

Competence — (1.04 Boundaries of Competence; 2.01 Evaluation, Diagnosis, and Intervention in a Professional Context; 2.02 Competence and Appropriate Use of Assessments and Interventions; 2.05 Interpreting Assessment Results).

As in the first case, competence is the critical issue in all clinical work. Had the neuropsychologist had inadequate training and experience in geriatric assessment, the results may have been different. It should be pointed out that one of the most common mistakes that inexperienced neuropsychologists make is diagnosing 'brain damage' or 'impairment' where there is none (personal communication, ABPP/ABCN examination committee). The patient's results, although clearly average, could certainly have been misinterpreted. One must know what the correct normative standards are and use them appropriately. In every case, with every patient, ethical practice must first be defined in terms of competence.

Professional Relationships — (1.20 Consultations and Referrals (b) "...psychologists cooperate with other professionals in order to serve their patients...effectively..."; 1.21 Third Party Requests for Services).
Dr. Smith worked appropriately with other professionals. Despite the intense pressure from Surgery and the hospital administrator, Smith acted ethically by not 'colluding' with them, despite severe pressure, and by correctly indicating Mrs. R's mental status. A neuropsychologist, or any psychologist for that matter, must act as an independent professional, in accordance with license/certification laws.

Principle D: Respect for People's Rights and Dignity
Smith correctly was concerned with Mrs. R's right to self-determination, especially considering her normal mental status. He did not directly challenge her or confront her decision, as he realized that he might have risked alienating her and losing her. Instead, he slowly developed a trusting relationship and won her over with his skill, while at the same time respecting her autonomy and right to determine her own future. He competently provided the most appropriate service to the patient and gradually won her over with counseling and the development of a professional relationship.

Case Study 3
What happens in the criminal forensic arena when an elderly man is referred for a neuropsychological evaluation by his attorney but refuses to participate? As are the others, this is an actual case from the author's practice. You are called one day by the State Public Defender's Office, Assistant Public Defender Gray. He asks if you would evaluate his client — a 76 year-old male, who has been indicted on charges of aggravated sexual abuse of a minor child, endangering the welfare of a minor, and public lewdness — he is accused of fondling his six-year-old granddaughter while baby-sitting for her. "I have to tell you, though, doc, this guy is not very cooperative...we all think something is wrong with him, but need to be sure." You accept the case.

The background information reveals that the client is a divorced male for over 25 years, whose ex-wife recently died. He has one daughter, the mother of the six-year-old girl who is the alleged victim of sexual assault. The client is out on bail, and he denies the charges against him. Further, despite the fact that his own attorney requested the evaluation, the client refuses. He stated, "...there's nothing wrong with me and I am innocent. Besides, I'm 76 years old; what do they want from me?"

You attempt to make an appointment with the client. He tells you that he knows nothing about this. He even denies hearing anything about it from his lawyer. You tell him you have a copy of a letter from his attorney, explaining that you would call to set up an appointment for the evaluation. He says he never saw any letter like that and he hangs up. Annoyed, you call Mr. Gray's office. Gray tells you again that his client isn't very cooperative and wonders if you could intervene, "...you're the doctor, maybe you could convince him he needs the testing to help him." Gray explains that *if* there is something wrong with him, it could benefit him, either by (1) taking a defense tack of insanity, if it actually comes to trial and *if* he's really that bad, or (2) diminished capacity, which might allow the court to not impose a jail sentence but to remand him to treatment, probation, etc. In either case, Gray says, the prosecutor has a good case and is not inclined to give him much leeway, despite his age, "unless we can prove he's not all there." To complicate matters even more, it is the client's *daughter* who otherwise could be instrumental in getting him to cooperate but who is refusing to even talk to him. "After what he did, never! Let him rot in jail!" She, the daughter, further confides in you that he (her father — the client) also abused her when she was little, but she said nothing about it. "Now it's all out in the open. I was too ashamed before, but not after what he's done to our daughter, too."

You have spoken to the client several more times but have not made much headway. You're not sure, but you do suspect that the man doesn't completely understand the very serious nature of the charges against him. In fact, you think that perhaps he has a mild dementia or a psychiatric disorder. "Sir," you say, "the testing that I have been asked to do might just help you. You don't seem to understand that you are in very serious trouble." "My daughter made the whole thing up to get my money," he says. He then hangs up on you again.

You report back to Gray that things are not going very well. Gray says that he absolutely needs the testing because it's the only avenue to any possible defense. "We'll just have to get a court order to make him do it", says Gray. "Oh great," you think, "he's not hostile enough!" But frankly, you aren't sure how to proceed. How would *you, the reader,* proceed at this point? What are the ethical issues involved in this sensitive matter?

If a court order is issued, you certainly do not need the client to sign an informed consent for the evaluation, and that is precisely the turn of events. The court order was issued and the client arrived for the scheduled appointment. However, he was un-testable, as he refused to even speak to the neuropsychologist. It is not possible to test someone without eliciting his cooperation. So the opportunity was used to speak with the client. After an hour and twenty minutes, the client is a little more cooperative. He is talking to you, though he still refuses the testing, and you are now convinced more than ever that he *really* doesn't get it. You are persistent, and finally a little later he blurts out: "You mean she would actually try to send me to jail for that? I love her, that's why I did it. I loved them both!"

You explain that he should tell Mr. Gray exactly what he just said to you. Now, on the basis of the interview, you believe he has some mental disorder, you are not sure what, and really need to test him. He continues to refuse. Next, having no other recourse, the Judge orders him to be admitted to the State Psychiatric Hospital for 30 days of observation. The discharge summary notes a diagnostic impression of "Rule-out Paranoid Personality Disorder; rule-out Dementia, NOS." Neuropsychological testing is requested.

The case is resolved when the judge orders the client, his attorney, and the prosecutor to his chambers for a confrontation. Essentially, the judge read the client the riot act: either cooperate fully with the doctor's testing or spend the next three months in jail! Testing began three days later.

Premorbidly, he was a High School graduate, born and raised in the Northeast, who worked his entire life as an insurance salesman. Test results revealed a mild dementia syndrome, but striking executive system deficits. He earned a WAIS-R Full Scale IQ of 89. He was unable to perform the Stroop. He was unable to achieve any categories on the Wisconsin Card Sort. He made 113 errors on the Halstead Category Test. He could not complete Trail Making B. He earned a CVLT total T-Score of 31. Boston Naming Test was 39/60. Animal Naming was 12; CFL was 19. He made numerous perseverations on fluency and memory tests. He was clearly impaired. On the basis of test results, an MRI was requested which revealed a large frontal neoplasm, consistent with a glioma. Even then, he had no neurological symptoms, none at all. He was given probation and remanded to psychiatric and medical care.[4]

Case 3 analysis and ethical resolution

You acted ethically in this case. You attempted to solicit cooperation from the client. You did not give premature feedback to counsel, or to anyone for that matter. And you waited for the client to consent and cooperate, albeit not without some severe pressure. You advocated for your client in a professional manner without crossing boundaries. Suppose, however, that you had decided to contact the client's daughter, in an effort to elicit her cooperation.[5]

---

[4]   As a clinical note, it is interesting that, diagnostically, he had a fairly rapidly growing tumor which may have been related to his alleged social impropriety with his granddaughter, if in fact it occurred. If the allegation by the client's daughter, that he abused her as well, many years before, is true, his present neurological condition likely had no bearing whatsoever.

[5]   Although contacting the patient's family is a logical and ethical decision in ordinary clinical cases, the fact that the client's daughter was on the opposite side of a felony indictment would have resulted in a clear conflict of interest and violation of Ethical Standards 1.17 Multiple Relationships and 7.03 Clarification of Roles in Forensic Assessments.

What are the ethical issues in Case 3?

Competence — (1.04 Boundaries of Competence; 2.01 Evaluation, Diagnosis, and Intervention in a Professional Context; 2.02 Competence and Appropriate Use of Assessments and Interventions; 2.05 Interpreting Assessment Results).
As in every case, experience in geriatric neuropsychology is crucial. Without sufficient training and experience, one may not have provided the appropriate tests and arrived at the conclusion to request neuroimaging in a man without any hard symptoms.

Professional Relationships — (1.21 Third Party Requests for Services)
It is incumbent upon the psychologist to clarify his or her role with the requestor of services at the very beginning (a). In this case, the psychologist was called upon by defense counsel to act as diagnostician and expert. The psychologist must further avoid the potential of conflicting roles and clarify the nature of his or her responsibility (b).

Forensic Activities — (7.02 Forensic Assessments)
Forensic assessments are based on techniques sufficient to provide appropriate substantiation to their findings (a). Such techniques should have an empirical basis and scientific credibility. In the present case, the forensic assessment is a neuropsychological evaluation. Appropriate tests and norms were utilized in the evaluation, and diagnostic conclusions were based on credible scientific evidence.

Conclusions

This chapter presented case examples of common ethical situations and dilemmas in practice with geriatric clients. Issues of sensitivity to the special nature of geriatric individuals were stressed, with an understanding that competence in geriatric neuropsychological practice requires special training and experience and acquisition of a special knowledge base. Seniors often have sensory, motor, cognitive, emotional, social, and/or behavioral changes which must be clearly understood by the neuropsychologist working in this arena. The competent neuropsychologist will utilize the most appropriate measures and norms and will make decisions and conclusions based on appropriate scientific evidence. Accommodating to the patient's needs, while at the same time securing the validity of the assessment process, is a most important factor.

Establishing rapport with geriatric clients, eliciting their full cooperation, providing informed consent where appropriate (or utilizing surrogates in cases where informed consent cannot be granted because of medical or mental conditions), and providing gentle feedback are crucial issues in geriatric practice. Respect and dignity for the elder client underlies all of these professional activities, where the welfare of the client is our top priority.

Clinical neuropsychologists who practice with geriatric clients are encouraged to familiarize themselves with these issues. In so doing, the avoidance of potentially damaging ethical dilemmas can be maintained in a rewarding and meaningful clinical practice.

References

American Psychological Association (1992). Ethical principles of psychologists and code of conduct. *American Psychologist, 47*, 1597-1611.

American Psychological Association (June, 2001). Proposed revision to the ethical principles of psychologists and code of conduct, Draft 5. Available at: www.apa.org/ethics/draft/html.

Heaton, R.K., Grant, I., & Matthews, C. G. (1991). *Comprehensive norms for an expanded Halstead–Reitan battery: Demographic corrections, research findings, and clinical applications.* Odessa, FL: Psychological Assessment Resources, Inc.

Mattis, S. (1988). *Dementia Rating Scale.* Odessa, FL: Psychological Assessment Resources.

Tuokko, H., & Hadjistavropoulos, T. (1998). *An assessment guide to geriatric neuropsychology.* Mahwah, NJ: Lawrence Erlbaum and Associates.

Chapter 7

ETHICAL ISSUES IN FORENSIC NEUROPSYCHOLOGY

Jerry J. Sweet, Christopher Grote, and Wilfred G. van Gorp

Introduction

The common dictionary definition of *forensic* notes the Latin source of the term *forensis*, referring to public or forum (the public square or marketplace of ancient Roman cities in which legal, political, and other business was conducted). Although so frequently associated in current parlance with formal civil and criminal court proceedings that some consider the term to be synonymous with such activities, the term forensic actually has a much broader meaning at present. In historical context, and true to common dictionary descriptions, the term forensic actually denotes public discussion, argumentation, and formal debate. In fact, the term 'forensic' has been used within educational systems to describe debating activities. For the purposes of this book chapter, *forensic neuropsychology* will be considered to be those activities of neuropsychologists that involve rendering an opinion that will be 'argued' or, in some manner, adjudicated by others. Thus, forensic neuropsychology includes cases that are seen within a context of potentially adversarial critique and discussion by individuals who are not healthcare providers. Some cases originally seen within a context of ordinary clinical referral will end up involving neuropsychologists in adversarial disputes, whereas other cases will involve neuropsychologists at a point that services are requested expressly for the purpose of aiding in the resolution of an adversarial proceeding. Neuropsychological activities related to criminal and civil proceedings, whether judicial (criminal, child custody, personal injury, medical malpractice, competency, product liability, worker's compensation, etc.) or administrative (educational 'due process,' disability determination, 'fitness for duty,' etc.) are all considered to be within the purview of the present chapter.

Forensic activities have risen to a place of prominence in the practices of clinical neuropsychologists since the 1980s. In fact, attorneys are the number one referral source for private practice neuropsychologists, who are now the majority of the field, and the number five referral source for institutionally-based neuropsychologists (Sweet et al., 2000). Given that our definition of forensic neuropsychology involves a greater number of cases than simply those referred by attorneys, the involvement of neuropsychologists in forensic activities is truly widespread. This fact explains the recent surge of practitioner interest in, and commensurate increasing numbers of relevant publications (e.g., McCaffrey et al., 1996; Guilmette & Hagan, 1997; van Gorp & McMullen, 1997; Sweet, 1999) regarding the topic of forensic neuropsychology. These publications include the *Journal of Forensic Neuropsychology*, which began circulation in 1999, and an April 2000 issue of *Journal of Head Trauma Rehabilitation*, exclusively on the topic of forensic neuropsychology, and a Summer 2000 issue of *Brain Injury Resource*, exclusively on the topic of relevant forensic topics.

Clinical neuropsychology has a relatively brief history compared to other health care specialties. For the most part, clinical neuropsychologists did not achieve a national presence in healthcare settings and in clinical psychology training programs until the 1980s, even though its formal roots in the United States could be traced back a few decades earlier. By comparison, many medical specialties and clinical psychology, the progenitor of clinical neuropsychology, are much older. How is it then that forensic activities relatively quickly have become so common place to neuropsychologists, and, conversely, that forensic neuropsychology has become so well integrated into the wide array of judicial and administrative processes? Sweet (1999) has contended that the rapid growth of clinical neuropsychologists rendering opinions in adversarial matters has in great measure resulted from the scientist traditions within the field and the self-selected tendency for neuropsychologists to provide a quantitative basis for their opinions. Moreover, these scientist-practitioner underpinnings also result in many clinical neuropsychologists being accustomed to the often intense scrutiny of peer review related to one's work. The scrutiny in forensic matters pertaining to 'what do we believe' to be true, 'how did we come to believe' it is true, and 'what is the evidence for and against' a particular proposition is recognizable and familiar to scientifically minded clinicians, such as clinical neuropsychologists. Judicial and administrative decision-makers need such dispassionate, objective information upon which to base their ultimate judgments. Importantly, the information provided by clinical neuropsychologists is typically different from and non-redundant, although sometimes complementary, to information from medical colleagues in neurology, psychiatry, radiology, and other specialties. Thus, there is also an important element of uniqueness in the information provided by neuropsychologists.

The present chapter will discuss the unique issues, conflicts, and potential resolutions pertaining to engaging in ethical forensic neuropsychological practice. This area of ethical concern has become an important one, as demonstrated by Pope and Vetter (1992) whose survey of American Psychological Association (APA) members resulted in forensic-related ethical concerns being ranked fifth highest for frequency of "ethically troubling incidents." As involvement in forensic activities has increased substantially in recent years, the relative frequency of forensic-related ethical concerns most likely has also increased since the Pope and Vetter survey. However, in general, neuropsychologists share many of the same concerns regarding ethical forensic practice as other healthcare and non-healthcare specialists, and in this regard bear no greater burden than these other professionals who strive to offer impartial information to triers-of-fact.

Readers may also be interested in the ethical guidelines promulgated by Division 41 (Psychology and Law) of APA (Committee on Ethical Guidelines for Forensic Psychologists, 1991), an earlier review by Binder and Thompson (1995), and illustrative ethics case examples in relevant textbooks (e.g., Nagy, 2000). For ease of enumeration and understanding, readers will note the listing in Table 1 of ethical conflicts pertinent to forensic neuropsychology, and in Table 2 of related ethical principles and standards.

Unique Ethical Aspects of Forensic Neuropsychological Activities

Role Differences: Clinician Versus Retained Forensic Expert Witness
Immediately recognizable to any experienced health care provider asked to render an expert opinion is the monumental difference between such a forensic endeavor and providing clinical care. The traditional role of a clinician

Table 1. Ethical conflicts that commonly arise in forensic matters.

Role differences: Clinician versus retained forensic expert witness
'Treating' expert (fact) witness versus retained expert (opinion) witness roles
Limitations or absence of confidentiality
Possible absence of informed consent to evaluate
Billing issues (liens, letters of protection or assignation, billing health insurance)
Pressing need for documentation and justification of opinion; bases of judgments
Test security and release of records
Practicing within limits of competency and within scope of practice
Undermining of objectivity due to influence of multiple pressures
Truthfulness
Balancing of forensic expectations, legal rules, and ethical responsibilities, which may
          at times conflict
Legitimate versus pseudo-credentials
Maintaining competency
Multiple relationships
Appropriate use of assessment instruments

Table 2. Specific ethical principles and standards that relate to common forensic issues.

Principle A:	Competence
Principle B:	Integrity
Principle C:	Professional and Scientific Responsibility
Principle D:	Respect for People's Rights and Dignity
Standard 1.02:	Relationship of Ethics and Law
Standard 1.04:	Boundaries of Competence
Standard 1.05:	Maintaining Expertise
Standard 1.06:	Basis for Scientific and Professional Judgments
Standard 1.09:	Respecting Others
Standard 1.21:	Third-Party Requests for Services
Standard 1.23:	Documentation of Professional and Scientific Work
Standard 1.24:	Records and Data
Standard 1.25:	Fees and Financial Arrangements
Standard 1.26:	Accuracy in Reports to Payors and Funding Sources
Standard 2.02:	Competence and Appropriate Use of Assessments and Interventions
Standard 2.05:	Interpreting Assessment Results
Standard 2.10:	Maintaining Test Security
Standard 3.03:	Avoidance of False or Deceptive Statements
Standard 5.01:	Discussing the Limits of Confidentiality
Standard 5.04:	Maintenance of Records
Standard 5.09:	Preserving Records and Data
Standards 7.01–7.06:	Forensic Activities (professionalism, assessments, clarification of role, truthfulness and candor, prior relationships, compliance with law and rules)
Standard 8.02:	Confronting Ethical Issues

is to provide a palliative or curative service to a patient, either directly or through the provision of a consultative opinion to another health care provider who is rendering care to the patient. In a forensic context, the person being evaluated is not a 'patient,' but rather an individual who is pursuing one of a number of possibly broad-ranging goals, which can be divided into *awards* and *favorable outcomes*. Awards include financial compensation (e.g., in the instances of personal injury litigation and disability determination) and treatment at no personal cost with the possibility of compensation and/or rehabilitation, if treatment fails (e.g., in the instance of a work-related injury). Favorable outcomes not involving financial compensation include educational accommodations (e.g., development of a special individual educational plan to meet non-routine educational needs, special test-taking considerations) permission to return to duty (e.g., after involuntary treatment for illness or drug addiction), avoidance of criminal responsibility or criminal punishment, or even avoidance of military service. In each instance, it is common that non-health care providers will rule on the final outcome. Before the individual's goal of receiving an award or favorable outcome can be reached, others must first be convinced of the necessity and appropriateness of any award. Health care providers, such as clinical neuropsychologists, provide valuable information to the administrators, lawyers, and judges involved in the specific forensic arena. Often this information is very similar to that which is the subject of neuropsychologists' common activities with traditional clinical referrals. However, unlike the traditional clinical context, the individual who is the subject of the evaluation is not the intended recipient of the service when the context is a forensic one. Instead, the recipient of the service is the party who retains the expert, which could be a plaintiff attorney or defense attorney engaged in a lawsuit, a disability insurance carrier, a parent of a school age child, a school system, a governmental agency (e.g., Social Security Administration, Veteran's Administration, Federal Aviation Agency), police department, or some other party.

'Treating' Expert Witness Versus 'Retained' Expert Witness

In litigated proceedings, an important distinction is made between a 'treater' and a 'retained' expert witness. Although both are considered experts, which is a matter of training and experience, a 'treater' is a witness who formerly has been or currently is in a role of providing clinical care to an individual who can be considered a 'patient' by virtue of the nature of the referral and the relationship with the professional. The term is used broadly to include clinicians who have provided interventions intended to ameliorate a condition, as well as those who may have performed only assessment activities. There has been much discussion of the possible bias on the part of a treating health care provider toward the plaintiff who was once, or is still, a patient of the provider (cf. Strasburger et al., 1997). It has been speculated that such a bias may have its roots in a positive therapeutic bond with the patient, within which rests the normally appropriate goal of wanting to *help* the patient. However, as a 'treating' expert witness, the intended goal of participating in the legal proceeding is to provide facts, as dispassionately as possible. This dual role of treater and subsequent expert has been described as inherently fraught with tension and pressures, which, particularly if not acknowledged, could act to alter an otherwise more objective expert opinion. Standard 7.05 (*Prior Relationships*) indicates that in forensic activities psychologists must take into account the ways in which prior relationships, such as therapist to patient, might impact their role as witnesses.

Limitation or Absence of Confidentiality

A fundamental aspect of forensic activities is that there are at least two possibly adversarial parties who deserve equal access to all information that might prove relevant to the issue(s) at hand. Within the American judicial system, representatives of both plaintiff and defendant are entitled to access pertinent information that will be used by either side. Thus, when a neuropsychology expert is retained by either side to evaluate the plaintiff, it is important to inform the evaluee of the absence of confidentiality for any information that is elicited. Similarly, when in the course of acting as a treating neuropsychologist it is discovered that litigation may be forthcoming, it is important to

discuss the eventual limits of confidentiality that may result from the litigation. Ultimately, if information gathered in the course of treatment is subsequently requested to be released for litigation purposes, the patient should
be informed. In situations in which the neuropsychologist believes it is inappropriate to release some or all of the information obtained in treatment, a
preliminary private inspection of the material, known as *in camera* review,
by the judge can be requested. The judge can then independently determine
whether the material should be released, despite the beliefs of the neuropsychologist, or that it lawfully can be withheld. If it must be released, the
patient should be informed, as the last remaining option for the patient would
be to drop the lawsuit to stop the information from being released. There
appears to be no instance in which it is ethically or legally acceptable for the
neuropsychologist to simply decide unilaterally to withhold, or alternatively
to deny the existence of, information about the patient because of the belief
that it was either not relevant or would be harmful to the patient, if released.
Moreover, when in the role of a retained expert, it is also inappropriate for a
neuropsychologist to exclude information that under normal clinical circumstances would affect one's opinion. Even if an attorney asks the psychologist
to exclude certain information from a report, it is still ethically unacceptable
to do so, unless the exclusion has been ordered by the judge. Attorneys are
advocates; their unilateral decisions (i.e., those that do not include the judge
and opposing attorney) cannot be considered objective. Neuropsychologists
should not be naïve in this regard; whether in the role of treater or retained
expert, neuropsychologists must strive to remain fully objective in their work
and opinions.

Possible Absence of Informed Consent to Evaluate

It has become commonplace in American health care to require *informed
consent* before proceeding with diagnostic and intervention procedures. By
obtaining a patient's signature on a sheet of paper that documents the type of
procedure to be undertaken, along with the risks and benefits to the person
undergoing the procedure, it is believed that both parties are informed and in
agreement with regard to what is to take place. Although not yet as universal
in psychological and neuropsychological practice, the trend of such accredit-
ing bodies as the Joint Commission of Accreditation of Healthcare Organizations, is that all patient care should involve informed consent as evidenced
by a signature on a clearly stated form that describes the diagnostic or treatment approach. Whether or not neuropsychologists believe such an expectation applies to their practices, the forensic context typically does not allow
for independent consent to undergo a procedure, including obtaining the
examinee's signature. For example, an individual referred by an insurance
carrier for a disability evaluation or by a police department for a 'fitness for
duty' evaluation, has not come of his or her own initiative to the office of
a neuropsychologist. In such a situation, the individual may or may not be
willing to sign an informed consent document. It may not even be appropri-

ate to do so, given that the condition of the evaluation may not be voluntary or under the control of the person being evaluated. Nevertheless, ethical
Standards 1.07 (*Describing the Nature and Results of Psychological Services*)
and 1.21 (*Third-Party Requests for Services*) require that the individual be
informed of the purpose and nature of the evaluation process, which can in
turn be documented by the neuropsychologist within the individual's file.

Billing issues

Billing for services rendered is required in most instances within our society. As clinicians, neuropsychologists are quite familiar with the importance
of establishing and maintaining fees and financial arrangements as early
and explicitly as possible, as indicated in Standard 1.25 (*Fees and Financial
Arrangements*). Within a forensic context, the early and clear establishment
of fees and financial arrangements is generally possible and comparable
to traditional clinical activities. However, there are a few exceptions that
deserve attention. First and foremost, there needs to be a clear understanding
that the neuropsychologist is being reimbursed for his or her time, *not* for his
or her opinion. An expert's opinion is not for sale; expert reimbursement is
only for the time invested in determining and presenting an opinion.

Second, time invested by the neuropsychologist can be paid for in advance,
in part or in whole, which is relatively rare in clinical activities. If the amount
of money initially accepted for forensic activities subsequently is not needed,
a refund can be provided. However, the converse is not viewed as acceptable.
Generally it is not appropriate for an expert to render services for which
reimbursement is dependent upon the ultimate forensic determination or verdict. For example, a plaintiff attorney may retain a neuropsychologist, but
not be able to, or perhaps not want to, reimburse the expert's time at the
outset. In such instances, the neuropsychologist may be asked to accept a
lien, *letter of protection*, or *letter of assignation*, all of which delay payment
until the eventual outcome of the litigation. Both because of the appearance,
and the actual possibility, that the expert's opinion could be tainted by such
a possible conflict of interest in the outcome of a forensic case, this situation
should be avoided. At the time of retention, the neuropsychologist should
explain the fees and financial arrangements that are acceptable. If necessary, the neuropsychologist can also note that delayed payments, payments
contingent upon litigation outcome, and any other financial arrangements
that might create a conflict of interest are not acceptable.

Third, and finally, our ethics code, in Standard 1.26 (*Accuracy in Reports
to Payors and Funding Sources*), notes that funding sources must be informed
accurately of services provided. Our society distinguishes between paying for
health care services and paying for the time of forensic experts. It is commonplace for some form of health insurance to reimburse a portion of neuropsychological services delivered within typical clinical scenarios involving
the concept of 'medical necessity.' However, health insurance carriers do not
view forensic activity as reimbursable under insurance provisions, as such

activity is not medically necessary for diagnosis and treatment. It is not credible that an attorney could independently determine necessity for evaluation or treatment of his client. Within the present managed care era, it is in fact difficult at times for professionally trained health care providers and insurance carriers to agree on medical necessity. In fact, insurance carriers can argue effectively that intentional billing of forensic neuropsychological services under health insurance represents fraud, which is illicit and unethical. Thus, if a plaintiff attorney asks a neuropsychologist to perform an evaluation for forensic purposes and send the bill to the plaintiff's health insurance carrier, an ethical response would be refusal accompanied by an explanation to the attorney of the salient issues. Most plaintiff attorneys will not expect to use their client's health insurance for forensic purposes and the remainder usually readily accept that it would not be appropriate to do so once the reasons are explained.

Pressing need for documentation and justification of opinion
Standard 1.23 (*Documentation of Professional and Scientific Work*) directs psychologists to provide appropriate documentation of professional and scientific work. Specifically, when it is believed that the services will be used in legal proceedings psychologists are to document with regard to "the kind of detail and quality that would be consistent with reasonable scrutiny in an adjudicative forum." Standards 1.06 (*Basis for Scientific and Professional Judgments*), 2.01 (*Evaluation, Diagnosis, and Interventions in Professional Context*), and 7.02 (*Forensic Assessments*) also note that psychologists should provide information necessary for substantiating diagnostic findings and recommendations. Standard 1.06 stipulates that psychologists rely "on scientifically and professionally derived knowledge" in making scientific and professional judgments. Specifically within forensic reports and testimony, Standard 7.04 requires truthfulness and candor, and 7.02 directs psychologists to note factors that may require a limited opinion, when appropriate. These directives are important parts of the Ethical Principles, and are completely consistent with both the scientist-practitioner foundations of clinical neuropsychology and current evidentiary standards represented in the *Daubert* standard and in *Federal Rules of Evidence* (cf. Lees-Haley & Cohen, 1999), which, in part, emphasize a scientific basis for expert opinions. Differently, as described in Standard 3.03 (*Avoidance of False or Deceptive Statements*), psychologists are to avoid false or deceptive statements regarding "...the scientific or clinical basis for, or results or degree of success of, their services..."

In general, with regard to the need for documentation, as noted in Standards 1.24 (*Records and Data*), 5.04 (*Maintenance of Records*), 5.09 (*Preserving Records and Data*), respectively, psychologists create, maintain, and preserve records in a manner consistent with the ethics code and law. Separately from the Ethical Principles, the American Psychological Association has promulgated specific record keeping guidelines for practicing psychologists, which are consistent with some regulatory agencies (American Psychological Association, 1993).

Test security and release of records

It is common when involved in litigated cases that neuropsychologists receive various requests for copies of any and all records that have been generated with a particular plaintiff. These requests may come in the form of legally sanctioned orders authorized by a court or less formal written or telephone requests from attorneys. Distinguishing what can be released requires an understanding of the relevant issues and the available options for responding. Basically, there are two general concerns that at a minimum should be considered. These are (1) test security and (2) balancing ethical concerns regarding release of records with pertinent state law.

If the questions and answers to tests of ability were released indiscriminately to attorneys and to the public, there would be at least two significant problems. The first is that the tests may not be useful in the future with patients or litigants (i.e., validity would be decreased). The second is that test authors and test publishers have a proprietary right to be protected from acts that would devalue their test creations. Years of work could be made worthless by release of information that was only intended for professional purchase and use, which is the very reason that test publishers have established guidelines that limit availability and use of their products. In fact, test publishers have asserted their intent (in sales catalogs and in test manuals) to protect their copyrighted property.

Although different with regard to the issues underlying each, test security and release of records are inextricably intertwined in practice. However, release of records does not always involve issues of test security, given that some patient records do not contain formal testing materials or results and, further, in those that do contain testing records, not all requests for release of records ask for copies of test protocols. Some requests ask only for reports and notes. When a psychologist is providing services for a third party (e.g., attorney), rather than a 'patient,' Standard 1.21 (*Third-Party Requests for Services*) suggests that the limits of confidentiality should be addressed initially. In forensic situations it is expected that the plaintiff who has been referred by his or her own attorney will sign a release to give the report to his or her own attorney, but that a signed release from the plaintiff who is undergoing a defense-mandated examination is not expected (i.e., many plaintiffs will not sign any document unless their lawyer is present). However, it is understood as part of formal legal and administrative proceedings that all findings will be made available to both sides. The intention to release all available information should be made clear at the beginning of a forensic evaluation, per Standard 1.21.

Ethical Standards 1.24 (*Records and Data*), 2.02 (*Competence and Appropriate Use of Assessments and Interventions*), and 2.10 (*Maintaining Test Security*) instruct psychologists to limit access to psychological test materials and results to those who are trained to use such information. Standard 1.02 (*Relationship of Ethics and Law*) instructs psychologists to resolve conflicts that occur between ethics and the law. The official statements regarding third party observers by the National Academy of Neuropsychology (NAN Policy and Planning Committee, 2000a) and the American Academy of Clinical Neuropsychology (American Academy of Clinical Neuropsychology, 2001) reinforce the fundamental premise that access to the questions and answers to our clinical instruments should be limited whenever possible to psychologists. A helpful guide regarding how to handle test security issues has also been published by the National Academy of Neuropsychology (NAN Policy and Planning Committee, 2000b). In the vast majority of forensic scenarios, psychologists are available to both sides of an adversarial proceeding, allowing for direct release of psychological test records from one psychologist to another. Often, educating the attorneys and judge regarding applicable state law (e.g., in Illinois a statute known commonly as the *Mental Health Code* directs psychologists *not* to release test protocols and manuals to non-psychologists), ethics guidelines, and official statements of professional organizations will be sufficient. When this is not the case, requesting the judge to enter an order of protection (which directs either the destruction or the return of test protocols at the conclusion of the legal proceeding) can also be a means of satisfying both legal and ethical responsibilities. When all else fails, a retained expert usually has the option of withdrawing from the case.

Professional Relationships

The prior iteration of ethical principles (American Psychological Association, 1981) contained a specific principle on *professional relationships* (see discussion by Sweet & Rozensky, 1991). Although less prominent, Principles B (*Integrity*), C (*Professional and Scientific Responsibility*), and D (*Respect for People's Rights and Dignity*) also refer to an obligation to have reasoned and constructive relationships with other professionals which seems to preclude what could be perceived as an antagonistic stance toward fellow psychologists. Standard 1.09 (*Respecting Others*) specifically states that psychologists should "respect the rights of others to hold values, attitudes, and opinions that differ from their own." Macartney-Filgate and Snow (2000) have discussed an illustrative forensic case example that illustrates the importance of carefully discriminating strong emotional responses to observed practice deviations from appropriate ethical responses. Importantly, these authors recommend that forensic experts avoid prejudging or condemning other professionals, leaving the ultimate judgment of practice standards to regulatory bodies.

The prior topic of test security provides a different type of example pertaining to professional relationships. In no instance is it ethically acceptable to use concerns of test security or release of records to obstruct the 'opposing' side of an adversarial proceeding. Specifically, a psychologist acting as an expert is not entitled to decide unilaterally whether a particular licensed clinical psychologist is competent to review test materials and results (Sweet, 1990). Only the State government has the authority to determine license to practice. In the midst of an adversarial proceeding it likely will be perceived as a conflict of interest for an opposing psychologist to assert that another psychologist is not well trained enough or, in some manner, to conduct an investigation into whether the psychologist is well trained and competent. Rather, upon notification that a psychologist licensed by the State has been identified to receive copies of records, the requested records should be copied and released without delay.

Practicing within limits of competency and within scope of practice
Fundamental to ethical practice is practicing within one's areas of competence, defined by Principle A (*Competence*) as those areas in which one is "qualified by education, training, or experience." Standard 1.04 (*Boundaries of Competence*) elaborates upon these ideas, which are extended in 1.05 (*Maintaining Expertise*) to a responsibility to maintain "a reasonable level of awareness of current scientific and professional information" in fields of activity. Quite clearly, psychologists are not to practice outside the areas of their licensed scope of practice.

"...nothing but the truth...": Avoiding multiple pressures that undermine objectivity
Principle B (*Integrity*) notes the importance of psychologists' promotion of integrity in science, teaching, and practice. This Principle states: "In these activities psychologists are honest, fair, and respectful of others. In describing or reporting their qualifications, services, products, fees, research, or teaching, they do not make statements that are false, misleading, or deceptive." The importance of maintaining objectivity and rendering an unbiased opinion cannot be stressed enough, and is mentioned in Standard 7.04 (*Truthfulness and Candor*). To suggest that remaining unbiased amidst various powerful forces can be difficult is an understatement. Responsibility for maintaining objectivity and minimizing bias rests with the individual neuropsychologist. Neuropsychologists are encouraged to rely on empirical approaches, such as use of normative standards for comparison of individual performance and reliance on relevant peer-reviewed literature, to anchor expert opinions. Regardless of amount of prior forensic experience, debiasing strategies, such as those recommended by Borum et al. (1993), Garb (1998), and Sweet and Moulthrop (1999), can also be useful to clinicians who are striving to maintain objectivity.

Balancing forensic expectations, legal rules, and ethical responsibilities
It should be apparent that the roles and activities of an expert witness are complex. There is a need to constantly balance forensic expectations (e.g., the need for 'black and white' statements), the need to meet evidentiary standards

(e.g., with regard to scientific merit versus unfounded opinion), and ethical responsibilities (e.g., third-party requests for services). At times these various factors are in conflict. Standard 1.02 (*Relationship of Ethics and Law*) states that it is a psychologist's responsibility to resolve conflicts between ethics and law in a responsible manner, which includes making known the conflict, when it is identified. Standard 8.02 (*Confronting Ethical Issues*) suggests that psychologists ordinarily should consult with other psychologists knowledgeable about ethical issues and with psychology ethics committees or other appropriate authorities when confronted with an ethical dilemma. In a forensic situation, it is important that a psychologist not simply rely on the advice of attorneys who have a vested interest in some aspect of the case that has spawned the ethical conflict.

Legitimate versus pseudo-credentials

Standard 3.03 (*Avoidance of False and Deceptive Statements*) indicates that psychologists are to avoid false or deceptive statements, including inaccurate statements about their credentials. This is particularly important in forensic situations, as the training, credentials, and experience of an expert can influence the 'triers of fact.' Relevant to particular credentials that imply special expertise with forensic activities, an American Bar Association Journal article describes the lack of value in credentials purchased from organizations such as the American College of Forensic Examiners and the American Board of Forensic Examiners (Hansen, 2000). These particular credentials have been and continue to be available to persons within a variety of disciplines, including psychology. Although not unethical to possess, as individuals are free to purchase any product or service not viewed as illegal, based on Hansen (2000), it seems unethical to suggest implicitly or explicitly in a forensic proceeding that this type of credential is associated with earned status or greater knowledge within a particular professional field. It would also appear unethical to imply or state that purchased credentials obtained without legitimate peer review were equal in merit to legitimate board certification in a particular specialty. Legitimate board certification commonly is achieved by way of an accepted, rigorous peer review process sponsored by a nonprofit professional organization that has standing within a given professional field.

Prevention and Resolution of Ethical Conflicts in Forensic Activities

Neuropsychologists may not have the experience of being exposed to 'adversarial' cases during their formal education and training. That is, in most training settings, cases given to trainees involve referrals of non compensation-seeking patients, typically sent by physicians requesting neuropsychological testing for the purpose of assisting with diagnosis and treatment of their patients. Data and opinions from such cases typically will not be critically reviewed or challenged as to their accuracy or veracity, nor will they be used to determine the financial impact or worth of possible injuries or diseases.

Upon entering practice, newly trained neuropsychologists are likely to receive referrals of individuals seeking compensation or other benefits. This is especially true for those whose primary work setting is in private practice (Sweet et al., 2000). In carrying out professional activities associated with potentially adversarial cases, there is a high likelihood that neuropsychologists will encounter unfamiliar professional or ethical quandaries, for which they had not been prepared while in graduate school. Some of these dilemmas might be especially difficult to resolve, especially if the neuropsychologist is practicing independently and has less access to consultation with colleagues. Indeed, it may be difficult to either anticipate, or know how to satisfactorily resolve, issues that might challenge the autonomy and integrity of expert neuropsychological opinions in such cases. This section will review four potential wellsprings of ethical dilemmas in adversarial cases: the referral source, the retained neuropsychologist, 'patients' versus 'plaintiffs', and 'other' psychologists involved in adversarial cases.

The Referral Source

For ease of presentation, we will continue to use the term 'adversarial' to refer to those contested cases in which the presence, significance and remunerative worth of an injury or disease is at issue, and in which a claim has been made for an award or other favorable outcome. Most often, these are cases in which a personal injury lawsuit has been filed, or in which payments or awards are being sought from workers' compensation or disability carriers. Typically, an attorney or disability case manager will be the person making the referral to the neuropsychologist, and will describe the type of patient being referred and the questions being asked of the evaluator. In many ways, the questions asked of the neuropsychologist in adversarial cases will not differ from those asked in non-adversarial cases. Typical questions in both types of cases might include: does the patient have any cognitive or behavioral deficits; if so, what is the etiology of these deficits; how can the person best be treated? However, there are at least three ways in which the relationship between the neuropsychologist and the referral source may vary, depending on whether or not the case is adversarial. These include 1) the range and specificity of questions asked; 2) the way in which questions are answered; 3) the intent or goal of the referral source. These three issues are neither exhaustive, nor do they necessarily occur in each referred adversarial case. However, 'forewarned is forearmed,' and awareness of these issues may be useful to neuropsychologists who wish to either avoid or satisfactorily resolve potential ethical dilemmas with referral sources. Regarding the first issue, neuropsychologists should anticipate being asked to answer both more, and more specific questions, in adversarial cases. This is especially true in cases referred by disability carriers who often present the neuropsychologist with a list of written questions. In contrast, many neuropsychologists are more familiar with much more general and/or broad requests from referring physicians in non-adversarial cases, which may be informal to the point of an open-ended request to simply 'please evaluate.' In such situations, it is often left to the discretion of the neuropsychologist to define the extent of what needs to be evaluated and how it should be carried out. Disability carriers and attorneys, however, may specifically direct the neuropsychologist to answer questions such as "How many sessions of psychotherapy, and at what cost, will be sufficient for the patient to recover from this trauma?", or "Can the person return to work and perform their usual duties; if not, when can they return?" The range, and specificity, of these questions present the neuropsychologist with at least two challenges. First, it may put the neuropsychologist in the relatively unfamiliar position of having someone else determine the purpose and goals of an evaluation, which some may find unpalatable. Second, and more importantly, neuropsychologists must remind both themselves and their referral sources as to the limits of their knowledge. After all, just because a question has been asked does not mean that it can be satisfactorily answered. Ethical Standard 2.05 (*Interpreting Assessment Results*) requires psychologists to indicate any significant reservations they have about the accuracy or limitation of their interpretations. Also relevant is Standard 1.06 (*Basis for Scientific and Professional Judgments*), which requires psychologists to rely on scientifically or professionally derived knowledge when making scientific or professional judgments or when engaging in scholarly or professional endeavors. Thus, when appropriate, psychologists should not refrain from stating that they are unable to answer a question.

Second, neuropsychologists may be asked to answer questions more succinctly and more plainly in adversarial cases. This can be difficult, as many neuropsychologists by virtue of temperament and training may prefer to equivocate or to qualify their replies to questions, if simple answers fail to convey the 'truth' of a complex set of variables. While this is often reasonable, given the complexities and subtleties of clinical neuropsychological work, it may not satisfy participants in legal proceedings who may be asking 'yes or no' questions, such as "Does the neuropsychological evaluation indicate that the patient has brain damage?" In keeping with ethical standards, when serving as expert witnesses, neuropsychologists need to be vigilant with regard to establishing the limits of their opinions and not allowing their statements to be distorted or manipulated.

Within the setting of a deposition or trial, many questions may be preceded with the phrase "Do you have an opinion within a reasonable degree of psychological certainty as to..." This then raises the important question of what is meant by 'reasonable certainty'? This usually is not defined for the expert witness. Left to their own interpretation, a psychologist might wonder if this means one should rely on Fisherian statistical analysis as a guideline, and that one should be at least 95% certain ($p<.05$) that something is true. Alternatively, most have also heard the phrases 'beyond the shadow of a reasonable doubt' (a very high level of certainty), as well as 'a preponderance of evidence' (something just greater than 50% certainty).

Confusion about what is meant by this phrase is not limited to psychologist expert witnesses. A recent review (Lewin, 1998) concludes that "no consensus exists among judges, attorneys or academic commentators as to whether 'reasonable medical certainty' means 'more probable than not' or 'beyond a reasonable doubt' or something in between" (p. 380). The phrase "medical certainty" appears to have originated in a Chicago trial, early in the 20th century, and later was widely disseminated via a best-selling manual on trial technique, without ever being precisely defined. Despite this lack of consensus, the outcome of litigation is often dependent on physicians' or psychologists' willingness to express opinions within a reasonable degree of certainty, and the Supreme Court of the United States has recognized "within the medical discipline, the traditional standard for 'fact finding' is a 'reasonable degree of medical certainty' " [Addington v. Texas, 441 U.S 418, 430 (1979)]. Indeed, "the phrase 'reasonable medical certainty' appears in roughly 4000 state court appellate opinions and nearly 1000 opinions from the federal trial and appellate courts while the equivalent expressions of 'reasonable (you-name-it) certainty' by non-physician experts appear in hundreds of other cases" (Lewin, 1984, p. 384). Lewin concluded, "Because these 'magic words' have achieved 'occult' or 'talismanic' status in the interrogation of medical witnesses, one would expect the phrase to have a definite and ascertainable meaning. Yet, the phrase seems to have various meanings in different jurisdictions and different contexts, generating substantial confusion among the bench and bar, as well as for physicians who are called upon to produce expert opinions" (pp. 385, 386). Physician experts have variously defined the term as meaning: 51% or greater probability (Danner & Sagall, 1977), "that level of certainty which a physician would use in making a similar clinical judgment" (Rappeport, 1985), and to indicate a near absolute certainty, on the order of 90% or even 99.9% probability (Rhoto v. Ribando, 504 So. 2d 1119, 1122 n.2 (La. Ct. App, 1987). Interestingly, the common definition, which is 'more probably true than not,' is consistent with 51% or greater probability, which, in most instances, is below the threshold that clinicians would use with their own patients.

In summary, neuropsychologists should be aware that they will be asked if they are reasonably certain of opinions they put forth in any given case. They should consult with attorneys beforehand as to whether a specific jurisdiction has defined what is meant by reasonable certainty. In the event that a jurisdiction has not precisely defined what is meant by 'reasonable certainty,' psychologists should consult ethical standards and have their own understanding of what is meant by this concept. Again, among others, the ethical standards that address reservations or limitations about ones' opinions should be considered.

Third, referral sources in adversarial cases will have many of the same reasons for making a referral, as would a physician in making a referral in a non-adversarial case. They are interested in the presence, severity and etiology of injury or disease, and how it might be treated. However, referring attorneys, disability insurance carriers, school systems, and other interested parties may also have a financial interest in a case. For example, plaintiff attorneys often receive a portion of a settlement or jury award, whereas defense attorneys or disability carriers may have an interest in minimizing the size of such awards. Accordingly, the attorneys and other interested parties may be under considerable pressure to produce a favorable outcome, and may express this directly or indirectly to the retained neuropsychologist. Therefore, it may be helpful for neuropsychologists to adopt prophylactic measures when retained in an adversarial case. Upon initial contact, a neuropsychologist might emphasize to the retaining attorney or carrier that they will be acting as an independent evaluator, and not as an 'advocate' for either the patient or the defense. That is, the neuropsychologist will 'tell it like it is,' regardless of whether the referral source considers these opinions favorable.

Neuropsychologists should be reluctant to deviate from their usual practices if requested to do so by a referral source. For example, it would be extremely uncommon for referral sources, such as physicians, to request an opportunity to review drafts of a patient report before a final report is generated. Yet, such requests might come from attorneys who hope to preview, and possibly even edit, a neuropsychologist's report to favor their position. It is not unreasonable to provide attorneys or carriers with verbal feedback about one's preliminary opinions, as long as it is clear that this is a chance to hear the expert's general impression, *not* a chance to argue for a different opinion from the expert. Fundamentally, neuropsychologists must not allow an attorney or other interested party to influence or, in any sense, become co-author of a neuropsychological report. Discussing the results of an evaluation before a report is written, and allowing the referral source to ask a series of questions as to why the neuropsychologist has come to certain opinions, even if it becomes obvious that the referral source is not pleased with those opinions, can be acceptable. After all, these evaluations often take place during the 'discovery' phase of legal proceedings, when it is the duty of the attorney to understand the strengths and weaknesses of their case. However, the referral source must be reminded that they should not attempt to change the opinions of the evaluating neuropsychologist. Attempts to badger or threaten the evaluating neuropsychologist, perhaps with non-payment of fees or failure to refer other cases in the future, should be pointed out by the neuropsychologist as a significant abridgement of their right to conduct an independent evaluation. In some cases, upon hearing the general impression, an attorney may then decide to forgo the neuropsychologist's opinion in a case, and might simply ask the neuropsychologist to not write a report and to submit a final bill. Of course, the neuropsychologist will also have the option of withdrawing from a case, not accepting additional cases in the future from a particular referral source, or even filing a complaint with the appropriate regulatory agency should it become necessary.

The 'retained' neuropsychologist

This section refers to the neuropsychologist who has been retained by the attorney or disability carrier to provide an independent evaluation in an adversarial case. Many of the relevant ethical guidelines have already been described earlier in this chapter, including several references to pertinent sections of the Ethical Principles of the American Psychological Association. However, these principles do not, and cannot, be expected to cover all possible sources of ethical dilemmas that may occur in adversarial cases. Some additional points to consider will be reviewed briefly.

Neuropsychologists need to remind themselves that it is natural to hope to please a referral source. After all, as social beings we do not wish to provide feedback that others might find disappointing. Additionally, neuropsychologists might be anxious that negative feedback will result in the referral source either not liking them or their work, and that this might prevent future cases from being referred. However, such desires and anxieties obviously do not excuse the neuropsychologist from providing an honest and impartial opinion, regardless of potential consequences. Conversely, neuropsychologists should not take much comfort when it is perceived that an opinion will be welcomed by the referral source. The primary goal of a consulting neuropsychologist is to provide information to a court or an administrative process, *not* to 'win' the case for either side. In this regard, Taylor (1999) has stated that neuropsychologists should be educators, rather than advocates, and "…become advocates for their own opinions, rather than advocates for particular litigants" (p. 437).

The authors of this chapter have had the experience of attorneys or carriers making derogatory, and sometimes profane, remarks about either patients or other medical witnesses. Under no circumstances should the retained neuropsychologist partake in such character assassinations. In some instances, one may find it necessary to make others aware that such remarks make you uncomfortable and may even impinge on your ability to provide an independent opinion. Finally, the authors suggest that when retained as an expert, a neuropsychologist should embrace the notion of an 'angel on your shoulder' throughout involvement in a case. That is, imagine that an esteemed neuropsychologist was listening in on your conversations with a patient or attorney. Would you phrase questions differently or would you reach different opinions, if you knew that an influential colleague was watching over you? What would you be saying or doing differently in this case had you been retained by the 'other' side? Utilization of these visual imagery exercises might prove illuminating! Further information on sources of bias and techniques that can be used by neuropsychologists to reduce subtle and obvious bias can be found in other contributions (Sweet and Moulthrop, 1999; van Gorp and McMullen, 1997). Fundamentally, neuropsychologists serving as experts need to challenge themselves consciously regarding the robustness of their opinions to ensure that the specific context at hand has not influenced opinions, negatively, in the form of reduced objectivity.

'Patient' versus plaintiff

Individuals referred in adversarial cases typically will have a different relationship with a retained neuropsychologist than that between patients in non-adversarial cases seen by 'treating' psychologists. As already reviewed, a 'doctor–patient' relationship typically will not exist in an adversarial case, so that the individual being evaluated (often aptly termed a plaintiff or claimant) typically will not get a report or feedback directly from the neuropsychologist. Second, the person being assessed is often compelled to appear for an evaluation by an expert who has been selected by a party who may be contesting the person's claims. As such, the patient may feel under duress at the time of evaluation. Some of this duress may relate to the belief that the neuropsychologist is not there to represent the plaintiff or claimant's interests. In fact, technically, this is true, as the retained neuropsychologist should present opinions irrespective of the plaintiff or defense party's potential benefits or losses. In any event, the person being evaluated should be reassured that the neuropsychologist will do everything possible to reach an impartial opinion. To accomplish this, common sense dictates that the patient should be treated with respect by the neuropsychologist and related staff, that bathroom, rest and lunch breaks should be offered, and that the patient should feel free to alert staff if they become too fatigued or stressed to produce cognitive efforts that represent their usual level of ability. In these respects, the same common courtesies afforded patients should be extended to plaintiffs and claimants.

Other psychologists involved in adversarial cases

It is common for neuropsychologists to be made aware that a compensation-seeking patient has previously been evaluated, or subsequently will be evaluated, by another neuropsychologist. As such, a neuropsychologist may be provided with, and in some scenarios should at least ask for, the reports and raw data from this other evaluations. Unfortunately, review of these materials at times may cause the retained neuropsychologist to perceive that the other psychologist has not acted in an ethical or competent manner. This topic has been reviewed extensively by the authors in another recent publication (Grote et al., 2000), and also in this volume in Chapter 13 Deidan and Bush comment on how to address perceived ethical violations of others. Therefore, only a brief summary of the authors' views is provided here, limited to the context of forensic neuropsychology.

Although the prevalence of unethical conduct among persons practicing neuropsychology cannot be determined, data from the Association of State and Provincial Psychology Boards (ASPPB) indicates that 'unprofessional/ unethical/ negligent practice' is the second most-common reason for disciplinary action against psychologists. Only "sexual/dual relationship with patient" was reported with greater frequency as a reason for disciplinary action, in the period between August, 1983 and July, 1998 (ASPPB, personal communication, December 15, 1998). A review of the APA ethical principles and a related commentary (Canter et al., 1994) indicates that it may be a violation of the principles *not* to take action when one suspects that another psychologist has acted unethically, unless the confidentiality rights of the patient preclude such action. Further, evaluation of legal precedent indicates that in certain circumstances a neuropsychologist who fails to report perceived unethical conduct of a colleague may be held legally responsible for harm that could have been avoided by an appropriate report. Analysis of other legal precedent also indicates that a reporting neuropsychologist's risk of liability appears to be low if the report was based on reliable information that the psychologist reasonably believed to be true and if the report was made only to an appropriate professional organization or public official. Subsequent commentary in the Grote et al. (2000) article concerns when and how psychologists should report perceived unethical practices of other psychologists, through a review of the following questions:

• What ethical principle may have been violated?
• How significant is the ethical violation?
• How reliable and persuasive is the evidence of the ethical violation?
• Have I taken into account any personal feelings that I may have toward this colleague?
• Can I act without breaching the confidentiality of a patient?
• Have I consulted with other colleagues about what to do?
• Am I prepared to contact the colleague informally?
• Am I prepared to contact organizations?

Obviously, the decision as to whether or not to contact or report a colleague concerning perceived unethical conduct should not be made lightly. Impediments to making this contact are many, and may include the fear of creating a hostile relationship with the colleague, or even that the colleague may attempt some type of reprisal. On the other hand, failure to address perceived unethical behavior could result in patients being misdiagnosed and mistreated, insurance companies being billed for unnecessary services, or the patient being denied compensation or treatment. Perhaps as important, the public's perception of the practice of neuropsychology may be diminished if unethical practices are ignored by psychologists who should have attempted to stop such practices.

Case Examples

The issues raised in this chapter reveal the complexity of day-to-day professional and ethical issues confronted by the neuropsychologist who is regularly — or even occasionally — engaged in forensic work. The complexity surrounding these issues is best illustrated through 'real life' case scenarios that delineate potential ethical challenges and appropriate resolutions. All the case examples that follow are composite examples based upon actual situations experienced by one or more of the authors in the course of their neuropsychological practices or described to the authors by colleagues who were seeking ethical guidance. In each instance, an attempt has been made to modify non-essential facts in order to protect the confidentiality of the parties involved. Whether in real life a resolution of the ethical conflict was attempted or not, we have outlined some of the possible means of conflict resolution for each of the examples. Readers should not assume that our suggestions regarding resolution are exhaustive.

Case 1: Psychoanalytic Neuropsychological Evaluation

Scenario
A 37-year-old professional writer and lecturer was referred for a neuropsychological evaluation by a treating clinical psychologist. The professional was in treatment for persistent anxiety associated with a history of relatively recent sexual abuse by a former treating psychiatrist. Following the last episode of the sexual abuse, the psychiatrist allegedly had prescribed (and the patient received) numerous treatments of electroconvulsive therapy (ECT) over a several month duration for symptoms of depression. The referring treating psychologist had come to believe that the patient's memory lapses and word finding difficulties extended beyond the expected effects of prolonged emotional distress and therefore referred the patient for a neuropsychological evaluation.

The patient came to her neuropsychological evaluation appointment with a copy of a 'neuropsychological evaluation' performed four weeks prior as part of ongoing litigation against the former psychiatrist. On the letterhead of the evaluation was printed 'psychoanalysis' next to the psychologist's name. Among the tests administered were the Wechsler–Bellevue intelligence test, the Babcock Story Recall, and the Rorschach Inkblot Test. In the discussion section of the report, the psychologist concluded "there is a hiatus in the thinking apparatus" of the patient, which was ascribed to the patient's difficulties with stress.

During the current evaluation, the woman exhibited numerous paraphasic errors, word finding problems, and verbal (but not visual) memory difficulties. She also exhibited notably poor performance on all measures of executive function (e.g., obtaining 0 categories on the Wisconsin Card Sorting Test), and normal performance on cognitive measures of other domains. Following the neuropsychologist's referral to a neurologist and subsequent brain imaging, an MRI scan revealed a left fronto-temporal lesion, which the neurologist believed may have occurred during one of the ECT episodes when the patient had a hypotensive crisis and an associated cerebral infarction.

The psychologist who performed the initial evaluation was contacted and told of the subsequent neuropsychological and medical findings. He was also informed of the concerns regarding his approach to the evaluation and his conclusions. He acknowledged he was in error, and indicated that he was semi-retired and would retire fully in the next two months.

Ethical Issues
The psychoanalytically oriented psychologist who conducted the initial evaluation was potentially in violation of a number of APA ethical standards,

including: 1.04 (*Boundaries of Competence*); 2.02 *(Competence and Appropriate Use of Assessments and Interventions)*; and 2.07 (*Obsolete Tests and Outdated Test Results*). The psychologist in question indicated expertise in psychoanalysis on his letterhead, not neuropsychology. He had used out of date and obsolete tests (e.g., Wechsler–Bellevue intelligence test), and had not made competent and appropriate use of assessments. His conclusion that "there is a hiatus in the thinking apparatus" was vague (and potentially misleading) and reflected his lack of expertise in neuropsychological assessment. Potential harm came to the patient, who was told that her difficulties were the result of stress, and would resolve if she could reduce her stress.

Resolution
In this instance, an informal resolution was attempted by contacting the psychologist directly. Given the acknowledgment of error and the indication of a decision to retire from the practice of psychology in the near future, no other action was taken by the neuropsychologist who performed the second evaluation. One might wonder what the next sequence of steps might be, if the psychologist had not indicated that he was retiring, or in the event that the person did not actually follow through with his stated retirement plans. In these instances, contact with the psychologist could again be initiated, with possible contact with the state psychological association ethics committee or state licensing board, if the matter was not considered resolved.

Case 2: The Disabled Professional in Rehabilitation

Scenario
A neuropsychologist conducted an examination of a middle-aged woman following an automobile accident in which she struck her head, resulting in a momentary (i.e., less than 30 second) loss of consciousness. The patient was taken to the hospital, evaluated in the emergency room, and released with a diagnosis of concussion. Although the patient returned to work the following week, she began to notice difficulty concentrating and was distractible, irritable with co-workers in her office, and could not tolerate loud noises. She had even been irritable with one of her own clients. During the feedback session subsequent to the testing, the neuropsychologist told her that the evaluation confirmed difficulty with attention/concentration, memory, and executive function. Although all results were in the high average range or above, the neuropsychologist believed that these scores in a high functioning professional represented a decline from premorbid levels. The neuropsychologist recommended the patient enroll in a twice weekly chiropractic rehabilitation program operated by the neuropsychologist's spouse, attend support groups for persons with head injuries that the neuropsychologist's son ran, and discontinue her work, applying for Social Security benefits. The patient saw a second neuropsychologist, as requested by Social Security, for an independent neuropsychological evaluation to determine if there was evidence of

work disability. Test results in the second evaluation of this woman were similar to that obtained by the first (treating) neuropsychologist, with all scores being high average or above. However, the second neuropsychologist concluded that, although the professional had sustained a post-concussion syndrome, with lowered scores on some tests, the failure to exhibit actual neurocognitive 'impairment' did not prohibit her from working.

Ethical Issues
The first potential ethical issue was the possibility of *multiple relationships* (Standard 1.17), in which an evaluating psychologist recommended the patient enter a spouse's and the son's rehabilitation programs. This may have potentially impaired the psychologist's objectivity in encouraging the patient to view herself as more impaired than was actually the case. This also may be potentially an example of a breach of Standard 1.19 (*Exploitative Relationships*) in which the patient's symptoms of post-concussion syndrome are used for financial gain of the psychologist. Finally, the psychologist may be in violation of Standard 1.14 (*Avoiding Harm*) in encouraging the patient to view herself as more impaired than was actually the case, and even to view herself as disabled. Such a communication may affect the patient's self-concept, her social role, her value to society, etc.

Resolution
A report was written by the consulting neuropsychologist for the insurance company indicating that, in his opinion, it was counter-therapeutic to view the individual as disabled and 'brain damaged.' The report was forwarded by the insurance company to the patient's attending physician, as well as to the original neuropsychologist. The consulting neuropsychologist could contact the treating neuropsychologist and inform her of the psychologist's concerns regarding the possible multiple relationships and the potential harm to the patient. In so doing, the treating neuropsychologist would then be able to respond.

Case 3: The Patient As A Treating Doctor

Scenario
A psychiatrist sustained a mild traumatic brain injury in an automobile accident one year earlier, and then sought cognitive rehabilitation. The psychiatrist consulted a neuropsychologist with special expertise in cognitive rehabilitation to make recommendations as to her rehabilitation needs. The neuropsychologist asked him to come in for a neuropsychological evaluation. The neuropsychologist administered a wide range of tests, most of which were developed and normed by the neuropsychologist some years ago on a local sample of normal individuals and patients with brain injuries; these measures did not appear to be widely used outside the neuropsychologist's own practice. The neuropsychologist asked the psychiatrist, as part of the

evaluation, to conduct a formal psychiatric interview of another prospective patient who had sustained a brain injury, and to determine a diagnosis and formulate treatment recommendations. The psychiatrist expressed trepidation at this task, stating concern about doing an adequate job, and whether or not the 'right' questions would be asked of the other patient. The second patient, who was to be interviewed, was not informed that the interviewing psychiatrist was, himself, a patient with a possible brain injury. The interview was conducted and videotaped, and the neuropsychologist — after subsequently reviewing the videotape — pronounced it adequate, but recommended a minimum of 12 months of daily cognitive rehabilitation in his treatment program.

Ethical issues
This is a highly unusual scenario. There are several ethical issues worthy of discussion. First, the neuropsychologist has potentially violated Standard 1.14 (*Avoiding Harm*), by having one patient subjected to a potentially upsetting diagnostic interview by another patient, who may or may not be competent to conduct such an evaluation. Not being present at the time, but merely recording the interview on videotape, the neuropsychologist increased the risk of harm to both patients by not being able to intervene immediately should the need arise. This neuropsychologist has also potentially violated Standard 4.02 (*Informed Consent to Therapy*). The interviewee has not been informed of, nor agreed to, an interview by another patient. This scenario also may violate Standard 5.02 (*Maintaining Confidentiality*), in that the neuropsychologist has failed to respect the confidentiality of the interviewee, by asking the patient to reveal details of their background, injury, psychiatric and medical history, substance abuse history, etc., to another patient.

Resolution
This scenario came to the attention of a second neuropsychologists when a law firm asked for an independent review of the patient file as part of ongoing litigation related to the patient's head injury. The first step toward a successful resolution would be for the consulting/reviewing neuropsychologist to contact the treating neuropsychologist and express concern regarding the measures used, as well as having placed the patient in the role of 'examining doctor' with the examinee not being informed of this. If unsuccessful in resolving the matter, pursuit of a complaint through formal state or national ethics committees, or through the state licensing board could be considered.

Case 4: The Observer
As part of a medical malpractice lawsuit, a neuropsychologist employed at a hospital is asked by the hospital's liability insurance carrier to conduct a neuropsychological evaluation on a 58-year-old man who sustained anoxic brain damage during cardiac surgery, at which time the anesthesiologist did not notice his oxygen levels dropping. The attorney retained by the plaintiff

demanded to be present during the evaluation, and wrote a letter to the court indicating that he has an ethical obligation to monitor the questions asked of his client. He also indicated to the court that he would be requesting that all copies of the resulting raw test data and test protocols from the evaluation be sent to him.

Ethical Issues

Requests by third parties to be present during neuropsychological evaluations are becoming more and more common in forensic practice. States vary with regard to allowing third party observations of medical and psychological evaluations. As noted previously in this chapter, the presence of a third party may violate *test security* (Standard 2.10), as well as threaten reliability and validity of findings (2.02, *Competence and Appropriate Use of Assessments and Interventions*; and 2.05, *Interpreting Assessment Results*). With regard to the latter point, unrelated to the ethics of the situation, research evidence has demonstrated the negative influence on test results of third party observers (e.g., Kehrer et al., 2000).

Resolution

The neuropsychologist could inform the attorney that he will not allow the presence of a third party observer in the examination and provide related organizational policy statements and research on the subject. If these actions do not resolve the issue, the two parties (plaintiff/defense) could go to the judge for a final determination. Based upon the Court's decision, the psychologist could either decline to accept the case, or institute certain provisions as to the presence of the observer. In no instance should a psychologist allow videotaping or audiotaping of an evaluation, as doing so violates copyright of the author and publisher, and increases the risk that necessarily test secure information could be widely disseminated and thereby invalidate the tests.

Case 5: Neuropsychological Evaluation Including Physical Examination

Scenario

A vocational rehabilitation counselor working with a worker's compensation claimant asked a neuropsychologist colleague with whom he had worked on many occasions to review a neuropsychological report. The claimant was a young adult female client evaluated by a neuropsychologist in the community. The vocational counselor requested feedback regarding the methods and conclusions of the report. Because of their work together on other cases, the request was informal and no remuneration was offered to the reviewing neuropsychologist.

The report presented for review was quite lengthy (16 pages) and reported results of very large amounts of testing that covered ten testing sessions spanning two months. The number of tests administered was the highest the neuropsychologist had ever encountered. The interpretations, writing style and report format were all idiosyncratic and dissimilar to other neuropsychological reports the consulting professional had encountered previously. The consulting neuropsychologist informed his vocational rehabilitation colleague that that the evaluation was unusual and noted the factors mentioned above.

During the discussion, the rehabilitation counselor asked if it was common for neuropsychologists to administer a physical examination to their patients. The counselor went on to inform his colleague that the neuropsychologist had asked the patient to undergo a physical examination. Although she had felt uncomfortable doing so alone with the psychologist, she eventually agreed to disrobe to her underwear in the presence of a female vocational counselor, and submitted to a physical examination focusing upon testing of neurologic functions (reflexes, etc.).

Subsequent to receiving feedback from the neuropsychologist, the vocational rehabilitation counselor informed the patient that this was improper. The patient indicated that she did not wish to file a complaint with anyone, however, and was pleased to be finished with the matter.

The consulting neuropsychologist, concerned about the behavior of his colleague, sought advice from the chair of the state psychological association ethics committee. A letter of inquiry was sent from the consulting neuropsychologist to the evaluating neuropsychologist, seeking clarification of the physical examination and the very lengthy testing. In return, the consulting neuropsychologist received a brief response attempting to justify the physical examination. This information was forwarded to the state ethics committee without, at her request, divulging the identity of the patient.

Ethical Issues
This case presents a number of unusual elements. First, the inclusion of a physical examination as part of the neuropsychological examination was unusual. This would seem to clearly violate ethical Principle A: (*Competence*). The neuropsychologist did not recognize the boundaries of his competency and limits of his expertise. This also represented a violation of ethical Standard 1.04 (*Boundaries of Competence*), for the same reasons. Because the patient could well be harmed by an unnecessary invasion of her physical privacy, this may represent a violation of ethical Standard 1.14 (*Avoiding Harm*). The evaluating neuropsychologist did not appear to recognize his error in conducting a physical examination. A psychological, physical and neurological examination might be requested to determine if there is a condition(s) present that might have affected the psychologist's judgment. If present, this might have violated ethical Standard 1.13 (*Personal Problems and Conflicts*). In reviewing the methods and report, the consulting neuropsychologist indicated that the methods and report were idiosyncratic. This may represent a violation of Standard 2.02 (*Competence and Appropriate Use of Assessments and Interventions*) and Standard 2.05 (*Interpreting Assessment Results*).

Resolution
The state ethics committee, after lengthy due process, found the evaluating neuropsychologist in violation of ethical standards. During the course of the state investigation, the American Psychological Association (APA), state licensing board, and American Board of Professional Psychology (ABPP) became involved. Ultimately, the evaluating neuropsychologist lost his license when it was determined that he had used poor judgment and that his professional behavior was unacceptable. As a result, he also lost his membership in APA and the state psychological association, and his ABPP diplomate in clinical psychology.

Case 6: The Reviewing and Expert Neuropsychologist

Scenario
A neuropsychologist is retained as an expert by a state licensing board to review work done by another neuropsychologist. This neuropsychologist expert is informed of multiple prior legal/ethical complaints against the neuropsychologist whose work he is reviewing. The neuropsychologist reviews the colleague's work, writes a report to the licensing board, and has no further contact with the board or the other neuropsychologist until two years later. This time, the two professionals are retained as experts on opposing sides in the same legal case. Although the neuropsychologist who reviewed the other professional's work did not divulge the prior review of the colleague, she asks the attorney retaining her: "Why don't you ask Dr. X about prior complaints regarding his professional practice by the licensing board and state psychological association ethics committee, though I can't tell you why I am advising you to ask this."

Ethical Issues
In many ways a violation of confidentiality, this breach violates Standard 7.03 (*Clarification of Role*). The psychologist is involved in conflicting roles by having reviewed the psychologist's prior work and then using that information to provide 'ammunition' to an attorney in an unrelated matter. There is evidence that the psychologist's professional judgment may be compromised by the disclosure and 'advice' given to the new, retaining attorney. Although a psychologist's past may be relevant to an attorney, it should have no relevance to the opposing psychologist's independent opinion regarding a particular plaintiff in litigation. This situation also violates Principle E of the Ethics Code, in that the role of reviewer for the state ethics committee is used for exploitation to gain a tactical advantage. Given the potential exploitation, Standard 1.19 (*Exploitative Relationships*) may have been breached. Importantly, Standard 5.02 (*Maintaining Confidentiality*) may have been breached, in that the consulting psychologist did not take precautions to respect the confidentiality rights of the person about whom he has consulted.

Resolution
When a psychologist learns of a potential breach or disclosure of confidential information by his or her colleague, a decision must be made regarding whether to file a formal ethics charge. In this instance, as in most such situations, the psychologist should first speak to his or her colleague regarding the disclosure, and express concern. Based upon the psychologist's response, the affected individual must then decide whether or not to file a complaint against the disclosing psychologist with the APA or state ethics committees.

Case 7: The Other Expert Took and Failed the Board Examination

Scenario
Two neuropsychologists are retained by opposing parties in a neuropsychological consultation that is now being litigated. When neuropsychologist A reviews neuropsychologist B's deposition, he recognizes the name of the colleague (neuropsychologist B) as an individual whose failure to pass the exam for board certification in clinical neuropsychology be witnessed. Neuropsychologist A reports this to the retaining attorney, and advises him to confront neuropsychologist B about this on the witness stand in court, as an attack on his qualifications.

Ethical Issues
This is *potentially* a breach of Standard 5.02 (*Maintaining Confidentiality*), in that the confidentiality of a colleague is being violated. Although Psychologist B has no formal confidential relationship with Psychologist A in the traditional sense, it is explicitly stated and all ABPP candidates are asked to sign a confidentiality statement at the beginning of the examination, detailing that both the process and presence of candidates at the exam are considered confidential. It is also a potential violation of Ethical Principle D (*Respect for People's Rights and Dignity*). Psychologist B has a right to expect that others will not divulge their attendance at an examination.

Resolution
This breach of confidential information can first be addressed with the colleague. If unresolved, complaints to APA and state ethics committees and to ABPP could be lodged.

Case 8: Please Don't Release That Part of the Records!
A neuropsychologist is retained by a plaintiff attorney to evaluate an adolescent who had sustained a moderate traumatic brain injury. In reviewing the records prior to the actual evaluation, the neuropsychologist noted the adolescent had a police record of several arrests, antedating the brain injury. When asked about this, the attorney pleaded with the neuropsychologist not to refer to this since nobody had noticed this and "it didn't matter." When the neuropsychologist stated that he believed it was relevant to his examination,

the attorney stated that the court might rule it inadmissible anyway, since it might be considered overly prejudicial, and asked the neuropsychologist to leave it out of his report. The neuropsychologist complied.

Ethical Issues
A neuropsychologist has a professional obligation to reveal all information that would materially affect his or another expert's opinion. This first speaks to Principle B (*Integrity*) which states that "psychologists are honest, fair, ..." Omission of this information could potentially be misleading, and could certainly be viewed as bias on the part of the witness. Moreover it is difficult to imagine that salient pre-injury behavior could be viewed as not relevant in a discipline concerned with the etiology and meaning of behaviors, and possible changes in behavior. This issue also pertains to Standard 2.05 (*Interpreting Assessment Results*) which states that "psychologists take into account the various test factors and characteristics of the person assessed that might affect psychologists' judgments or reduce the accuracy of their interpretations." Unless the psychologist indicates significant reservations s/he has about the accuracy or limitations of his/her interpretations, this could be a violation of this ethical standard. It is important for neuropsychologists to remember that in a litigated case only a judge is allowed to determine what is relevant. An attorney can decide to ask a judge to bar certain information from being disclosed to the jury, based on legal precedents and rulings. It is not appropriate for expert witnesses to pre-empt a judge, or other trier-of-fact, and attempt to make this legal decision.

Relevant to this point, new information regarding a litigant may be introduced during a deposition. If it is normally the case in non-litigated cases that a factor being introduced, such as prior criminal or educational history, would be taken into account in formulating diagnostic opinion, then, when asked during a litigated matter whether the same factor influences present opinion, a neuropsychologist is expected to answer honestly, regardless of how the information reflects on the plaintiff. During discovery depositions, the neuropsychologist's response to new information (to the extent that is legitimate and reliable) brought to his or her attention comes under Standard 7.04 (*Truthfulness and Candor*).

Resolution
The psychologist should inform the attorney that, as long as legally admissible and relevant to his/her expert opinion, the information cannot be withheld from the report, because doing so would create a potentially misleading situation. At times, as indicated above, information might be withheld if a ruling of the court renders the information inadmissible. When relevant legal statues are in conflict, or when the law and ethical standards are in conflict, a psychologist needs to pursue expert advice from colleagues, lawyers, and judges before proceeding. For example, it is unlawful to release information related to HIV and AIDS status without permission. If during the course

of a forensic evaluation it was previously unknown and discovered by the neuropsychologist that a plaintiff was HIV positive or had AIDS, an apparent conflict is present. Given that it is difficult to imagine a litigated case involving potential psychological or neuropsychological damages that would render such information irrelevant, it seems extremely unlikely that this information could simply be viewed as not relevant to an expert opinion. In such an instance as this example, the importance of having provided initial absence of confidentiality is underscored. However, even having informed the examinee of the absence of confidentiality, with such powerful and personal information as this, it seems prudent to gather further support for one's actions as an expert by seeking independent legal counsel and perhaps directly asking for the presiding judge's opinion. Ultimately, one must seek resolutions that balance ethical standards and the law.

Summary

Forensic neuropsychology is a relatively new and demanding practice area that, in most cases, requires exacting attention to detail. Ethical standards, while in most instances clearly stated, most often deal with situations that are not clear-cut (i.e., situations that are not 'black and white,' but rather varying shades of gray). Ethical behavior on the part of practitioners of forensic neuropsychology is expected, and can be of utmost importance in determining outcomes of related adversarial proceedings. It appears that accompanying the increase in involvement in forensic neuropsychology, there is an increase in concern among practitioners regarding ethical conflicts. As has been depicted within this chapter, a fair number of unique, and some of these very specific, ethical concerns arise from forensic activities. It is expected that this practice area of clinical neuropsychology will continue to gain prominence. In fact, it appears very likely (and would be our recommendation) that both forensic practice and related ethics issues will become commonplace components of academic preparation in graduate training programs. Ethical issues in forensic neuropsychology will also continue to be prominently debated in professional journals and increasingly become the topic of relevant scientific research. As the evolution of civilization leads to greater complexity and the need for more exact laws and ethical codes of conduct among citizens, so to with neuropsychology's growth of knowledge and practice there is a growing need for an understanding of relevant laws and ethical codes among practitioners.

References

Addington v. Texas, 441 U.S. 418, 430 (1979).
American Academy of Clinical Neuropsychology (2000). Statement on the presence of third party observers in neuropsychological assessments. *The Clinical Neuropsychologist, 15,* 433–439.

American Psychological Association (1981). *Ethical principles of psychologists.* Washington, D.C.: American Psychological Association.

American Psychological Association (1993). Record keeping guidelines. *American Psychologist, 46,* 984–985.

Binder, L., & Thompson, L. (1995). The ethics code and neuropsychological assessment practices. *Archives of Clinical Neuropsychology, 10,* 27-46.

Borum, R., Otto, R., & Golding, S. (1993). Improving clinical judgment and dicision making in forensic evaluation. *Journal of Psychiatry and Law, 21,* 35–76.

Canter, M., Bennett, B., Jones, S., & Nagy, T. (1994). *Ethics for psychologists: A commentary on the APA ethics code.* Washington, DC: American Psychological Association.

Committee on Ethical Guidelines for Forensic Psychologists (1991). Specialty guidelines for forensic psychologists. *Law and Human Behavior, 15,* 655-665.

Danner, D., & Sagall, E. (1977). Medicolegal causation: A source of professional misunderstanding, *American Journal of Law and Medicine, 303,* 305.

Garb, H. (1998). *Studying the clinician: Judgment research and psychological assessment.* Washington, D.C.: American Psychological Association.

Grote, C., Lewin, J., Sweet, J., & van Gorp, W. (2000). Responses to perceived unethical practices in clinical neuropsychology: Ethical and legal considerations. *The Clinical Neuropsychologist, 14,* 119-134.

Guilmette, T., & Hagan, L. (1997). Ethical considerations in forensic neuropsychological consultation. *The Clinical Neuropsychologist, 11,* 287-290.

Hansen, M. (2000). Expertise to go. *American Bar Association Journal, 86,* 44-52.

Kehrer, C., Sanchez, P., Habif, U., Rosenbaum, J.G., & Townes, B. (2000). Effects of a significant-other observer on neuropsychological test performance. *The Clinical Neuropsychologist, 14,* 67-71.

Lees-Haley, P., & Cohen, L. (1999). The neuropsychologist as expert witness: Toward credible science in the courtroom. In J. Sweet (Ed.) *Forensic neuropsychology: Fundamentals and practice* (pp. 443–468). Lisse, Netherlands: Swets & Zeitlinger.

Lewin, J. (1998). The genesis and evolution of legal uncertainty about "reasonable medical certainty." *Maryland Law Review, 57,* 380-504.

Macartney-Filgate, M., & Snow, G. (2000). Forensic assessments and professional relations. *Division of Clinical Neuropsychology Newsletter, 18,* 28-31.

McCaffrey, R., Williams, A., Fisher, J., & Laing, L. (1996). *The practice of forensic neuropsychology.* Dordrecht, Netherlands: Kluwer Academic.

Nagy, T. (2000). *Ethics in plain English: An illustrative casebook for psychologists.* Washington, DC: American Psychological Association.

NAN Policy and Planning Committee (2000a). Presence of third party observers during neuropsychological testing. *Archives of Clinical Neuropsychology, 15,* 379-380.

NAN Policy and Planning Committee (2000b). Test security. *Archives of Clinical Neuropsychology, 15,* 383-386.

Pope, K., & Vetter, V. (1992). Ethical dilemmas encountered by members of the American Psychological Association: A national survey. *American Psychologist, 47,* 397-411.

Rappeport, J. (1985). Reasonable medical certainty. *Bulletin of the American Academy of Psychiatry and the Law, 5,* 8-23.

Rhoto v. Ribando, 504 So. 2d 1119, 1122 n.2 (La. Ct. App., 1987)

Strasburger, H., Gutheil, T., & Brodsky, B. (1997). On wearing two hats: Role conflict in serving as both psychotherapist and expert witness. *American Journal of Psychiatry, 154,* 448-456.

Sweet, J. (1990). Further consideration of ethics in psychological testing: A broader perspective on releasing records. *Illinois Psychologist, 28,* 5-9.

Sweet, J. (1999). *Forensic neuropsychology: Fundamentals and practice.* Lisse, Netherlands, Swets & Zeitlinger.

Sweet, J., Moberg, P., & Suchy, Y. (2000). Ten-year follow-up survey of clinical neuropsychologists: Part II. Private practice and economics, *The Clinical Neuropsychologist, 14,* 479–495.

Sweet, J., & Moulthrop, M. (1999). Self-examination questions as a means of identifying bias in adversarial assessments. *Journal of Forensic Neuropsychology, 1,* 73-88.

Sweet, J., & Rozensky, R. (1991). Professional relations. In M. Hersen, A. Kazdin, & A. Bellack (Eds.), *The clinical psychology handbook* (2nd ed.) (pp. 102–114). New York: Pergamon.

Taylor, S. (1999). The legal environment pertaining to clinical neuropsychology. In J. Sweet (Ed.), *Forensic neuropsychology: Fundamentals and practice* (pp. 421–442). Lisse, Netherlands: Swets & Zeitlinger.

van Gorp, W., & McMullen, W. (1997). Potential sources of bias in forensic neuropsychological evaluations. *The Clinical Neuropsychologist, 11,* 180-187.

Chapter 8

ETHICAL ISSUES IN NEUROPSYCHOLOGICAL REHABILITATION

Dennis P. Swiercinsky

Introduction

Rosenthal (1996) provides a summary of the evolution of brain injury rehabilitation which he describes in four-year segments representing the era of
enlightenment (beginning in 1975) through eras of proliferation, refinement,
and accountability. In about a dozen years, brain injury rehabilitation came
into being as a legitimate discipline, became largely entrepreneurial-focused
in for-profit rehabilitation entities, received scientific scrutiny and skepticism,
and quickly reached ethical notoriety for allegations of consumer fraud and
abuse. With the escalation of 'health care reform' around 1995, brain injury
rehabilitation (or, more precisely, the *availability* of brain injury rehabilitation services) entered a new era where economics of health care organizations, and health care reforms in general, led to a consolidation (i.e., down-
sizing) of brain injury rehabilitation. What began as enlightenment — that
neuropsychological impairment from brain injury *can* be treated — has been
squelched for the sake of short-term economics.

The new mandate — how to deliver quality (i.e., effective) rehabilitative
care within significant (i.e., efficient) cost constraints — forces a comprehensive and critical examination of the scientific, theoretical, *and ethical* foundations of neuropsychological rehabilitation. The ways, means, and long-term
benefits of neuropsychological rehabilitation must be defined by bridging
humanistic, scientific, and economic concerns. The industry's rapid growth
quickly opened many ethical issues, the antecedents of which need careful
scrutiny in order to recover (or, redefine) and sustain the quality and quan-

tity of treatment that people and families in neurological crisis need and deserve.

The foundational issue confronting neuropsychological rehabilitation is to define and prove what works. As Prigatano (1997) points out, "If a proposed therapy works, ... the cost is worth the outcome. Society is likely to agree that an investment of $50,000 to $60,000 is cost-efficient if a patient can return to and maintain work after brain injury.... The increasing pressure to justify rehabilitation efforts from a financial perspective again points to the need for clear evaluations of the successes and failures of neuropsychological rehabilitation" (p. 499).

In just one-quarter of a century *neuropsychological* rehabilitation — significantly intertwined in the larger, multidisciplinary field of brain injury rehabilitation — has experienced a tumultuous coming of age. The rapid and energetic growth, coincident with enormous changes in health care delivery, has raised and continues to raise many unsettling questions about the importance, validity, place, and delivery of cognitive and psychological (i.e., collectively and comprehensively, *neuropsychological*) services along side the medical, physiatric, vocational, and mechanical-functional (i.e., physical, occupational, and speech therapy) aspects of brain injury rehabilitation.

From exceptionally innovative and professionally respected programs developed by Diller (1976), Ben-Yishay (1978), and Prigatano (1986) to thinly conceived mass-marketed brain injury rehabilitation based on promise (and financial gain for the provider) but little on neuroscientific foundation, the call to competency, integrity, professional responsibility, dignity, dedication to the welfare of others, and commitment to social responsibility (the six general ethical principles of psychologists; APA, 1992) confronts the survival of neuropsychological rehabilitation and the reclamation of its crucial value to those who need it.

Brain injury rehabilitation recently has shifted its focus, per Rosenthal's (1996) chronology, to short stays in treatment programs, to the use of skilled nursing care as opposed to inpatient post-acute (and more aggressive) rehabilitation, and to generally little concern for quality (i.e., outcome) of care over cost savings. (This is evidenced by the paucity of research demonstrating functional outcomes of the type relied upon by Prigatano and others.) The rapid fluctuations in brain injury rehabilitation, particularly its current stage of de-emphasis, despite the continuing life-altering agony of brain injury (nearly a million new cases every year the result of automobile accidents; Berube, 2000), require a sensitive analysis of the ethical backdrop. By examining ethical concerns at key junctures, similar to those discussed by Malec (1993) nearly a decade ago, in the brain injury rehabilitation paradigm, perhaps the erratic pendulum can be coaxed to an arc of stable responsibility — all on behalf of persons with brain injury whose quality of life is at stake.

System Challenges in Neuropsychological Rehabilitation

Some of the "system" issues are listed and discussed, in no particular order, that present potential ethical challenges in the complex scientific, economic, research, consumer protection, professional competence, and humanistic dynamics of brain injury rehabilitation.

Accountability for high costs of services

Ethical Principle F (Social Responsibility): "Psychologists are aware of their professional and scientific responsibilities to the community and the society in which they work and live."

Accountability to those who pay for and to those who utilize rehabilitation services presents issues of moral and scientific responsibility. Every cost for service presents a potential burden to patients and families, directly and indirectly. The cost of services must not achieve success in neuropsychological rehabilitation at the expense of financial ruin for the patient and family. High health-care costs drive up deductibles as well as insurance premiums, adding financial burden. High costs without empirical demonstration of benefits heralds the doom of covered services altogether and the threat of insurance policy exclusions for rehabilitation coverage, particularly those services that focus on behavioral (and, hence more elusive) treatments. There must be a balance between optimization of services and cost to all parties. Cost must be examined in both short- and long-range benefit. What an insurance company and a family spend on neuropsychological rehabilitation must be viewed in a broad context, including the benefit of the cost to society as a whole.

Accountability is tantamount to ethical responsibility. It is based on an unbiased blend of interpretation of scientific research and recognition of the clinical needs of impaired persons; this in the face of quite inadequate research (High et al., 1995) and quite significant need for services (Berube, 2000). Accountability is not merely the unmasking of dishonesty but the complex creation of reasoned justifications, accounting for humanistic as well as economic needs. As stated in the Ethics Code's Preamble, "Psychologists work to develop a valid and reliable body of scientific knowledge based on research."

Emotional commitment to long-term rehabilitation

Another form of accountability, aside from but linked to the high dollar costs of rehabilitation, is the moral and emotional accountability to patients and families. Indeed, patients and families are devastated by initially life-threatening, and later life-constricting, brain injury. The cost, in terms of money as well as in the cost of time and emotional commitment that are absolutely necessary in long-term rehabilitation of brain injury, is often addressed only tacitly, if at all. There is a moral (i.e., honesty) obligation to respect the emotional as well as financial cost in planning and implementing a comprehensive and long-range rehabilitation program, of which the neuropsychological aspect typically is the most lengthy. Family, employer, insurer, and patient education is critical in planning a lengthy and often arduous treatment regimen — one necessary to accommodate slow neurological recovery and even slower neuropsychological adjustment to a permanently altered lifestyle.

It is anathema, in the extreme, for neuropsychological rehabilitation to be suddenly halted when cognitive gains can no longer be measured, only to leave the emotional devastation un- or incompletely addressed. Neuropsychological rehabilitation requires a lengthy commitment, one that family and provider(s) must be prepared to honor.

Requirement for comprehensive treatment

Related to dollar and emotional costs of neuropsychological rehabilitation is the issue of treatment efficiency, couched in complementary services to achieve comprehensive gains with minimal, or at least manageable, emotional expense. The emotional toll of months and even years in rehabilitation, while the patient usually clings to (unrealistic and defeating) pie-in-the-sky goals, creates frustrating yet persistent rehabilitation needs. Personal acceptance and broad accommodation for functional change due to permanent brain injury lags for the sake of expected cognitive recovery. But neurocognitive remediation cannot be effective in the vacuum of the patient's expectations because neurocognitive remediation rarely, if ever, means *total* recovery to pre-injury functionality.

As the pioneers in comprehensive neuropsychological rehabilitation have created and refined their programs, the need has been identified for a simultaneous and interactive focus on cognitive rehabilitation, psychotherapy, establishment of a therapeutic milieu, broadly targeted education, patient and family alliances, and work trials (Prigatano, 1992). Psychotherapy, the credibility of which appears maligned in the era of managed care, because it is so often excluded from insurance coverage, is critically connected with success in cognitive and functional gains in rehabilitation (Heinemann et al., 1995). Treatment must be comprehensive — *multifaceted* — for the sake of effectiveness as well as for long-term efficiency. There is no denying this, yet programs forsake comprehensiveness for shortsighted economics.

Formulation of realistic rehabilitation goals

Another issue that commands attention and which is linked to the above issues is the quality of care needed in order to achieve reasonably expected and clearly defined outcomes. Realistic goals must be established based on neurological, neuropathological, and injury mechanism models as well as on psychological theory and fact, followed by the appropriate treatment, irrespective of 'ability to pay' or other socioeconomic constraints, to achieve those goals. Unfortunately, somewhere in the era of proliferation the link between implicit (if not vague) goals for neuropsychological rehabilitation and explicit means for such rehabilitation became disengaged. The means of rehabilitation (which are reimbursable) became the end, not the goals. The ethical responsibility of linking scientific understanding of normal and pathological brain mechanisms to comprehensive therapeutic intervention (Prigatano, 1997) has fallen short.

Moral mission of neuropsychological rehabilitation

Cost control and lengthy rehabilitation became simultaneous issues as brain injury treatment programs were proliferating in the for-profit sector. How many patients' therapies were terminated in the name of recovery or having attained maximum (although, incomplete) benefit for the sake of exhausted insurance policy benefits? Rehabilitation professionals turned to an incomplete science to help defend against such practices. Insurance companies turned to ruthless case managers to help support such practices. Patients and families turned to support organizations (e.g., the National Head Injury Association, created in 1980, recently re-named the Brain Injury Association, and the State and local affiliates) to help them through the unfinished business when the helping profession abandoned them. So far, anyway, it is the cost control issue in the hands of powerful insurance companies that is winning the competition while science and patient advocacy play catch up. Adversarial roles mask common moral responsibility. All the players in brain injury rehabilitation need to come to the bargaining table with realistic and selfless expectations, scientific facts, well-conducted case and outcome vignettes, social conscience, and respect that cooperation, not competition, will provide the most humane foundation for solving a problem that isn't going to go away otherwise.

Social accommodation as a critical component of neuropsychological rehabilitation

> *Ethical Principle C (Professional and Scientific Responsibility): "Psychologists...adapt their methods to the needs of different populations."*

Retrofit curb cuts graced sidewalks in the 1970s to accommodate persons in wheelchairs. Braille imprint accompanied letters and words in signage in elevators and on vending machines in the 1980s to accommodate accessibility for persons with visual impairments. But, society has found few ways to accommodate the slower thinking, unrelenting impulsivity, memory lapses, shallow learning curves, and socially ostracizing emotionality characteristics that permanently limit the 'competitive' social reintegration of persons who have sustained moderate to severe brain injury. While this is more of a 'societal' as opposed to 'system' problem, the gap between lofty goals for rehabilitation and the stark reality of a cold, cruel world cannot be denied. Neuropsychological rehabilitation programs must account for this limitation. If increased patient autonomy is to be achieved (Hanson et al., 2000), remediation must go hand-in-hand with social accommodation, and adjustment to lack of social accommodation.

Responsible use of technology in neuropsychological rehabilitation

Burgeoning technological applications, especially with the development of general purpose personal computers in the late 80s and early 90s, ruled by fascination rather than by objective validity. Do hours spent at a computer screen practicing scanning and reaction speed generalize to anything practical, much less facilitate neural repair? While technology may contribute to cost control, what has it contributed to effective rehabilitation? (Forty hours on a computer equals the cost of eleven hours billable speech therapy. Beyond the forty hours, it's free!) Wilson (1997) makes a strong case that despite its continuing use such isolated cognitive retraining has no clear evidence for its effectiveness and lacks theoretical and practical foundation in a model of neuropathology.

Of course, not to throw out the baby with the bath water, technological applications may have a *complementary* place in a comprehensive rehabilitation program — providing focused activities, providing satisfaction in controlled mastery of new skills, laying the foundation for coping with a society that is ever-more becoming technologically based. With well founded and outcome studied programming, technology may, indeed, provide some generalizability to the real world experience. Technology in neuropsychological rehabilitation must provide *one* means to complement *several* ends, not *the* means to *an* end.

Treating brain injury involves a whole *person*

> *Ethical Principle E (Concern for Others' Welfare): "Psychologists seek to contribute to the welfare of those with whom they interact professionally."*

Brain injury typically leads to personal as well as family and sometimes community catastrophe. This destabilizing event, at a humanistic and holistic level, is overshadowed by system components that divide and denigrate rehabilitation rather than keep it necessarily integrated and person-focused. From hospital administration to therapy team meetings, to sleepless and agonizingly worrisome nights for a spouse or parent, to the cold necessity of replacing an injured worker who can no longer cut it, brain injury rehabilitation becomes like the blind men and the elephant. When and how does the elephant become, once again, an elephant?

It is no minor task (i.e., responsibility, ethical and moral obligation) to maintain the 'big picture' in helping an individual, his or her family, and the community of friends, employers, teachers, service agency personnel, insurance company representatives, hospital and treatment resource providers and administrators, bus or taxi drivers, personal attendants, and the myriad others who will interact with the person who has sustained a brain injury stay focused on 'the person.' References to the 'TBI in room 205' (or variations on the theme) are heard all the time in acute care and rehabilitation facilities. This is symbolic of the barrier society creates right off the bat that denigrates and relegates the person to an object rather than sustains him or her as a person. The use of order-imposing narratives is proposed by True and Phipps (1999) to help maintain an ethical focus on the *person*.

Unfortunately, while it is the neuropsychologist who ought to be orchestrating the preservation of the real *person*, this function in the big scheme of things is often lost. It is, however, the ethical responsibility of anyone who knows that this needs to be accomplished in order to attain the kind of holistic outcome deserving of anyone who experiences catastrophic change to the brain.

The first ten years of growth in brain injury rehabilitation provided the definition and place of neuropsychological rehabilitation and of the clinical neuropsychologist. With puberty approaching, the innocence of youth gave way to the turmoil of adolescence. As identity continued to evolve, amongst social confusion, the hard questions of science caused pause from the energy and enthusiasm of patient advocacy — the "consumer movement" as Rosenthal (1996) describes it. Clinical art, encroached upon first by entrepreneurial enthusiasm then reigned in by powerful economic conservatism, turned to science to address questions of brain function theory, treatment efficacy, and standards of care rooted in demonstrated outcome. Now, with emergence into adulthood, neuropsychological rehabilitation faces the challenges of learning from the past, making appropriate use of accelerated technologies, and always focusing on asking 'Are we doing the right thing for the *person*?'

Ethical Junctures in Neuropsychological Rehabilitation

Decreasing the chaos and containing the focus on system issues, while addressing ethical concerns, may be aided by identifying key concerns at logical junctions in the neuropsychological rehabilitation paradigm depicted in Figure 1. Such a schematic aids in identifying some of the ethical issues found in the broad realm of neuropsychological rehabilitation. Of course, as Rosenthal (1996) implies, the foci of ethical issues are dynamic and depend on the Zeitgeist — the social, economic, technological, and consumer factors driving the social and clinical milieu.

Understanding neural substrates and their roles in neuropsychological rehabilitation is understandably complex — and humbling. As in any emerging field, the ambiguity inherent in blending partial knowledge, hypotheses,

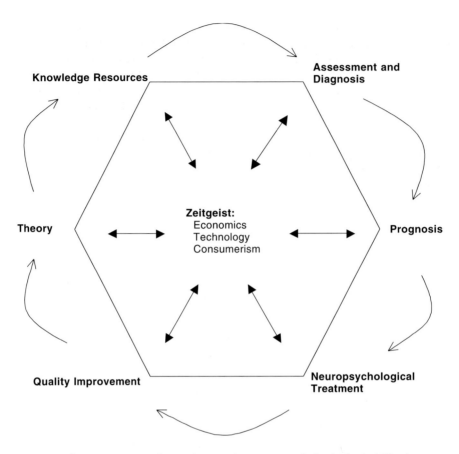

Figure 1. Ethics stopovers at key points on the neuropsychological rehabilitation paradigm.

suppositions, hopes, and guesses for the sake of human service invites ethical dilemmas, let alone introducing economic, regulatory, cultural and other factions into the equation. The link between limited objective knowledge and subjective need to treat is blurry. Just how this overlap between partial knowledge and desired treatment outcome plays out contributes to issues of ethical (i.e., professional) responsibility. Tight integration of knowledge, clinical needs, and neurologically desired outcomes just does not yet exist.

The six stages in the paradigm (i.e., knowledge resources, assessment and diagnosis, prognosis, treatment, quality improvement, and theory) represent interactive and complementary domains. All exhibit interactional influence and focus, modulated by economic climate, technological development, and consumer advocacy — the Zeitgeist.

Each point in the neuropsychological rehabilitation paradigm depicted here is examined for what it should represent within an ethically ideal society, and where the profession stands given our status of scientific development. By establishing ethical sensitivity and moral obligations for each juncture in the paradigm, potential dilemmas might be identified and ameliorated. Examination of each stage in the paradigm allows the profession to gauge such issues as the pressure to treat (despite lack of outcome data, thus not really sure what we are doing), to save money on treatment methods (versus waste money — we yet just don't know), to incorporate new technologies (or not), to train professionals thoroughly (versus quickly and economically to meet consumer demands), to invoke scientific standards and scrutiny (or get to market quickly), to weigh quality of life against financial burden (to whom), and to write standards of practice (versus 'winging it' for the sake of immediate clinical needs).

Knowledge Resources

Principle A (Competence): "Psychologists strive to maintain high standards of competence in their work. They recognize the boundaries of their particular competencies and the limitations of their expertise. They provide only those services and use only those techniques for which they are qualified by education, training, or experience. Psychologists are cognizant of the fact that the competencies required in serving, teaching, and/or studying groups of people vary with the distinctive characteristics of those groups."

Essential and comprehensive knowledge resources that feed clinical endeavors come from research in neuroscience and cognitive psychology as well as from a host of related disciplines and clinical practice. Scientific enlightenment provides the basis for education and training of rehabilitation professionals. The profession of neuropsychology has endeavored for years to establish standards of scientific training and, hence, standards that underlie clinical services. Suggestions in the Policy Statement from the Houston Conference on Specialty Education and Training in Clinical Neuropsychology (Hannay et al., 1998) include: a broad knowledge base that includes biological bases of behavior, psychopathology, neuroanatomy, neurological disorders, neuropharmacology, and neuropsychology of behavior; and a broad range of skills that emphasize or imply communications, outcome assessment, recognition of multicultural issues, and holistic team efforts in assessment and treatment. Thus, the availability and accessibility of a comprehensive knowledge base provide the foundation for everything else in neuropsychological rehabilitation. To acquire and apply this broad knowledge base is essential and ethically responsible.

Ethical Standard 1.06 (Basis for Scientific and Professional Judgments): "Psychologists rely on scientifically and professionally derived knowledge when making scientific or professional judgments or when engaging in scholarly or professional endeavors."

Scientific foundation must continue to be the cornerstone of neuropsychology, unrelenting in response to pressures to eke out treatment justifications for which minimal objective foundation often exists. The manner in which scientific research, case studies, outcome statistics, and other data are combined in order to lay the foundation for neuropsychological rehabilitation depends on a means for cataloging and making that knowledge readily available. Currently, that database is technologically weak, contributing to the lack of coherence in achieving research-to-market credibility.

Neuropsychological rehabilitation depends on a broad cross-disciplined and scientific knowledge base. Melding research and practice is the profession's traditional way to achieve responsible development. Combining sensitive observations, measures of clinical outcomes, personal and social expectations, and formal scientific studies is essential to address specific clinical treatment development and to provide the training and on-going education of neuropsychologists. So far, the profession uses a technologically antiquated method for knowledge dissemination, making its use for clinical practice not particularly easily.

An evolving, accessible knowledge depository, based on sound, multidisciplinary science and clinical observation is the foundation for excellence in contemporary clinical practice and for defining the parameters of many ethical situations. Basic and essential outcomes of scientific studies provide the bedrock upon which procedures in clinical practice are defined. Methods for accessing such knowledge, however, have not kept pace with the proliferation and varying degrees of professional standards that characterize the knowledge base.

Full text Internet publication (universally available, free to individual users, and on demand) with links to signed peer reviews and commentary could provide open access to knowledge and knowledge evolution. Topical continuity, chronological follow-up, refinement studies, and branching to related information might characterize this form of growing, searchable, organized, peer-commentary database. The technology to achieve such a repository and catalog of knowledge exists today but is not utilized in neuropsychology. As the technology is implemented, neuropsychological rehabilitation will have an easily accessible knowledge base.

An example of developments that neuropsychology might adopt is reflected in 'WebBrain,' a hierarchical and hyperlinking system that categorizes topics and provides neural net-like jumps to related peer subcategories and topical entries (examples of companies providing such technology include TheBrain Technologies Corp. and Synergietics). Such a sophisticated system as WebBrain eliminates users' needing to learn the restrictions of a complex thesaurus of cataloging terms — the terms are on-screen and guide the user. Diverse sources of information may be integrated into one huge database with hierarchical and peer links that evolve as the system is utilized — providing a dynamic linking system not dependent on a fixed cataloging that may exclude an important datum from connection with relevant other data. New links, in the form of new research studies, outcomes, and peer professional evaluations can be added at any time — making the data and cataloging a real time knowledge base.

A problem with applying scientific knowledge to clinical applications lies in the fragmented manner in which clinical research is often accomplished and presented for professional consumption. Too often studies conclude with the caveat that more research is needed to refine discoveries or confirm statistical probabilities. Yet, rarely are follow-up studies performed. Or, if they are performed their link to the instigating research is not easily apparent within the existing cataloging system. A searchable database in the style of WebBrain, or something similar, would greatly enhance the collection, use, and evaluation of the knowledge that forms the foundation of clinical practice. Just as the American Psychological Association ethical guidelines (American Psychological Association, 1992) prescribe the use of up-to-date norms, current editions of tests, and contemporary practices that have been shown superior to older practices, so must the profession's collection and presentation of knowledge be based on contemporary technology. This will help erase the secrecy behind clinical practice and ease the access to providing otherwise elusive knowledge. Such a knowledge base must be free to researchers and to anyone desiring access in order to evaluate a clinical strategy.

Methodological limitations in neuropsychological rehabilitation research

The impact of scientific knowledge on clinical delivery systems to assure a reasoned and substantiated basis for what is done has been slow in coming and veiled, if not inconclusive. The abundance of published studies relative to neuropsychological knowledge, and rehabilitation, specifically, is fragmented and often founded on dubious methodology (High et al., 1995). There is precious little complementary knowledge on which to build models and theories, let alone commercially offered practical rehabilitation. Ethical problems abound in medical research, in general, including neuropsychological, when a suspected treatment benefit can be evaluated only by withholding the treatment from a group of persons who *might*, otherwise, benefit. Applying the rigors of scientific method to study the most complex system known to man leaves a huge risk for unaccounted variance. Hence, given the ethical and methodological constraints, research has yielded only limited 'hard' facts on which to model neuropsychological rehabilitation treatment methods. What published study does not conclude with the caveat and recommendation that '...more research is needed?'

The works of Ben-Yishay, Diller, Prigatano, and others provide case vignettes that support long-term, comprehensive neuropsychological rehabilitation. The autobiography by Claudia Osborn (1998) provides an insightful testimonial to the success of comprehensive, multidisciplinary, long-term neuropsychological rehabilitation for brain injury. Despite the ethical and methodological constraints in performing outcome studies that follow strict

I'm not so sure

scientific guidelines, the mounting case evidence provides ample foundation for a guiding direction in constructing neuropsychological rehabilitation.

Assessment and Diagnosis

Ethical Standard 2.01 (b): "Psychologists' assessments, recommendations, reports, and psychological diagnostic or evaluative statements are based on information and techniques (including personal interviews of the individual when appropriate) sufficient to provide appropriate substantiation for their findings."

Neuropsychological assessment (of brain–behavior relationships) provides the foundation for diagnosis, for understanding injury dynamics, for drawing prognoses, and for designing treatment. A cursory initial assessment may direct entry-level rehabilitation efforts while on-going assessments fine tune interventions and prognoses. Driven, in part, by the availability of neuropsychological examiners, funds to pay for examination, and integration of *useful* assessment information into the rehabilitation matrix, the assessment aspect of neuropsychological rehabilitation may consist of anything from nothing or token peripheral assessment to comprehensive examination highly integrated within the total scope of multidisciplinary rehabilitation.

Whereas neuropsychologists were integrally involved in brain injury rehabilitation in the 1970s and 80s, their presence by the mid-90s gradually diminished. Some brain injury rehabilitation centers do not employ neuropsychologists at all anymore. While the definitive role of the neuropsychologist is, ostensibly, to be the expert in brain–behavior relationships, and whereas the ultimate concern of permanent consequences of brain injury is inevitably social-behavioral (not treatment merely restricted to talking, walking, using the hands, or the like), the absence of the neuropsychologist in an integrated role is antithetical — at least conceptually, and is unethical. Why is the designated expert no longer, or more essentially, present?

The ethical issue involved here is, What has caused the shift in focus away from utilization of neuropsychology in brain injury rehabilitation, much less in its leadership role? The answer is related to cost–benefit. Cost is always empirically defined. Benefit, on the other hand, is at least somewhat subjective. Unless the benefit of neuropsychological assessment (and neuropsychological rehabilitation, in general) is deemed high, the cost–benefit ratio will be too great to justify.

Lynch (2000) points out that lengthy and comprehensive neuropsychological assessments are gradually yielding to shorter, 'screening' approaches, largely driven by pressure from third-party payers. Again, powerful economic players dominate the lack of scientific foundation for what is evolving in neuropsychological assessment practice.

Therapists, doctors, families, case managers, lawyers, and others often speak of needing a "good" neuropsychological evaluation. A situation exists

in the profession — an ethical issue in a broad sense — in that such a quali-
fier as 'good' should never be needed. *All* neuropsychological assessments
should be 'good,' that is, they should address the assessment questions in easily readable language based on ecologically valid tests, offer useful outcome
research-based diagnostic understanding, relate assessment results to practical daily living and vocational concerns, and provide as much specific long-
range rehabilitation guidance and outcome expectation as a sound, contemporary model of neuropathology and neurorecovery will allow. Perhaps the
paucity of 'good' neuropsychological assessment has led to the paucity of
neuropsychology in general.

While it has been pretty much standard to obtain a neuropsychological
assessment as a part of brain injury rehabilitation, the quality and integration
of the assessment is typically variable. Without diagnosis (need it be qualified
as a 'good' diagnosis — one based on practical diagnostic understanding,
not merely labeling?), the treatment it guides can only be shotgun at best,
damaging at worst. If assessment (and diagnosis) guides treatment that leads
to demonstrable outcomes, cost–benefit will take a hefty leap forward. Not
only is the general issue of 'good' neuropsychological diagnostics at stake, so
is the issue of ecological (i.e., practical) validity of neuropsychological tests
from which to guide practicality and generalizability of treatment.

An ethical concern in this regard is suggested by the fact that in the present
era of rehabilitation services consolidation, obtaining the contribution of a
neuropsychologist is ever more restricted by the mandates of managed care
(Sweet et al., 1995). As long as there is no (good) foundation on which to
prescribe (useful) treatment, there is no justification for (expensive?) treatment, according to the scientific paradigm, *as well as no justification by the
managed care paradigm.*

The issue poses the question: Does a 'good' neuropsychological assessment
provide a valid link between what is seen and interpreted in test performance
and the gains that might be expected from specific treatments to address
specific deficits? If the answer is yes, then neuropsychological assessment, and
serial re-assessments, would be essential for prediction, treatment monitoring, and quality control. Neuropsychological assessment would not be an
optional luxury but an essential foundation for neuropsychological rehabilitation. It is ethically concerning that the link between assessment and
treatment has been so flagrantly denied, or minimized. It is up to the neuropsychology profession to fix this link not only to restore neuropsychology's presence but also to make its presence *essential* for effective, useful,
comprehensive, maintainable, generalizable, economical, and psychologically
satisfying rehabilitation.

Neuropsychologists traditionally have been assessment and diagnostic
specialists. The tradition began with Ward Halstead and has continued with
burgeoning refinement in just the past thirty or so years. Unfortunately,
the neuropsychological assessment of whether or not a person has brain
damage, the significant goal of assessment in 1960, is far from being that

simple today. Achieving neuropsychological diagnostic understanding is exceedingly more complex and tied to important issues in prognosis and treatment planning.

It is interesting that in litigation cases, more money may be spent on the neuropsychologist, as the key expert witness in defining damage and functional consequences of brain injury than was spent by insurance providers on neuropsychological services within the context of clinical care and coordination. It is also interesting that considerable professional education has recently been aimed at training *forensic* neuropsychologists to provide this litigation service because the neuropsychologist cannot financially survive through standard reimbursement for clinical services. Advertisements for training workshops in forensic neuropsychology have used this pitch to enroll attendees. Does *this* pose any ethical issue? At the least, it underscores the important and even critical contribution available from the neuropsychologist.

Competency — being a 'good' neuropsychologist — means integrating, at a high level of understanding, all the knowledge domains suggested by the Houston Conference statement. Professional (i.e., ethical) responsibility of the neuropsychologist lies in his or her maintenance of a broad perspective of the art of human service while basing decisions on hard scientific foundation. This argument must be emphasized over and over again to reintegrate the neuropsychologist into a (if not *the*) key role in brain injury rehabilitation.

Prognosis

Outcome, ideally, drives the cost–benefit aspect of rehabilitation. While such a highly important aspect of assessment and of rehabilitation, it is typically handled cautiously and conservatively by most practitioners. *Prediction* of outcome (i.e., prognosis) depends on adequacy of knowledge of neuropathology, thoroughness and validity of assessment, clinical experience and the systematically documented outcome experiences of other neuropsychologists, and measurement of objective outcomes from initial treatment. The effort, intensity, kind, and success of treatment that a patient receives depends on precise specification of treatment, based on prognosis, that will realistically address specific needs (i.e., acquired deficits) to attain specific goals. The worth and dignity of a patient and the willingness to commit to treatment is reflected in the accuracy and scientific merit of prognosis. It is the link that binds assessment, treatment, and outcome and, in part, defines 'good' neuropsychology. Good neuropsychology respects the person who needs the right kind of treatment.

It would be inhumane to impart treatment that carries outcome expectations on a rehabilitation client that would be virtually impossible to attain, something that very likely may happen without a reasonably determined prognosis. It would be equally unconscionable to deny treatment because the question of benefit cannot be objectively presupposed within a reasonable probability, something that may be done by fiat by third-party payors. Prediction of benefit from neuropsychological rehabilitation depends on ecological validity of neuropsychological tests (Sbordone & Long, 1996) and integration with other areas of diagnosis: such as brain imaging, neurological status, social and family resources, and other health and injury characteristics.

While perhaps only occasionally related to the scope of issues presently considered, an obvious example of an ethical dilemma in brain injury rehabilitation related to prognosis is that of the practice of coma stimulation. Coma stimulation or coma arousal *presumes* that brain recovery depends on an optimum availability of sensory stimulation in order to encourage the brain to re-establish or re-map stimulus–response connections (Baker, 1988). The benefit of coma stimulation has never been defined in terms of reliably linking specific procedures with pre-defined (and useful) outcome or the antecedent brain condition that would make coma stimulation work. Coma stimulation is based on theory, limited knowledge, and heavy hope. To do coma stimulation is probably high on the humane dimension but low on the cost-benefit dimension, at least as we currently understand it. Its *ecological* validity is still questioned. The ethical dilemma lies in the challenge of blending available, and admittedly incomplete, knowledge about brain plasticity and recovery with the cost of treatment that may or may not benefit the patient.

Another and related ethical problem, closer to the heart of neuropsychologists, yet extremely complex, is the issue of generalizability of treatment based on prediction of potential benefit of specific neuropsychological rehabilitation techniques. Can a 'good' neuropsychological assessment identify the impaired brain–behavior domain(s) that will benefit from specific treatments (e.g., computer-based stimulus attention training, practice on a specific task to increase psychomotor speed, or cognitive exercises that require graduated multitasking) to ease the impact of the deficit and generalize improvement in real-world functionality?

If the answer is 'yes' to the above question, will it make a difference in ultimate functionality (say, 3–5 years post injury)? Would spontaneous recovery over the course of 5–7 years yield slower but just as adequate an outcome? Is it the interpersonal benefit of intense rehabilitation or the actual training modality (say, delivered by real person or by computer) that makes any difference, presuming there is a difference? Depending on that answer, are high cost therapists more beneficial than low cost social enrichment endeavors (e.g., recreational and social support programs)? Many questions can be asked that challenge the treatment versus spontaneous recovery issue. Yet, prognostication must account for potential spontaneous recovery, especially in view of limited availability of formal neuropsychological rehabilitation in many cases.

If serial neuropsychological assessment demonstrates that there has been benefit from neuropsychological rehabilitation, does the difference in test scores have a qualitative meaning for the patient's practical day-to-day, family-related, or work-related functionality? In other words, once rehabilitation techniques demonstrate functional gains on neuropsychological tests, what is the utility of test scores for determining practical, real-world expectations? This is not only a question of generalizability but also one of criterion-related significance in test scores. What does absolute level of performance mean for prognosis, for real-world significance? How much change in absolute performance over serial testing is necessary to suggest a real-world functional benefit? Will frontal disinhibition still present a practical challenge for the patient regardless of scores on so-called 'frontal lobe tests,' even if the score becomes 'normal'?

As these questions imply, both broad and specific predictions from neuropsychological assessments are essential and tough to come by in 'good' neuropsychological rehabilitation. To accept less than scientifically- or empirically-based or, at least, strongly theoretically-based predictions leads to messy, if not impossible, statistical as well as ecological validation of the assessment–treatment–outcome paradigm. Such a state underlies disagreements as to the value and benefit of any component in the paradigm. Payers have no moral obligation to pay for recommended services that have no objectively demonstrated benefit. Consumers (patients and families) have no responsibility to partake of treatment that could, in the end, offer anything from no functional benefit with increased frustration and irritability to relearned skills enabling return to work, with considerable variation in between those extremes.

The links from assessment to prediction to treatment to outcome typically have been focused on hope and guess, based on empathy, compassion, and personal experience and bias. With the emerging demand for 'good' (i.e., objectively determined cost beneficial) outcomes, evaluation, enhanced theory, and knowledge will more and more drive the paradigm.

Theoretical bias, counter-transference, and frank lack of clinical sophistication and objectivity can contribute immensely to missed (or erroneous) diagnosis and obscure prognosis. Here is a composite, but familiar, scenario that illustrates obstacles to comprehensive (i.e., 'good') neuropsychological rehabilitation.

Vignette

A 48-year-old high school teacher is involved in a high speed, three-vehicle (one a semi-tractor rig) accident on an interstate highway. Her vehicle is violently spun nearly 360 degrees. She was shaken but not frankly, or only briefly, unconscious and had to be extracted from her vehicle by the jaws of life. Her emergency room CT was normal, and she was treated only for severe headache and numerous body aches and sent home. The typical 'mild' post-concussion syndrome ensued (persistent headache, irritability, depression, continued aches, some gait awkwardness, fatigue, startle response, poor ability to sleep, forgetfulness) subjectively preventing her from returning to the classroom. The patient became socially withdrawn due to unremitting hyperacusis. Her preserved native penchant for self-pride, bouffant hair dos, make-up, and tasteful dress obscured the nature of her disability and won her little sympathy from doctors, family, and ultimately jurors — she didn't *look* impaired. The familiar post-concussion syndrome, the typical pattern of mild memory and attentional impairment with preserved intelligence on neuropsychological tests, the mechanical understanding of violent twisting of the brain and brain stem during the spinout (causative of shearing lesions), and the virtual lack of conversion, factitious or malingering evidence are well accepted neuropsychological and neurophysiological tenets pointing to 'organic brain injury.' Hyperacusis and startle response are well documented related to injury to cranial nerves VII and VIII feedback circuits within the brain stem. Yet, the patient was treated only in psychotherapy for anxiety disorder, with suspicion of posttraumatic stress disorder related to her vague memory of the impact. Two years later, she lost her day in court. She lost her job, without disability benefits. Yet, she still carries the diagnosis of mild postconcussion syndrome.

Beliefs among neuropsychological practitioners about causation and ultimate resolution of post-concussion syndrome and mild traumatic brain injury are contradictory. Unquestionably, there is significant variation in brain injury severity, post-concussion syndrome, rate of recovery, and outcome. Some mild brain injury patients return to work within a few months, others are never able to return to their former occupations. It is simplistic to decree any potential brain injury as having some kind of clearly expected outcome; the myriad components of mild brain injury differ dramatically from case to case. Unresolved hyperacusis is neurophysiologically understandable yet virtually undetectable by neuropsychological tests. Yet, hyperacusis can virtually and totally impair a person's functioning in many environments, let alone noisy high school classrooms. It may be a determining variable in the expression of mild traumatic brain injury.

Given the hypothetical that treatment X has shown some (but not perfect) benefit in clinical studies with a range of degrees of neuropsychological deficit, Y, where the trend is for greater benefit measured on Z when Y is strongly deficient than when it is only weakly deficient, how should this knowledge component, derived from *group* data, be applied in the next *individual* case? Should the patient receive X regardless of the level of Y, or should there be some cutoff criterion? Since even weak deficit on Y has shown some (if even minimal) improvement on Z, should X be applied in every case, regardless? Of course the solution is easy. Since the knowledge base was not obtained with a control group due to the ethical dilemma in clinical research of denying a group of patients (i.e., controls) a *potential* (presumed) treatment benefit, the knowledge base is correlational and not causative. Payers say 'no' in the name of cost–benefit. But, clinicians recognize the link of empirical research (correlational or otherwise) to theoretical relationships and humanistic benefits of treatment (irrespective of the mechanical, objective treatment paradigm) and say 'yes' in the name of moral obligation. (As Walton [1998] reflects, "There are still many incurable neurological disorders but none are untreatable.") So, what makes the decision easy depends on who is in charge of the treatment, payer or clinician.

Prognosis depends not on a categorical diagnosis of mild brain injury to which generalized research findings apply but on an accounting of multifarious individual components of the person and the injury mechanism. Assessment, and treatment, of brain injury is addressing the most complex biological system. It cannot be simplified. Kaufman et al. (1995) ask, although within a somewhat different context: Should all patients be treated for the sake of benefit to a few, or should the emotional and economic cost (to patients, families, and third-party payers) be spared by not offering treatment that might not be effective at all?

If the state of knowledge resources, assessment, diagnosis, and prognostic acumen were insufficient, the minimization of the high school teacher's 'brain injury' by the uninformed might be understandable. But, the sophistication of clinical neuroscience research is sufficiently well advanced to understand trapezoid body injury, frontal disconnection causing serotonergic channel interruption, incomplete basal ganglia-cerebellar interruption, reticular activation system bruising with interruption of attention and sleep–wake cycles, and cervical strain, that can account very logically for every one of her post-concussion symptoms. If the profession cannot understand clinical presentation at this level of knowledge then we have violated the Hippocratic axiom, "first, do no harm." In other words, do not declare an individual 'uninjured' or even vaguely injured on the basis of a select set of neuropsychological tests that fail to take into account a much broader range of data, including data untapped by existing neuropsychological assessment tools. If prognosis suffers at the hand of inadequate assessment, treatment suffers.

While often and usually reduced to one or two words (e.g., 'good,' 'guarded,' 'poor') prognosis is so much more than this. Comprehensive prognosis is the extension of comprehensive assessment and diagnosis. Without a reasoned, detailed prognosis, treatment becomes generalized and non-specific, outcome becomes a shot in the dark.

Neuropsychological Treatment

Benefit from treatment is, of course, the quintessential purpose of neuropsychological rehabilitation. Treatment is, at least, methodologically multifaceted, hierarchical, milieu-dependent (e.g., home-based versus facility-based), multimodal, technologically associated, and temporally evolving. Because of such diversity in the definition, conceptualization, and process of neuropsychological treatment, doors are ever opening to challenges of efficacy, cost–benefit, scientific validity, appropriateness of application, functional benefit, and so forth. Many of these challenges carry diverse ethical considerations regarding informed consent and other therapy standards, confidentiality involving patients who are marginally capable of understanding such concepts, competencies, documentation, dealing with third-party payers, and public statements regarding treatment efficacy.

Neuropsychological treatment, variously including strategies of cognitive remediation, cognitive rehabilitation, cognitive training, and psychological support, is performed for two reasons. Variations of neuropsychological rehabilitation strategies are performed to enhance functioning across as broad a spectrum of domains as possible for the sake of enhancing 'quality of life,' in general — the 'non-specific treatment approach.' Additionally, neuropsychological treatment is intended to attain specific goals and specific functional recoveries (based on assessment of functional weaknesses and inference of acquired impairment), in order to return the individual to his or her job, school, driving, and so forth — the 'applied treatment approach.'

Ethical issues potentially arise in several contexts. The available armament of neuropsychological treatment strategies range from specific to general, research-based to theory-based (or, merely, idea-based), widely to narrowly accepted within the profession, and validated to virtually untested. Yet, for the sake of a 'non-specific treatment' approach, any and all strategies, regardless of focus, that invigorate and enhance the psychological well-being of the patient might be used for the sake of rebuilding confidence. In order for the neuropsychologist to advocate on behalf of the patient, in order to justify purchase of such services, the neuropsychologist occasionally finds himself or herself pitted against managed care restrictions, insurance limitations, and scientific foundations or lack thereof. Banja (1999) reviews the provider's ethical dilemma in his or her role as patient advocate — being the bridge between specific scientific merit of a treatment and treatment for quality of life at any cost.

Issues of 'medical necessity' and lack of empirical outcome studies (i.e., issues of treatment justification) lie at the heart of ethical conflicts in advocating for the patient versus restraining intervention based on scientific merit. A non-specific treatment approach based on theory must still link treatment with current understanding and theory of neural plasticity and neural recovery. And, it needs to be linked to documented psychological (emotional as opposed to cognitive) benefit within the total scheme of things.

A generalized neuropsychological rehabilitation treatment program intended to facilitate spontaneous recovery needs to be lengthy (often extending for years), appropriately varying in intensity, involving of family, broad-based, and yet affordable. Such a treatment program must be individualized, accounting not only for the financial resources of the patient, but for the availability of a mix of insurance, environmental, social, family, and community resources that can be mobilized to augment spontaneous recovery. Without scientific proof of any treatment's ability to augment spontaneous recovery or guarantee production of outcome, such treatment must be designed economically, making use of diverse resources that spare, particularly, patient and family financial drain. Coma stimulation is an appropriate example of a generalized treatment that can be very expensive if not designed to involve family and friends in cost-reducing ways.

The applied treatment approach to neuropsychological rehabilitation is designed to achieve a narrower, more specific outcome. It needs to be, perhaps, of shorter duration and to target specific applications proven to effect specific, desired outcomes for specific purpose(s). Ethical issues arise in providing neuropsychological treatment in this regard similar to those discussed regarding neuropsychological assessment. Ecological validity continues to be the essential concern. In the face of limited objective validity, is subjective validity sufficient justification for service delivery, generalization across patients, and expectation of reimbursement? Third-party payers have emphatically said 'No'.

The weary neuropsychologist who dismisses his or her patient from a rehabilitation therapy session thanking God for the gift of spontaneous recovery hasn't sorted out the full range of assessment and prognostic variables that will determine the specific mix of therapeutic interventions needed and the limitations of reasonable outcomes. Neuropsychological rehabilitation is complex and multifaceted. It has non-specific (generalized) and specific (applied or targeted) foci, both of which have specific (e.g., limited) outcome expectations based on prognostic understanding.

Informed Consent

Ethical Standard 4.02(a): "Psychologists obtain appropriate informed consent to therapy or related procedures, using language that is reasonably understandable to the participants....informed consent generally implies that the person (1) has the capacity to consent..."

Another dilemma in providing neuropsychological rehabilitation to persons with brain injury is the issue of 'consent for treatment.' Anosognosia, or a lesser variation, is typical of persons with brain injury, particularly involving frontal injury (Prigatano & Schacter, 1991). Associated with a lack of appreciation of deficit(s) is organically based amotivation and inattention. How does the neuropsychologist intervene on behalf of a patient who may actively oppose the treatment needed to address deficits or that will prevent additional functional deterioration?

What happens when a patient does not have the capability to process information about his or her brain injury and appreciate the intended benefit from rehabilitation? Often, the neuropsychologist becomes the advocate for a patient that cannot address, let alone willingly accept, his or her own needs. The neuropsychologist must understand the comprehensive biopsychosocial diagnostic picture of the patient, the 'non-specific' and the 'applied' treatment needs and goals, conservation of resources that will meet needs irrespective of money, availability, and the role of family in defining and justifying treatment needs. Once again, the role of the neuropsychologist is pivotal in comprehending and defining treatment needs and orchestrating its access and delivery. When a patient appears to lack the cognitive capacity to provide informed consent, "psychologists obtain informed permission from a legally authorized person," if permitted by law [ES 4.02(b)]. Additionally, the psychologist should inform the patient about the proposed interventions in a manner that may be understood, seek the patient's assent to participate, and consider the best interests of the patient [ES 4.02(c); Bush & Sandberg, 2001].

The Rehabilitation Industry
In an ideal world, neuropsychological rehabilitation should not be directed solely by available financial resources and limiting institutional-based resources. Instead, rehabilitation should be broad-based, culled from many resources, and be integrated within the sociocultural milieu. Unfortunately, resources to facilitate spontaneous recovery, and even more so to effect specific, targeted rehabilitation goals (e.g., return to a specific job) are centralized (and usually isolated) within the walls of the formal rehabilitation industry, minimizing or limiting the role of the neuropsychologist. When conflicts surface between organizational demands and ethical neuropsychological practice, the practitioner should make known his or her commitment to ethical practice and attempt to resolve the matter "in a way that permits the fullest adherence to the Ethics Code" (ES 8.03).

Malec (1996) offers discussion of a perspective of neuropsychological rehabilitation based on human relationships at the core of decision-making about rehabilitation interventions. Both Malec (1996) and Banja and Johnston (1994) imply a neuropsychological rehabilitation system that is truly comprehensive, going well beyond the scheduled therapy hours of cognitive remediation sitting with a therapist or sitting in front of a computer screen. It is the ethical responsibility of the profession to assert a primary role in treatment, to advocate based on scientific and neurophysiological foundations for comprehensive treatment, to identify and hold to meaningful outcomes, and to monitor and refine treatment as biological, social, and psychological factors demand it.

Education — of the patient, family, payers, and other professionals — is essential. The neuropsychologist, as the designated expert in brain–behavior relationships, provides the leadership in understanding the dynamics of treatment, and the integration of biopsychosocial treatments. The responsibility is great. Without this educator-leader role of the neuropsychologist, however, fragmentation in rehabilitation will likely prevail.

Quality Improvement
Quality improvement (QI), or variously called quality of care, quality assessment (QA), quality management or maintenance (QM), or quality control, is the overseer process that, theoretically, provides feedback for modification or justification of the direction taken by any of the other points in the representation of the six-dimensional rehabilitation paradigm depicted in Figure 1. The foundation of QI is precision, the one component that supposedly

adds credibility and refinement to all other aspects of the neuropsychological rehabilitation paradigm.

Through the evolution of neuropsychological rehabilitation over the past three or four decades, motivation for QI has been driven by various external factors: economics (i.e., insurance companies wishing to find ways to justify cost cutting or service limitations), regulatory and governmental agencies (e.g., setting standards in response to consumer complaints or concerns), and private enterprise (e.g., cloaking marketing of rehabilitation programs in something appearing more scientific and objective that it really is). By virtue of its recent coming-of-age in the neuropsychological rehabilitation paradigm, QI is the least developed component. Paradoxically, QI has been misused and self-serving rather than objective and credible. Because of this, and owing to regulatory pressures, objective financial justification of treatment programs, reimbursement authority, and consumer confidence, QI is under the gun and has become one of the most central aspect of rehabilitation, in general, neuropsychological rehabilitation, specifically. It is time to take QI seriously.

Any component of the system under scrutiny, and whose actions impart virtually all other aspects of the paradigm, has the potential to lose sight of objectivity. Hence, potential and significant ethical issues emerge. Instead of being methodologically driven, QI is often need-driven. Instead of finding out things about the stages and effects of rehabilitation and how well it is performed, QI becomes an arm of ulterior motives, to be twisted and manipulated in order to *justify* rather than to *improve* services.

If a program component must justify its existence within a larger helping or social system, the criteria for its existence will be identified, followed by the selection of measurable variables which, *a priori*, will yield results that fit the criteria. While this amounts to pulling the wool over the eyes or creating a smoke screen, it denigrates the rehabilitation paradigm. The weak link pulls down the credibility of all the rehabilitation components. Quality improvement must represent the super-ego within the rehabilitation paradigm. It must be the independent supreme court that lays the foundation for justification of everything done.

Quality improvement is hard to do methodologically and is often seen as a nuisance among service providers. Since the trend in health care generally, and neuropsychological rehabilitation specifically, is to be outcome-driven, QI becomes the key component on which the industry, or aspects of it, will survive with integrity. Marketplace survival pressure has the potential to obscure moral judgment and reduces the soundness of QI. Issues of precision in measuring and establishing quality controls on program or outcome measures may become blurred. Are measures valid in that they exhibit contextual relationship to the component of rehabilitation that is under the QI scope? Are measures reliable and standardized? Do the measures reflect customer satisfaction with services as well as scientific merit?

Within the larger scope of the rehabilitation paradigm, quality improvement is the validity marker for assessment, diagnosis, prognosis, and treatment. The quality of QI methodology depends on objectivity, total absence of conflicting motives (i.e., dual relationships of those conducting QI studies), and synchrony with evolving knowledge, developing theory, and social values.

Functional Independence Measures (FIM) in acute rehabilitation and Minimum Data Set (MDS) in skilled nursing facilities may provide a retrospective database from which QI may be addressed. But, these outcome measures depend on inter-rater reliability and criterion-related validity specified for the categories on these instruments that are rated. Banja and Johnston (1994) offer several suggestions or guidelines to improve 'outcome information systems.' Their emphasis on refined criteria for services, who needs services, treatment guidelines, and roles and obligations of case management depends on a data system consistent with an open, accessible, peer-reviewed, network-linked database discussed above (under 'Knowledge Resources').

Indeed, quality improvement is in its infancy and is the newest member of the rehabilitation paradigm. Given the Zeitgeist, however, it is becoming the most essential for the evolution of 'good' neuropsychological rehabilitation.

Theory

Theory integrates and binds knowledge, proposes reasonable explanations to fill in the knowledge gaps, and forecasts trends and developments in knowledge evolution. Theory (or, unfortunately, often just a loose idea) is the abstract form from which clinical service programs emerge. While theory is complex, its foundation is supposed to be explicated in assessment, treatment, and related applied functions in neuropsychological rehabilitation. Theory (i.e., what we think) begets practice (i.e., what we do). The more practice (assessment and treatment) is accomplished and refined using quality (i.e., outcome) improvement measures, the more theory (and, hence, practice) can be improved. What we think and how we do things based on that thinking must hang together, complement each other, and evolve together.

Because the knowledge base in neuropsychological rehabilitation has burgeoned exponentially in the past twenty years, as a combination of empirical as well as theoretical interests, there must be some effort at coherence. Otherwise, research findings become isolated bits and pieces that do not contribute to the emergence of theory, let alone clinical practice, that unifies and makes credible aspects of what we do. The profession becomes a quagmire of data without integration yielding coherent concepts. An information management system proposed earlier will allow a natural evolution of theory by finding the multiple ways bits of information become meaningfully linked together.

When practitioners differ regarding the legitimacy of, for instance, the diagnostic understanding and treatment needs of 'mild traumatic brain injury,' a knowledge and theory gap is obvious. The difference between theory and opinion becomes obscured. Controversy exists because of insufficient empirical knowledge, incomplete integration of diverse knowledge, or poorly constructed theory that binds together available knowledge. In part this dilemma may stem from the failure of knowledge management systems. At least, the situation reflects the need for careful inspection of knowledge deficiencies, not the need for more vigorous opinion, bias, and rhetoric.

Theory is the glue that binds together a diverse knowledge base, which then directs assessment, prediction, and treatment. Without linking the cause (of brain damage) with what is done about it (assessment and treatment), there is no credible way to fill in the gaps that arise in prediction. Without theory, there is no reasonable method for choosing quality improvement variables — variables that truly make a difference in the grand scheme of things.

Zeitgeist (Cultural Milieu)

Throughout history, the cultural milieu has determined the basis for values. Science is not immune, although it supposedly is not biased by the Zeitgeist. The ethical responsibility of neuropsychologists is to minimize a biasing Zeitgeist and maximize scientific objectivity while maintaining respect for the worth and dignity of each individual. While even the court system — the highest law of the land — is vulnerable to the vicissitudes of social winds, there is still the lofty goal of science. To maintain a 'big picture' perspective on the work of neuropsychological rehabilitation, the Zeitgeist must be considered secondary to science and ethics. The psychologist who places the economic needs of his or her employer before objective knowledge and ethical tenets in planning and implementing a treatment program is violating the standard of behavior in situations of multiple relationships and third-party influence. The neuropsychologist's first and foremost obligation is to his or her patient in the name of objective assessment, accurate diagnosis and prognosis, and effective treatment — and advocate only as scientific knowledge and reasoned theory substantiate it, not as fractional social whims attempt to drive it.

In summary, neuropsychological rehabilitation is the multifaceted process of (1) understanding the biopsychosocial status of an individual (premorbid, comorbid, and postmorbid) who has sustained a brain injury; (2) understanding the appropriate cognitive, behavioral, psychodynamic, physiological, and neurological interventions that may be variously and coincidentally employed in addressing the biopsychosocial status; (3) knowing the experimental and scientific research data that demonstrate favorable and unfavorable outcome links between comprehensive diagnostic characteristics and treatment interventions, and how the mix of intervention strategies, progressive diagnostic updates, prognoses, and serially established outcome goals coalesce into an efficient continuity of multiple-resource utilization; and (4) refining each clinical case with known theory and clinical practice and knowing how each individual case outcome refines the common knowledge for the sake of the next individual with brain injury (in terms of assessment refinement, diagnostic understanding, prognostic accuracy, treatment techniques, and outcome measures and determinations). It is the responsibility of the neuropsychologist to submit for public record data on outcomes in order to build such a knowledge base.

If the above sentence is overwhelming, it is a snap to comprehend compared with the reality of a patient's life whose catastrophic disentanglement the neuropsychologist is responsible for helping reassemble to a more satisfactory state (however vague that may be). Utmost in the mind of the neuropsychologist must be the (possibly contradictory) tentative marriage of unbiased scientific objectivity (redundancy intended) and compassionate empathy (ditto). While financial, self-serving, irrational thought (associated with both neural and sociocultural catastrophic disentanglement of brain injury) creates biases from many directions, someone — the neuropsychologist, at least — must maintain and constantly renegotiate the 'big picture.' Such an integrative viewpoint for the neuropsychologist is necessary to catch ethical and moral snags at any point in the process, dynamics that are pulled in and from many directions by isolated (i.e., non-integrated) forces unable to impose decisions and influence without bias. Brain injury has been characterized as the 'silent epidemic.' This is because the often subtle impact on cognitive, emotional, and personality functioning is usually not obvious to the untrained observer. Any functional failures of the injured person are attributed to volitionally-driven or psychodynamic shortcomings, even though these failures may have been heretofore uncharacteristic of the individual and may, postmortem, lead to devastating consequences such as job loss, divorce, social alienation, or criminal behaviors. Whereas physical or (maybe) speech impairments are recognizable (but, even so, marginally tolerated) as neurological impairments, the attitude amongst the uninitiated (family, friends, employers, teachers, and many professionals who should know better) is one of '...if only the person would try harder....' Even neuropsychological rehabilitation professionals sometimes resort to this thinking when the shortcomings of matching diagnosis, treatment, and outcome become too frustrating.

The roles and positions among patient, specific provider (of *a* rehabilitation service, such as occupational therapist), payer (for specific services and to specific providers, such as insurance company), family, employer, educator, and associated 'gate keepers' (such as social worker, case manager, social security claims determiner) yield divergent and sometimes quite conflicting perspectives of the situation and, by consequence, produce fragmentation in and resistance to a comprehensive and complementary package of help and intervention. Values, beliefs, expectations, and foundations for decision-making and/or process influence differ coincidentally with perspective, background influences, training, experience, and personal biases. Even the 'big picture' (and, presumably, minimal bias) held by someone (the neuropsychologist, perhaps) can conflict dramatically with the personal experience of the patient him- or herself. Thus, providing just and socially concordant neuropsychological rehabilitation can be an overwhelming challenge. Irrespective of how 'good' an outcome may be, there is left the dangling aspect of permanent (i.e., irrecoverable) change due to brain injury.

Just as the use of silicon implants or diet pills, offered to meet consumer demands, eventually led to cases of harm, offerings of the rehabilitation industry are in as precarious a position. The vagueness of outcome expectations and measures, the very large factor of unknown variance couched especially in 'spontaneous recovery,' and the also large factor of irrecoverable deficits despite treatment provide a smoke-screen immunity for the rehabilitation industry. Outcome vision and assessment must be careful, unbiased, and targeted toward improving (not *a priori* justifying) treatment. (Is outcome couched in quality management or quality *improvement*?)

Outcome assessment is excruciatingly difficult yet essential as the glue that binds techniques and services, payers, providers, and recipients. Correlational studies are, by nature, weak in allowing extrapolation of causative associations. Experimental studies, requiring control and experimental groups, are few. Case studies fail to identify the common independent (across individual) variables that affect dependent variables. And, as suggested earlier, outcome assessment is often maintenance oriented, identifying measures that are already known affected by 'independent' variables, instead of improvement oriented, selecting variable measures that may not be inherently associated with treatment but which bear on an overall desired outcome.

The moral vision that must drive neuropsychological rehabilitation must remain above the constraining factors prevailing in medical care, financial accessibility of rehabilitation, and social expectations. Additionally, there is moral obligation within neuropsychological rehabilitation to influence the removal of unfair, disenfranchising, and exclusionary practices of providers and payers, which exist even in the face of emerging enlightening scientific foundation, and, at least, humanistic duty.

Recommendations

Based on the foregoing, some recommendations for neuropsychological rehabilitation are offered which should help preserve and strengthen the ethical, scientific, and objective foundation of the discipline.

Owing to the complexity and the complexity-reducing simplification (and inherent biases and ethical compromises) that occur within individual multidimensional and multidisciplinary components of rehabilitation, someone, notably the neuropsychologist, ought to be able to step back and formulate a narrative picture that reveals "...competing values and perspectives of those involved in the patient's life. ...Narratives and ethics go hand in hand in promoting patient-centered care...." (p. 506) (True & Phipps, 1999). Instead of falling victim to fragmentation, the neuropsychologist must make concerted effort to advocate for an honest, objective, scientifically based, humanistic, holistic understanding of the person affected by brain injury.

Neuropsychological rehabilitation (i.e., comprehensive cognitive and psychological rehabilitation of brain injury) must include psychological services in order to enhance functional outcomes (Heinemann et al., 1995). Indeed, it is the underlying emotional and personality resources that often determine the success or failure of any intensive rehabilitation effort. Unfortunately, it is excluded from many insurance plans as well as 'comprehensive' rehabilitation programs because of high cost and, ostensibly, unproven benefit.

Payers often (usually) omit various forms of psychological services coverage in rehabilitation. Yet, psychology typically aims to preserve the 'big picture' in its involvement, understanding the hidden depths of emotional, personality, family, social, and other dynamic factors that play a crucial role in the appropriateness and success of treatment. Any rehabilitation effort must assess the need for and relative importance of psychological services in rehabilitation and insist on that component as crucial to a comprehensive program's success.

Assessment, the foundation for diagnosis, prognosis, and treatment planning, must not be 'black box' based. Each and every datum in an assessment must have explainable ties to available neurofunctional criteria, mechanical forces and physiological factors producing bran injury, impact of psychological (as opposed to strictly physiological) determinants of test performance, native cognitive style, brain plasticity, and practical (i.e., ecological) effect of treatment schemes. This is a big bill to fill but one that the profession must aim toward. There are inherent ethical problems in 'black box' (i.e., brain–behavior for brain–behavior sake) thinking. Assessment techniques must be ecologically valid and tied to *specific* diagnostic and functional performance.

The issue of 'full' versus 'screening' approaches to neuropsychological assessment must be resolved. The barrier, presently, is the incomplete understanding of what any given neuropsychological test actually does and how importantly any given test contributes simultaneously to neurological, neurofunctional, and ecological diagnosis.

Research geared toward understanding the relationships among treatment effects; spontaneous recovery; and effect of pace of recovery on personal, family, and vocational outcome will aid in producing cost–beneficial programs. This goal may not be possible without significant expansion of an easily accessible national brain injury database.

Considering the best possible resources to benefit recovery, treatment planning must include cultural, financial, and personal factors in defining long-range goals. Such variables as the age of the patient, stress impact on family, premorbid characteristics, community resources, and (changing and emerging) patient and family expectations help to define the 'big picture' and provide the respect for the rights, dignity, worth, and welfare of rehabilitation recipients. Again, a comprehensive picture, in the form of a narrative, appropriately shared amongst the rehabilitation players, would enhance the contributions of the neuropsychologist.

Quality improvement measures and studies must be methodologically driven (not regulatory, outcome-desired, or instrument driven) in order to tie in with accumulating knowledge and developing theory. Quality improvement typically stands alone to the disdain of the profession as evil baggage of institutional regulation. It need not be so if its motivation is honest and ethical, and methodology is scientific.

References

American Psychological Association (1992). Ethical principles of psychologists and code of conduct. *American Psychologist, 47,* 1597-1611.

Baker, J. (1988). Explaining coma arousal therapy. *The Australian Nurses Journal, 17(11).*

Banja, J. (1999). Patient advocacy at risk: Ethical, legal and political dimensions of adverse reimbursement practices in brain injury rehabilitation in the US. *Brain Injury, 13,* 745-758.

Banja, J., & Johnston, M. V. (1994). Outcomes evaluation in TBI rehabilitation. Part III: Ethical perspectives and social policy. *Archives of Physical Medicine and Rehabilitation, 75*(12 Spec No), SC19-26; discussion SC 27- 18.

Ben-Yishay, Y. (1978). *Working approaches to remediation of cognitive deficits in brain damaged persons.* New York: New York University Medical Center.

Berube, J. E. (2000). The auto choice reform act. *Journal of Head Trauma Rehabilitation, 15,* 1063-1067.

Bush, S., & Sandberg, M. (2001). Utilizing 'assent' to determine 'consent': Proposed ethical revisions and their implications for TBI rehabilitation. *Archives of Clinical Neuropsychology, 16,* 807 [abstract].

Diller, L. L. (1976). A model for cognitive retraining in rehabilitation. *Clinical Psychologist, 29,* 13-15.

Hannay, H. J., Bieliauskas, L.A., Crosson, B.A., Hammeke, T.A., Hamsher, K. deS., & Koffler, S.P. (1998). Proceedings: The Houston conference on specialty education and training in clinical neuropsychology. *Archives of Clinical Neuropsychology, 13,* 157-249.

Hanson, S. Guenther, R, Kerkhoff, & T. Liss, M. (2000). Ethics: Historical foundations, basic principles and contemporary issues. In R. Frank and T. Elliott (Eds.), *Handbook of rehabilitation psychology* (pp. 629–643). Washington, DC: American Psychological Association.

Heinemann, A., Hamilton, B., Linacre, J. M., & Wright, B. (1995). Functional status and therapeutic intensity during inpatient rehabilitation. *American Journal of Physical Medicine and Rehabilitation, 74,* 315-326.

High, W. M., Boake, C., & Lehmkuhl, L. D. (1995). Critical analysis of studies measuring the effectiveness of rehabilitation following traumatic brain injury. *Head Trauma Rehabilitation, 10,* 14-26.

Kaufman, H. H., Levy, M. L., Stone, J. L., Masri, L. S., Lichtor, T., Lavine, S. D., Fitzgerald, L. F., & Apuzzo, M. L. (1995). Patients with Glasgow Coma Scale scores 3, 4, 5 after gunshot wounds to the brain. *Neurosurgical Clinics in North America, 6,* 701-714.

Lynch, W. J. (2000). Brief neuropsychological batteries: A review and preview. *Journal of Head Trauma Rehabilitation, 15,* 1172-1178.

Malec, J. F. (1993). Ethics in brain injury rehabilitation: Existential choices among western cultural beliefs. *Brain Injury, 7,* 383-400.

Malec, J. F. (1996). Ethical conflict resolution based on an ethics of relationships for brain injury rehabilitation. *Brain Injury, 10,* 781-795.

Osborn, C. L. (1998). *Over my head.* Kansas City: Andrews McMeel Publishing.

Prigatano, G. P. (1986). *Neuropsychological rehabilitation after brain injury*. Baltimore: Johns Hopkins University Press.

Prigatano, G. P. (1992). Neuropsychological rehabilitation and the problem of altered self-awareness. In V. von Steinbuchel, D.Y. von Ctamon, & E. Poppel, (Eds.), *Neuropsychological rehabilitation* (pp. 55-65). New York: Springer-Verlag.

Prigatano, G. P. (1997). Learning from our successes and failures: Reflections and comments on 'Cognitive Rehabilitation: How it is and how it might be'. *Journal of the International Neuropsychological Society, 3*, 497-499.

Prigatano, G. P., & Schacter, D.L. (Eds.) (1991). *Awareness of deficit after brain injury*. New York: Oxford University Press.

Rosenthal, M. (1996). 1995 Sheldon Berrol, MD Senior Lectureship: The ethics and efficacy of traumatic brain injury rehabilitation — Myths, measurements, and meaning. *Head Trauma Rehabilitation, 11*, 88-95.

Sbordone, R. J., & Long, C. (Eds.) (1996). *Ecological validity of neuropsychological testing*. Delray Beach, FL: St. Lucie Press.

Sweet, J. J., Westergaard, C.K., & Moberg, P.J. (1995). Managed care experiences of clinical neuropsychologists. *The Clinical Neuropsychologist, 9*, 214-218.

True, G., & Phipps, E.J. (1999). Narratives in rehabilitation. *Journal of Head Trauma Rehabilitation, 14*, 505-507.

Walton (1998). Decade of the brain: Neurological advances. *Journal of Neurological Science, 158*, 5-14.

Wilson, B. A. (1997). Cognitive rehabilitation: How it is and how it might be. *Journal of the International Neuropsychological Society, 3*, 487-496.

Chapter 9

a lot difficulties on research [handwritten annotation]

ETHICAL ISSUES IN NEUROPSYCHOLOGY IN PSYCHIATRIC SETTINGS

Ruben C. Gur, Paul J. Moberg, and Paul Root Wolpe

Introduction

Clinical neuropsychologists have been steadily abandoning the differentiation between 'organicity' and 'functional' disorders (Gur & Gur, 2000). Indeed, a majority of neuropsychologists and other health care practitioners currently conceptualize 'mental illnesses' as diseases of the *brain*, which are biologically based. That is, mental disease and brain disease are interchangeable terms (Szasz, 1996). The literature now strongly supports the assertion of fundamental biological underpinnings for neuropsychiatric disorders. While this conception is well recognized by researchers, in day-to-day clinical practice it often is forgotten. It is still quite common for neuropsychological reports to record statements such as: "the patient is suffering from a *functional* psychiatric disorder as opposed to an *organic* disorder," suggesting that psychiatric disturbances cannot be attributed to disruption in brain structure or function. It is now well known that psychosis and depression represent dysfunction in brain regions and neurotransmitter systems (Grant & Adams, 1986).

There have been enormous gains in our understanding of the brain dysfunctions contributing to neuropsychiatric disorders. Yet, there is still often a tendency among clinicians and lay people to view mental illness as fundamentally different than other brain disorders such as stroke, epilepsy or tumors, and to see the mentally ill patient as less capable than similarly impaired patients with such disorders. President Clinton signed the Mental Health Parity Act of 1996 (PL 104-204) on September 26, 1997, emphasizing that psychiatric disorders are indeed brain-based and deserving of the same status as other medical illnesses. The legislation is intended to ensure that coverage for mental health services is in parity with coverage provided for other serious physical disorders. Nonetheless, there are still disparities in how mental illness is treated, conceptualized, institutionalized, and reimbursed.

Mental disorders commonly affect feelings of personal well-being and of how one is viewed by others, so patients not only have to cope with the symptoms of their disease but also with the stigma associated with it (Lucassen, 1998). The major difference between the patient with a stroke and the patient with major depression may be the *perception* of their competence. While most patients suffering from stroke, Parkinson's disease or other neurologic disorders are presumed to be competent until proven otherwise, patients with psychiatric illness are often presumed to be incompetent. Clinicians and the lay public still see the patient with mental illness as more frail and vulnerable than a patient with other brain disorders.

While this difference in perception may not seem substantial, it can have significant impact on how these patients are treated by clinicians. A patient suffering from a melanoma is assumed to retain the capacity to make decisions concerning their treatment and care, yet many patients with mental illness are assumed *not* to have this capacity. For example, in general, a patient with psychiatric illness who is demonstrating disordered behavior is more likely to be hospitalized or treated against their wishes compared to a brain tumor patient demonstrating the same type of behavioral disruption. While there are special considerations to be made when dealing with patients with neuropsychiatric disorder, they are not incompetent *by default*. To be sure, patients with psychiatric illness may require additional safeguards and approaches that may not be appropriate for patients suffering from other types of neurologic or medical illness. However, they *do not* typically have unremitting and non-remediable decision-making deficits. For example, patients with schizophrenia often suffer from perceptual distortions, thought disorder, reduced motivation, and poor emotional responsivity. These clinical symptoms are commonly accompanied by deficits in neuropsychological function. In concert, these deficits do place the person at higher risk for impairment in decision-making ability. Yet these patients are often capable of making reasoned and informed decisions.

Patients with schizophrenia *as a group* do tend to have impaired ability to make decisions about their treatment and care compared to healthy people or patients suffering from other psychiatric or medical illness (Grisso & Appelbaum, 1995; Grisso et al., 1997). In most clinical situations, however, these patients are not incompetent and can handle their day-to-day affairs, such as managing their finances and self-care activities. Many individual patients, even when acutely ill, perform at the level of the general population on tasks of decision-making ability (Carpenter et al., 2000).

The ethical principles outlined by the American Psychological Association (1992a, 1992b) should be applied to patients suffering from psychiatric illness, as they are to any other patient population, while keeping in mind the unique characteristics of this population. There are a multitude of issues which can confront the neuropsychologist when assessing patients in a psychiatric setting, including refusal of patients to participate in testing, disagreements between the neuropsychologist and psychiatrist over treatment issues or results of testing, etc. Many of these issues are, however, endemic to most settings. In this chapter we will focus on two specific aspects of the Ethical Standards most relevant to patients suffering from psychiatric illness: informed consent (research and clinical) and competence.

Informed Consent

Studies conducted over the last three decades have generally found that patients with mental illness are capable of consent, but have greater difficulties than medically ill or healthy participants (Appelbaum et al., 1982; Lidz et al., 1984; Meisel & Roth, 1981; Roth et al., 1987; Stanley et al., 1987; Sugarman, 1999). Patients with mental illness are frequently thought to fall in the 'vulnerable' classification when it comes to informed consent, primarily due to the significant emotional and behavioral disruption experienced by these patients. However, they have never been officially classified as a vulnerable population for regulatory purposes.

Informed consent deals with the ability of an individual to comprehend information about a research project or treatment, process and manipulate that information, apply the information to their current situation or status, and use this information to make a reasoned and rational decision. As noted in Standard 6.11 of the APA Ethics Code (APA 1992a, 1992b):

(a) Psychologists use language that is reasonably understandable to research participants in obtaining their appropriate informed consent (except as provided in Standard 6.12, *Dispensing With Informed Consent*). Such informed consent is appropriately documented.

(b) Using language that is reasonably understandable to participants, psychologists inform participants of the nature of the research; they inform participants that they are free to participate or to decline to participate or to withdraw from the research; they explain the foreseeable consequences of declining or withdrawing; they inform participants of significant factors that may be expected to influence their willingness to participate (such as risks, discomfort, adverse effects, or limitations on confidentiality, except as provided in Standard 6.15, *Deception in Research*); and they explain other aspects about which the prospective participants inquire.

Overall, this standard highlights five standards of information that should guide informed consent discussions with research participants. Many of these same principles hold to consent practices in clinical situations as well (see Standard 4.02). The real difference between consent in research and clinical situations is in the implied incentives. For example, you cannot coerce some-one into research, even if it would benefit them or if they are a threat to themselves or others. Also, while most clinicians defer to a lower threshold for competence for research (i.e., if the subject does not seem able to consent, the researcher moves on to another subject), competence and consent for treatment is different when the proposed intervention is conceptualized as being to someone's direct benefit. The five standards of information that should guide informed consent discussions with research participants are:

1. *The nature of the research.* A general statement should be offered about the purpose and goals of the research, including a description of the spe-cific activities required of the subject, amount of time required, any mon-etary or other compensation for their participation, possible applications or use of the research results, possible adverse implications for popula-tions that might be affected by the research results, and any other informa-tion that the investigator deems necessary and important for a potential participant to know.

2. *The participants' freedom to decline or withdraw.* The subject must under-stand and be instructed that they may choose to participate in the study or not, and may withdraw from the research at any time, with no prejudice or penalty. The investigator must not prod, coerce, threaten or intimi-date potential research participants when discussing the optional nature of their involvement in research. This is especially important when the investigator is (or is perceived by the participant to be) in a position of authority over the participant.

3. *The foreseeable consequences of declining or withdrawing.* The investiga-tor is mandated to explain any foreseeable consequences to the partici-pant who has decided not to become involved in the research or who has decided to withdraw from a protocol once started.

4. *Factors that may influence willingness to participate.* Known or suspected factors that may impact on a participant's willingness to participate in research should be clearly communicated, including a full disclosure of possible risks, unpleasant experiences, or use of chemical substances intro-duced into the body. Other relevant factors may include exposure to expe-riences or activities that may conflict with a person's values or are outside the realm of the normal range of experience causing distress to the par-ticipant, fear or anxiety that may be connected to the research activity, sensory deprivation, unpleasant sensory stimulus, unpleasant psychosocial stimulus, autonomic arousal, sexual arousal, physical exertion, or any other factor or experience which may affect an individual's willingness to participate. Psychiatric patients may find certain tasks or procedures that are innocuous to other participants to be quite significant. For exam-ple, involving a patient with thought disorder and hallucinations in a protocol requiring sensory deprivation would likely exacerbate psychotic symptoms. These types of risks should be explicitly stated. As psychiatric

conditions may be more stigmatizing than other types of medical conditions, risks to anonymity should also be discussed. Lastly, clear and unambiguous language should be used to ensure adequate comprehension and understanding of all explanations and descriptions of the research. This is especially crucial in patients with psychiatric illness as both affective and cognitive impairments stemming from their illness may interfere with their clear understanding of research procedures.

5. *Answers to inquiries.* Researchers should be available to answer questions or address concerns raised by prospective research participants. No distortion, misrepresentation, omission of important factual information nor minimizing or 'watering down' of risks should be made. Subjects should be given information as to who the responsible party is and how to contact them should additional questions or concerns arise, both during and after the research. Subjects should also have access to emergency mental health care at all times, should their participation in the research somehow initiate or exacerbate symptoms.

The necessary elements of informed consent have been elaborated by Roberts & Roberts (1999), who detail three overarching components of the informed consent process (see Figure 1).

1. *Information* deals with the clear and accurate communication of: (a) the purpose of the research, (b) the possible risks or benefits of the protocol, (c) any alternatives to participation (including choosing not to participate), (d) who the responsible or principal investigator is for the experiment, (e) the procedures and arrangements for any possible serious side effects or complications that may be caused by the experiment, (f) experimental procedures to be utilized and any salient design features, such as drug wash-out, placebo, etc., (g) any incentives to be given, and (h) any legal considerations, such as liability for adverse events.

2. *Decisional Capacity* of the participant, which includes: (a) the ability to express a preference or communicate a choice clearly, (b) the ability to comprehend information, (c) the ability to think through, manipulate and utilize this information in a rational and deliberate way, and (d) the ability to appreciate or attach meaning to this decision and how it may impact the person on a subjective level.

3. *Autonomy*, or the ability of the person to choose freely without any pressure or coercion, is the third component. As noted in Figure 1, a 'vulnerable' participant lacking any of the above components may be more susceptible to exploitation in the research (or clinical) situation. Vulnerability may arise from intrinsic factors, such as cognitive impairment due to psychiatric illness, or from extrinsic factors, such as the limits or restrictions imposed by psychiatric hospitalization. Lastly, interpersonal or relational factors resulting from the researchers' relationship with the subject may increase subject vulnerability (e.g., a prisoner being asked to participate

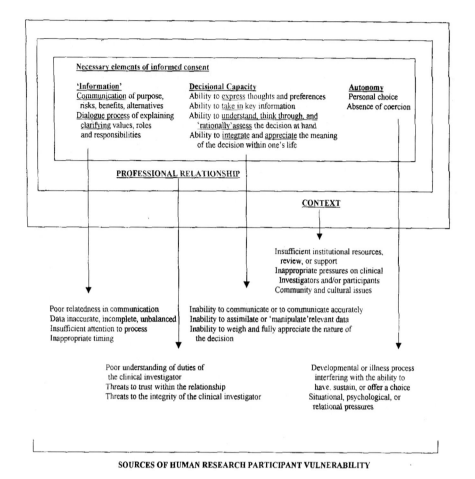

Figure 1. A schematic of the informed consent process and sources of human research
         participation (Roberts & Roberts, 1999).

in research by the warden). As can be seen in this discussion, informed
consent is a very dynamic and complex process, tapping a number of cognitive, emotional and interpersonal variables. In patients with psychiatric
illness, all three of these variables may be compromised, complicating
attempts to communicate adequate informed consent. However, the difficulty is not qualitatively different from the process in patients suffering
from other medical illnesses.

In recent years, there has been controversy over the circumstances required
for the ethical involvement of patients suffering from serious mental illness
in clinical research. Those opposed to such involvement have argued that the
current safeguards, such as institutional review boards and informed consent,

are not sufficient to protect people suffering from major mental illness (Hilts, 1998; Shamoo, 1997). Proponents, in contrast, speak of the intense need to improve our understanding of mental illnesses, the immediate and future benefits of research involvement, and the injustice and disrespect associated with scientific neglect of vulnerable populations (Dresser, 1996; Roberts, 1998; Shore, 1996). In general, studies of informed consent that have compared patients with psychiatric disorder (i.e., schizophrenia, depression) to patients suffering from medical illness (i.e., cardiac disease) have shown that patients with psychiatric illness do have greater difficulty with consent decisions both in clinical care and research (Appelbaum & Grisso, 1995; Roberts, 1998; Roberts & Roberts, 1999). However, the mechanism responsible for this greater degree of impairment in decision-making capacity is unclear. Specifically, significant neuropsychological deficits could underlie these impairments or they could be the results of clinical symptoms that accompany these disorders.

More recent research has championed the division of informed consent into an *information-based* component and a *subjective* component. Both components are thought to be important in assessing the capacity to give informed consent. The information-based approach attempts to provide practical responses to the applied ethical questions facing the neuropsychologist in day-to-day practice. That is, it attempts to gain information about the patient's capacity through the use of objective testing measures. The subjective component addresses other aspects of the consent process such as hope, or desire to please the clinician or to escape suffering. These aspects are harder to quantify. Given the emphasis on objective measures and the perceived relationship of the information-based approach with neuropsychological practice, the information-based component will be discussed first, followed by the more subjective aspects of informed consent.

Information-Based or Neuropsychological Components of Informed Consent

In one of the earliest studies by Stanley et al. (1988), the reasoning abilities of 45 elderly patients suffering from major depression, 38 patients with dementia, and 20 healthy elderly controls were studied. Results showed that the performance of both patient groups fell below that of healthy controls, with the cognitively impaired dementia patients showing the most pronounced deficits on measures of 'functional competency,' followed by patients with major depression. In a more recent study with younger patients, Schacter et al. (1994) administered objective clinical assessment scales including the Brief Psychiatric Rating scale (BPRS; Overall & Gorham, 1961) to 38 patients with schizophrenia and found that conceptual disorganization and psychotic thought content were related to poorer performance on information-based tasks of treatment consent. These data were subsequently confirmed by the landmark MacArthur Treatment Competence Study (Appelbaum & Grisso, 1995). In this comprehensive, multicenter protocol, 498 subjects comprising three patient groups were assessed with regard to clinical decision making skills: patients with schizophrenia or major depression, patients with ischemic heart disease, and healthy community-dwelling volunteers. From this set of studies it was shown that, in the acute phase, patients with schizophrenia and depression had greater decision-making problems on some structured cognitive measures than people with cardiac disease and healthy volunteers. Within the psychiatric groups, patients with a diagnosis of schizophrenia performed more poorly than those suffering from depression. Notably, once the psychiatric patients were treated, their decision making skills were noted to greatly improve, more closely resembling the comparison groups.

Not all studies, however, have found deficient abilities to give informed consent. Two early studies by Kleinman et al. (1993) and Soskis (1978) found that patients with schizophrenia showed an excellent understanding of the procedures, risks, benefits, and side-effects of neuroleptic medication. Another study by Stanley et al. (1981) examined risk assessments and risk taking by 27 psychiatric inpatients and 38 inpatients with medical illness. Subjects were asked to evaluate protocols of varying designs and procedures. Results revealed that patients with mental illness were not any more likely to participate in risky hypothetical human experiments than were subjects with medical disorders. Interestingly, the severity of general psychopathology was not found to be significantly related to poorer risk assessment in the vignettes provided.

In one of the most recent studies, Carpenter and colleagues (2000) attempted to directly address the competency issue by formally assessing decision-making skills along with neuropsychological and clinical status in a sample of patients suffering from schizophrenia. In addition, they sought to assess the effectiveness of an educational informed consent process in remediating any deficits in decision-making skills. They sought to address three questions: (1) Do patients with mental illness have the necessary decisional capabilities to provide informed consent? (2) Does psychiatric symptom severity affect this capacity? (3) Is there any way to therapeutically treat these deficits? Participants included 30 patients with a diagnosis of schizophrenia and 24 healthy controls. Decisional capacity was assessed with the MacCAT-CR, a structured assessment tool that assesses four areas of decisional capacity related to generally applied legal standards for competence and consent to treatment and research (Appelbaum & Grisso, 1996). These four areas include: (1) Understanding relevant information, (2) appreciation of the implication of the information for one's own situation, (3) reasoning with the information in a decisional process, and (4) evidencing a choice. In addition to the MacCAT-CR, each participant also underwent a brief neuropsychological battery to assess overall level of cognitive ability. Tests included: (1) the Reading subtest from the Wide Range Achievement Test (Wilkinson, 1993), (2) the Repeatable Battery for the Assessment of Neuropsychological Status (RBANS: Randolph, 1998), (3) the Letter-Number Sequencing subtest from the Wechsler Adult Intelligence Scale-III (Wechsler, 1997), (4) a modified version of the Gray Oral

Reading Test (Weiderholt & Bryant, 1992). Each patient was also administered the BPRS in order to assess degree of general psychopathology. The
investigators undertook a second experiment examining the use of remediation
techniques for decisional impairments. An educational remediation intervention was undertaken in patients with significant impairment of decision-making ability as assessed by the MacCAT-CR (scores below 20), and subsequently
confirmed by poorer performance on the Evaluation of Signed Consent (ESC;
DeRenzo et al., 1998). Each participant came in for two additional 30-minute
sessions in which the study information was reviewed, information was provided again, questions were asked, and prompts were used to help the participant understand and master the material. Other instructional techniques, such
as using an interactive computer program for reviewing basic study components or using 'flip-charts' for reviewing relevant study information, were also
utilized.

Results revealed that, with the exception of the Choice variable, patients
with schizophrenia scored significantly below controls on measures of Understanding, Reasoning, and Appreciation from the MacCAT-CR (see Figure

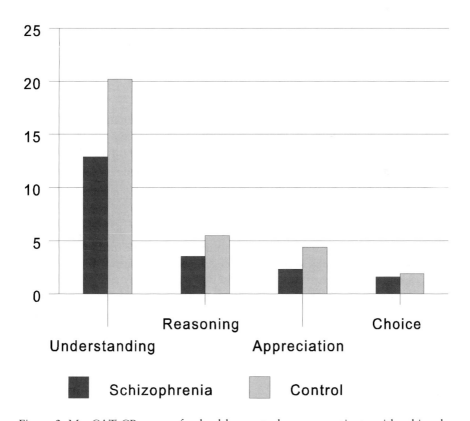

Figure 2. MacCAT-CR scores for healthy controls versus patients with schizophre-
    nia.

2). These data underline a general impairment in decision-making ability in patients with schizophrenia as a group.

Correlations of the four MacCAT-CR variables with BPRS scores revealed moderate negative correlations across all scales, with poor performance on the Understanding and Reasoning scales being associated with higher levels of psychopathology on the BPRS. Consistent with most studies of neuropsychological functioning in patients with schizophrenia, patients demonstrated significantly lower scores on the neurocognitive measures relative to healthy controls. Specifically, the following relationships were observed between RBANS scores and MacCAT-CR indices: (1) Understanding scores in the patient group were best predicted by the RBANS total score and by the Gray Oral Reading Test; (2) reasoning performance was best predicted by the RBANS total score and the RBANS immediate memory index; and (3) appreciation performance was best predicted by Letter–Number Sequencing from the WAIS-III and by the Visuospatial scale from the RBANS. As can be seen from the results of this study, while decisional capacity was moderately correlated with psychotic symptoms, measures of neuropsychological function were generally better predictors of decisional making capacity as assessed by the MacCAT-CR. These data mirror clinical observations that the degree of psychotic symptoms, except at the extreme, do not robustly predict patients' functionality in daily life (Appelbaum, 1998). That is, while clinical symptoms may impact these decisional processes, this effect is not of the magnitude of those seen on measures of neuropsychological functioning. Notably, the investigators also assessed the effects of an educational intervention on deficits in decisional making capacity in a subgroup of 20 patients and found significant improvements in Understanding ($p = .001$), Reasoning ($p = .04$) and Appreciation ($p = .001$). Additionally, the results of this study suggest that when offered additional opportunities to learn the necessary data, most schizophrenia patients who scored below the cutoff on the MacCAT-CR were able to bring their scores at least into the range of the control group.

The crux of this study is that many psychiatric patients may not understand research or treatment options using a single-session approach. Rather, a more interactive approach that is conducted over multiple sessions may provide better comprehension and appreciation of the information presented. Indeed, several authors have argued for empirically based strategies to ensure understanding by the participant. As outlined by Roberts et al. (2000), such procedures may include: (1) Better disclosure, including written materials, teaching aids (e.g., videotapes, diagrams), and translators; (2) fostering a consent dialogue over time, especially in the case of higher risk decisions; (3) identifying and responding to the psychological issues that may adversely affect decision making; (4) involving family members and trusted significant-others in the consent process; (5) use of self-report instruments such as The Values History (Gibson, 1990) to clarify the factors which may be affecting health care decisions; (6) use of pharmacologic and other treatments; and (7) providing other situational supports.

Carpenter and colleagues' (2000) comprehensive study highlights the fact that in patients with psychosis, severity of *clinical* symptoms generally did not dictate the decisional abilities of the patients with schizophrenia (at least as assessed with the MacCAT-CR). These data argue that, to a point, even patients with active psychosis (e.g., hallucinations, delusions) are capable of deciding whether to participate in treatment or research. These same investigators, however, also found that *cognitive* deficits were strongly related to poor performance on the MacCat-CR. While this may not be entirely surprising, as the MacCat-CR was designed to assess information- and cognitive-based aspects of decision-making ability, the substantial negative impact of cognitive deficits on the decision-making process poses a special problem for some neuropsychiatric patient groups.

For example, very significant neuropsychological deficits are seen in patients with schizophrenia, even at the first onset of psychosis (Saykin et al., 1991; Saykin et al., 1994) (see Figure 3).

Despite significant reductions in *clinical* symptoms following treatment with antipsychotic medications, patients with schizophrenia are commonly left with significant residual cognitive deficits (Censits et al., 1997). This impairment does not tend to be progressive, but rather remains fairly static and persistent over the course of illness (Goldberg et al., 1993; Gur et al.,

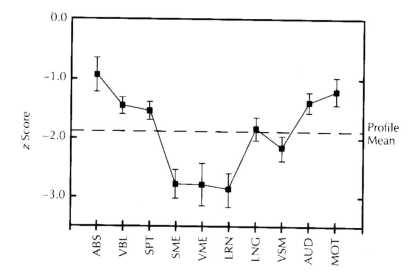

Figure 3. Neuropsychological profile (±SEM) for patients with schizophrenia (*n*=36) relative to controls (*n*=36) whose performance is set at zero (±1 SD) Functions are abstraction (ABS), verbal cognitive (VBL), spatial organization (SPT), semantic memory (SME), visual memory (VME), verbal learning (LRN), language (LNG), visual-motor processing and attention (VSM), auditory processing and attention (AUD), and motor speed and sequencing (MOT) (Saykin et al., 1991).

1997). As for the impact of clinical symptoms on neuropsychological abilities, static measures comparing neuropsychological performance and clinical scales have tended to report that negative symptoms (i.e., flat affect, anhedonia) explain more of the variance in neuropsychological performance, with the relationship between positive symptoms (i.e., hallucinations, thought disorder) and cognitive change being less clear (Bilder et al., 1985; Gur et al., 1997). While some variation exists, cross-sectional studies have generally concluded that the profile of neuropsychological deficits remains stable over time (see Goldberg et al., 1993 for review). For example, the stability of neuropsychological performance in patients with schizophrenia and its relationship to clinical change was compared in 60 patients with schizophrenia (30 first-episode, 30 previously treated) and 38 healthy controls, utilizing a comprehensive neuropsychological battery and clinical scales at intake and at a 19-month follow-up (Censits et al., 1997). Results showed that patients with schizophrenia had significant impairment in neuropsychological functioning at intake relative to healthy controls, and that this impairment did not change appreciably over the follow-up period (see Figure 4).

The failure to show neurocognitive improvement is notable given the fact that patients had a statistically significant improvement in clinical symptoms (i.e., positive and negative symptoms) with treatment. These studies generally support a significant neuropsychological deficit in patients with schizophrenia that is largely unaffected by treatment with neuroleptics or other interventions. That is, while neuroleptic treatment effects significant changes in clinical symptoms, there are still residual cognitive deficits that may impinge on the patient's ability to make informed decisions about research or treat-

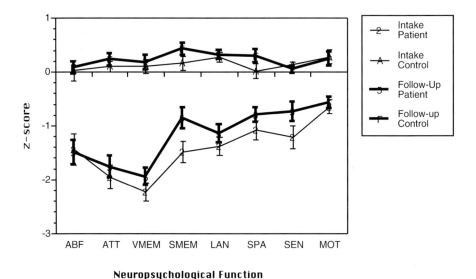

Figure 4. Censits follow-up.

ment. Given the data by Carpenter and colleagues (2000) and others showing links between cognitive performance and ability measures of decision-making capacity (Marson et al., 1995; Workman et al., 2000), these data provide strong arguments for the prominent role of neuropsychological testing in the assessment of decision-making capacity and ability to consent to research or treatment. Unfortunately, there is still no solid understanding of how different neurocognitive functions relate to these processes, and the ecological validity of neuropsychological testing is still in its infancy. Despite this fact, neuropsychologists can make a significant contribution in this area by defining the requisite neuropsychological abilities and tests that underlie decisional processes.

Subjective Components of Informed Consent
In addition to the neuropsychological, information-based, and cognitively propelled aspects of informed consent, it appears that subjective factors also play a significant role in this process. For example, personal attitudes, values, motivations and context seem to greatly affect research enrollment decisions in patients with mental disorders (as they do in patients with medical disorders and healthy controls) (Roberts, 1998). Despite the ongoing dialogues of various groups concerning ethics in psychiatric research, few studies have actually queried patients with mental illness on their perceptions and beliefs about research participation. In an early study by Benson et al. (1985), the consent disclosure sessions of 24 patients with schizophrenia, 24 patients with depression, and investigators involved in clinical mediation protocols were assessed. Results indicated that the participants in these protocols had limited knowledge of the protocol methods, and their understanding of its purpose was quite poor. Specifically, they did not have an understanding of the *meaning* of the study designs and did not seem to *appreciate* the features of the study, including the possible risks and benefits. Most subjects reported being unaware of the randomization and double-blind procedures, and only 4% fully realized that their participation in the study limited their access to other treatment strategies. Most surprisingly, 71% of the patients with depression and 42% of the patients with schizophrenia indicated that they had decided to participate in the protocol *prior* to receiving *any* information about the study. Subjective aspects of the decision making process are thus quite powerful, often overriding the informed consent process in treatment or research.

Similar to the Benson study, Grossman and Summers (1980) examined 20 outpatients with schizophrenia who underwent a careful consent disclosure session for a fictitious experimental medicine. In an assessment immediately following the session, three (15%) of the 20 subjects were judged to be 'fully informed,' nine (45%) were 'partially informed,' and eight (40%) were 'not informed.' Despite this fact, 60% of these individuals had consented to participate in the hypothetical experiment. Whether this uninformed willingness reflected subjective factors (hope of getting better, altruism) or external factors (desire to please the researcher, coercive pressure) was not clear from the data. In a direct assessment of coercive pressures, Lidz and colleagues (1984) conducted a four-year naturalistic observation study of consent interactions across three sites: (1) a diagnostic evaluation center; (2) a research ward; and (3) an outpatient clinic. The factors affecting patient decision-making and consent practices differed significantly across the three settings. For example, the research ward was judged to allow the least expression of autonomous choice, whereas the outpatient clinic afforded patients the greatest degree of autonomy.

In an elegant study of informed consent in patients with schizophrenia, Roberts et al. (2000) assessed the views of 63 patients with a diagnosis of schizophrenia and 73 psychiatry faculty and residents. Results revealed that the responses to 23 rated attitudes revealed remarkably similar rank orders and areas of agreement between patients and psychiatrists. Both groups strongly endorsed the importance of research in schizophrenia as well as autonomous decision making by all participants. Both groups indicated that participation in research was important for science as well as helping others. Where the two groups differed, however, was in the feeling of hope that went along with research involvement endorsed by patients with schizophrenia. In contrast, psychiatrists tended to underestimate this more 'optimistic' perspective. Both schizophrenia patients and clinicians valued autonomous decision making in research, but the patients were much more accepting than were the psychiatrists regarding influences of physician-investigators, personal physicians and family members on participation decisions. Both groups opposed participation in dangerous research, and they agreed that subjects who were unwilling to participate and/or undergoing involuntary treatment should also not participate in studies. In general, psychiatrists felt more strongly than patients that vulnerable populations should be included in research. The most compelling outcome of this study, however, was the fact that patients with schizophrenia offered highly discerning views concerning research participation. Notably, these opinions were quite consistent with those of the investigators. While there were some differences in their views, both groups underscored the importance of research participation. These data affirm the role of altruism, trust in science and clinical professionals, and the inspiration of hope as leading to research participation.

Overall, the aforementioned studies indicate that patients with mental illness generally resemble other traditionally defined vulnerable groups with regard to informational and cognitive problems with informed consent. Notably, a theme that seems to run across these studies is one of a relationship between acuity of illness and greater deficits in comprehending and acting upon information important for decision making in both clinical and research environments. That is, patients at the acute stages of illness with severe clinical symptomatology (e.g., psychosis, marked delusions, vegetative depression) appear to be those at higher risk for not providing valid consent. This statement mirrors the findings of studies examining consent in *medically ill* patients. For example, Schaeffer and colleagues (1996) assessed a sample of 127 participants in clinical experiments from a variety of disease types and severity (ranging from completely healthy to acutely and life-threateningly ill), within 24 hours of consenting to their respective protocols and 4–6 weeks later. Results showed that healthy participants retained the most information about risks and side effects at the initial assessment, whereas severely ill patients retained the least. These data indicate that the stage of illness, severity and type of illness all play important roles in the ability to provide informed consent. As for subjective factors in the consent process, both positive (e.g., optimism, hope, altruism) and negative (e.g., despair, susceptibility to coercion, incorrect expectations) influences seem to have considerable impact on the process.

Both cognitive and subjective factors, however, contribute significantly to this process, highlighting the complex and rich process that occurs when gaining consent from a subject. These factors are not yet clearly delineated, but it is evident that the neuropsychologist must balance the quantitative aspects of this process (i.e., objective neuropsychological and clinical assessment) with the less easily defined needs and hopes of the participant. As can be seen in this literature, the subjective component of the process is less studied and yet may provide insights into the decision-making processes of patients suffering from psychiatric illness. The task for the assessment of such subjective aspects lies in the hands of neuropsychological researchers to develop more objective methods to assess the "non-cognitive" aspects of consent.

The Right to Engage in, or Refuse, Treatment (Competence)
Competence is primarily a legal, rather than clinical, term and so bears a somewhat awkward relationship to clinical judgments about levels of psychological and cognitive functioning. Competence implies an all-or-nothing capability; a person is either competent or incompetent according to the law. However, in clinical settings, a person may have the capability to make certain kinds of decisions (such as whether to ask for PRN medication, for example) while not being competent to make other kinds of decisions (such as whether to have major surgery). Bioethicists, therefore, often speak of capacity, rather than competence. Capacity has a task-specific orientation that competence may lack. Another virtue of the concept of capacity, from a bioethical standpoint, is that it justifies granting decisional authority to some individuals who might not be considered competent under the law.

Patients deemed legally competent have the right to decide whether to accept or reject proposed medical care (Appelbaum & Grisso, 1988). When a patient is deemed incompetent, they are denied this right and others make decisions for them. As the concept of competence is a legal one, it can only be formally determined through legal proceedings. In the day-to-day practice of most neuropsychologists, however, we are frequently confronted with questions of ability to make rational and reasoned judgments about such matters.

While the definition of competence varies from state to state, most researchers have accepted the criteria elaborated by Appelbaum and Grisso (1988),
who identified four general capabilities that define competence:

1. *Communicating choices.* In this case, the patient must be able to communicate a choice that is stable and consistent over time. That is, the
   person must maintain and communicate a choice long enough for it to be
   implemented. The abilities may be affected by impairment in consciousness, thought disorder, impairment of short-term memory, or fluctuations
   in decision-making faculties. For example, in the case of a patient with
   severe depression, fluctuations in mood, memory abilities and cooperation
   may cause the person to communicate inconsistent choices about their
   care or other matters. It should be noted that this 'inconsistency' differs
   from that of the person changing their mind, and could be characterized
   by repeated and perhaps rapid alterations of choice.

2. *Understanding relevant information.* The ability to understand the facts
   underlying a treatment decision is central to most legal definitions of competence. That is, if patients cannot understand what they have been told
   about treatment, they are not in a position to rationally accept or reject
   it. There are several neuropsychological functions relevant to this category. Impairment in general intellectual skills, attention, working memory, auditory–verbal comprehension, memory, and problem-solving all
   can impact patients' abilities to understand what is told to them by the
   treating clinician. In the patient with psychiatric illness, information needs
   to be presented in a manner that is appropriate to the person's intellectual, educational and cognitive level. For example, if a patient is suffering
   from significant impairment in verbal memory ability, presentation of the
   information in another format (i.e., charts, video, demonstration) may be
   a more effective way to convey this information.

3. *Appreciating the situation and its consequences.* The difference between
   this category and the preceding one is the ability to grasp what the information given *means to the patient.* That is, if patients are told the specif-
   ics and possible risks and benefits of a treatment, can they understand
   the implications for their future. The factors going into these judgments
   include: acknowledging illness when it is shown to be present, evaluating
   the effect of the illness and the effect of the treatment options presented,
   and acknowledging that the general probabilities of risks and benefits
   apply to the situation. In this case, deficiencies are usually the result of
   pathologic distortion, denial due to cognitive or affective impairment or a
   delusional perception of the nature of the patient's condition, the probable
   outcome of treatment, or the motivations of those caring for the patient.
   A notable example of an inability to appreciate the impact of one's illness
   has been described in patients suffering from schizophrenia. Amador et
   al. (1991) have reported significant deficits in awareness in this patient
   group, with some patients attributing the symptoms or problems from
   their illness to other external factors or people. These deficits in aware-

ness are thought to represent alterations in brain anatomy and physiology (Flashman et al., 2000; Flashman et al., 2001), and can often present as significant barriers to treatment and treatment compliance.

4. *Manipulating information rationally.* This category pertains to the ability to use logical processes to compare and contrast the benefits and risks of various treatment options; that is, the patient's ability to weigh different types of information and reach an informed decision. As noted by Freedman (1981), rational manipulation entails the ability to reach conclusions that are logically consistent with the starting premises. This process requires that the patient weigh the risks and benefits of a single option, and the more complex process of weighing multiple options simultaneously, in a manner that reflects the weights previously assigned to them. Several neuropsychological and emotional factors may impinge on this process, including thought disorder, delirium, dementia, extreme phobia or panic, anxiety, euphoria, hypomania, depression and anger. For the neuropsychologist, there must be an assessment of the patient's 'chain of reasoning' or the ability to state the major factors in a decision and the importance assigned to them. In general, the clinician should be able to see that the outcomes reflect some weighing of these factors.

With the exception of the most severe mental disorders, a neuropsychologist would be hard-pressed to accurately assess decision-making capacity in a patient who is not appropriately (or is inadequately) informed. That is, the earlier discussion of informed consent has direct bearing on the issue of competence. If patients do not have the information and options concerning treatment, they cannot be expected to make a competent decision, even if their decision-making processes are intact. With regard to neuropsychiatry, however, there is a fundamental problem with the aforementioned Appelbaum and Grisso (1988) criteria for competence. In general, these four criteria ignore the way affective disorders can influence judgment. For example, a person who is clinically depressed may actually fit all four of their criteria — they may be able to communicate their choices clearly, to understand the relevant information and give it back to you accurately, and to manipulate the information rationally; the third criterion, to appreciate the situation and its circumstances, is where you would think the criteria would fail, but the depressed patient may be able to tell you "I perfectly understand that if I don't do this I might die. I can repeat the mechanism that would kill me. I just *don't care* if I die or not." It is this type of situation that the Appelbaum and Grisso criteria cannot accommodate.

As with most issues dealing with such thorny ethical dilemmas, a purely neuropsychological focus does not address other issues known to impact consent and other decision-making capabilities in patients suffering from neuropsychiatric or neurologic disorders. Such "non-rational" factors include: (1) trust in the clinician, (2) experience of suffering, (3) coercion, (4) desperation, (5) altruism of the ill person, and/or (6) hope. Roberts and Roberts

(1999) as well as others (Charland, 1999; Elliott, 1997; Roberts, 1998; Roberts et al., 2000) have shown that these factors also weigh heavily on the decision-making processes of psychiatric patients and need to be given as much attention as is given to neuropsychological and other clinical matters.

Neuropsychological testing does not traditionally assess such non-rational aspects of the decision-making process. In this case, the neuropsychologist must strike a balance between the neuropsychological testing data and those factors gleaned from the clinical interview and interactions with the patient. While most neuropsychologists intuitively do this, there is little in the way of research to help support the clinician's decisions in cases where frank psychosis or massive behavioral disruption is not evident. As noted earlier, there are objective measures which have been used to gauge a patient's ability to take in, process and comprehend the information needed to make a competent and rational decision. Few neuropsychologists, however, are aware of such instruments and even fewer use them in their daily practice with psychiatric patients.

As is well known to most neuropsychologists, the 'real-life' translation of neuropsychological tasks (ecological validity) is still in its early stages, and the extent to which deficits translate into real-life decision-making processes is even further behind. Marson et al. (1995) first attempted to address the issue of competence in patients suffering from Alzheimer's dementia by developing a scale to assess competency using a defined legal standard. This same group subsequently used this measure along with a neuropsychological battery to attempt to identify the neuropsychological predictors of competency performance and status in patients suffering from Alzheimer's disease using a specific legal standard model. Applying a reasonably large battery of neuropsychological tests that were theoretically linked to brain functions implicated in competency, the authors assessed 15 healthy elderly participants and 29 patients with AD. The investigators used two clinical vignettes (i.e., neoplasm and cardiac) designed to assess each subject's ability to consent to medical treatment under five different medical standards. Of the five standards assessed, the authors examined only one: the capacity to provide 'rational reasons' for a choice of medical treatment (LS4). Results revealed that measures of word-list generation, specifically deficits in semantic word-list generation (i.e., Animal Naming, which requires generation of as many animal names as possible in a given time) were the best predictors of poor performance on LS4 for both controls and AD patients. Notably, neither memory measures nor verbal reasoning skills were significantly associated with performance on LS4. This pattern of performance suggests that a higher level of verbal abstraction or reasoning was not necessarily as important as more 'basic' verbal generation skills. Using the neuropsychological data, the authors found that measures of semantic word-list generation, executive function and simple attentional skills correctly classified 93% of the subjects into 'competent,' 'marginally competent' or 'incompetent' categories. The authors stated that these data support the idea that poorer frontal system functioning may result in a reduced ability to generate rational reasons to either engage or not engage in medical interventions. While limited in sample size and perhaps somewhat confounded by the fact that patients with language disturbance were asked to respond to the vignettes orally, this study represents an important first step in defining the brain regions and functions most important for rational decision-making processes as well as tying this to normative performance. It also may give a theoretical foundation for the use of capacity (with its implication that decision-making ability is not an all-or-nothing proposition), rather than competence, to describe a person's decision-making ability. Also, if such neuropsychological deficits can be specifically linked to decision making skills, such linkage paves the way for developing behavioral strategies to circumvent these deficits (e.g., use of a recognition format when assessing comprehension). The use of this type of methodology in patients with psychiatric disorders will be important to help discern the neuropsychological deficits (and strengths) most important for competent and rational decision-making.

It should be noted that decision-making capacities can also fluctuate with changes in a patient's underlying mental disorder (e.g., increase in depression or delusions) or with other factors, such as the effects of medication, fatigue, lack of sleep, or the occurrence of an unpleasant or distressing incident just prior to the examination. Therefore, the neuropsychologist may wish to assess over different time points to ensure stability of the clinical picture before competence is judged impaired (or unimpaired). For example, if assessing a patient with major depression just after the introduction of a new antidepressant, any deficits that may be uncovered could reflect either a static organic impairment *or* medication-induced disruption of cognitive or emotional processes. In this situation, another evaluation when the patient is stabilized on their medication would be important to rule out such extraneous factors. Most often, the evaluation of competence does not result in an unambiguous rating of 'intact' or 'impaired' on all dimensions. In most cases, patients fall somewhere in the middle ground. For the neuropsychologist, there are no clear clinical benchmarks for determining competence or incompetence. Such judgments are made by the courts and are based on an attempted balance between protecting a patient's autonomy and the desire to shield them from the consequences of bad decisions. While most cases do not reach the court system, the neuropsychologist is faced with the decision of whether to pursue such action when substantial neuropsychological impairment is evident. In some cases, when the neuropsychologist feels that the patient would be found incompetent by the court, the use of a substitute decision by family members may be acceptable to the court, thereby avoiding actual court proceedings. Such a method has been endorsed by the President's Commission (1982) as a way to avoid excessive numbers of competency cases in the court system. In patients with psychiatric illness, even if the patient is found incompetent, the process does not end there. For example, if a patient with bipolar disorder is deemed incompetent due to an acute psychotic episode, effective treatment may reverse these impairments, thereby justifying the restoration of their decision-making rights.

In order to better understand how these principles may be engaged in everyday practice, we present two cases where the issue of ability to consent to treatment and competence were raised.

Case 1

Mr. B was a 24-year-old man referred for neuropsychological assessment by his mother and a consulting psychiatrist concerned about recent 'strange' behaviors. Specifically, the patient's mother noted that approximately three weeks prior to the examination her son had informed her that he possessed paranormal ('psychic') abilities, which allowed him to communicate with the dead, as well as to read other people's thoughts. He stated that he had had these abilities since around the age of 15 but only recently felt the need to tell anyone about them. Mr. B's mother stated that her son had alluded to such abilities several years ago but just recently began speaking openly about them. Mr. B recently quit his job working in the family business in order to pursue his interest in this area, although his mother stated that he was quite guarded about what exactly his plans consisted of. Both of Mr. B's parents were interested in getting their son into psychiatric treatment, which he apparently felt was 'unnecessary.' He had undergone a prior psychiatric exam as well as an MRI and EEG at the behest of his parents. His MRI and EEG were interpreted as normal. The psychiatric exam was felt to be consistent with a bipolar disorder, but a neuropsychological examination was requested to probe the possibility of a schizoaffective disorder. Regardless of diagnosis, Mr. B was noted to resist any idea that he would need to be treated for his reported experiences. In addition, while he felt it was not necessary, he agreed to the neuropsychological testing as he thought "it might be interesting."

At the time of the assessment, Mr. B was living alone in an apartment and was being supported by his parents. Mr. B had 16 years of education and was described as an A-B student throughout his school experiences. He lived on his own both in and after college and was reportedly able to manage his budget and pay his bills with no difficulty. Socially, Mr. B reported that he had always been a 'popular person.' He related that he was active in sports at school and continued to play sports socially. He stated that he dated sporadically but that he was not interested in a serious relationship at this time, instead wishing to devote his time to his 'psychic business.' With the exception of a broken index finger at age 17, his medical history was unremarkable. He denied any alcohol or drug use in the past or currently. No family history of neurologic or psychiatric illness was endorsed.

Upon interview, Mr. B stated that he knew that his parents thought there was something wrong with his "mind and emotions," but that they did not understand his unique abilities. He, in contrast, stated that he "never felt better" about his skills and future prospects. Mr. B felt the reason his parents were so concerned about him was because he was currently unemployed. He stated that this would change in the near future, as his psychic business would "take off" and the "money would be rolling in." Specifically, Mr. B stated that he had paranormal abilities to communicate with the dead, predict the future, and heal the sick. He stated that he had clients all over the country asking him to communicate with their deceased relatives and friends. Mr. B stated, "I am the only person with this blessing. I am unique and I have never met anyone else who can do what I do." He stated that his parents did not know about his business plans because they did not understand or support his paranormal abilities. As a result, he was reluctant to let them know the full extent of his plans. He also expressed a desire that the results of the exam not be shared with his parents or the consulting psychiatrist. He provided the examiners with details of his business plan and told of his recent contact with a client in a neighboring city who was going to provide him with "start-up money" for an office.

With regard to his symptoms, Mr. B reported that his ability to communicate with the dead began as a young boy. He stated that dead people communicated with him through his thoughts (i.e., he often had the experience that he knew what spirits were "thinking"). He reported that these thoughts were generally benevolent, but sometimes overwhelming because they demanded a great deal of his attention. He reported that the thoughts came to him several times a day, sometimes almost continuously. Mr. B stated that the thoughts had increased in intensity and frequency over the past three years. He had learned to control the thoughts through meditation and studying Tarot cards. He stated that he rarely heard voices, and he "saw spirits" a few times a year.

Mr. B's thoughts were generally clear and goal-directed, but delusional thinking and thought disorder were evident. Speech was rapid and tangential, with frequent derailments. Verbal expression and comprehension appeared to be intact. Mr. B's mood was elevated, and he seemed quite excited and animated.

Results of the intellectual assessment revealed abilities in the High Average range of functioning, with verbal and non-verbal skills appearing to be equally developed. Tests of achievement were commensurate with his obtained intellectual skills and occupational attainment and were not suggestive of gross learning disability. Neuropsychological testing revealed intact abilities in verbal and non-verbal problem-solving, verbal reasoning and comprehension, attention and memory, visual-perceptual ability, language and related abilities, and sensory-motor function. The only exception to his generally intact performance was seen on a visual vigilance task (Continuous Performance Test), where his reaction times were in the mildly impaired range. Notably, his scores on the Minnesota Multiphasic Personality Inventory-2 showed elevations consistent with a diagnosis of bipolar disorder (spike 9). His scores on the Beck Depression Inventory and State-Trait Anxiety Inventory were not suggestive of significant depression or anxiety. The results of the neuropsychological evaluation in conjunction with his clinical history and presentation were felt to be most consistent with a diagnosis of Bipolar Disorder.

Outcome

Overall, Mr. B demonstrated generally intact neuropsychological abilities with only very subtle difficulties in visual attention processing speed being noted. There was no clear evidence of any cognitive impairment that might be clouding his judgment and reasoning. That is, while his choice to pursue his career as a psychic would be considered by most clinicians to be out of the mainstream, he did show adequate reasoning as to how he made his choice and how he would go about this business, and he could understand that other people might question the existence of such abilities. He was able to maintain his activities of daily living and did not show any clear indications or potential of harm to himself or others. In all, there was no neuropsychological evidence to challenge his competence. He did, however, demonstrate significant thought disorder, a complex delusional system and other symptoms of bipolar disorder, potentially of psychotic proportions. Specifically, his delusions and thought disorder did prevent him from *appreciating* the nature of his illness as well as any potential consequences of his illness. While it was clear that Mr. B would probably benefit from pharmacologic and psychotherapeutic management, there was not sufficient grounds either clinically or neuropsychologically to compel him to do so. Consistent with the opinion of the consulting psychiatrist, Mr. B was judged not to be at significant risk of harm to himself or others, and was able to handle his personal finances, self-care and other activities of daily living. There was no strong data in his psychiatric or neuropsychological assessment to support incompetence, certainly not such that would stand in a court of law.

In a feedback session, the results of testing were shared with Mr. B, including the diagnostic impression of bipolar disorder and subsequent treatment recommendations. Mr. B acknowledged the examiner's conclusions, but "politely disagree(d)," stating that he was "a genuine psychic" and that there was no need for treatment of any sort. After some discussion, he did report that seeing a therapist might be helpful in better understanding his abilities, and that he would consider taking such action. Mr. B stated, however, that he would not see the consulting psychiatrist again nor would he take any medication for his symptoms. He also stated that he did not want the results of this exam shared with his parents or the consulting psychiatrist. Given the fact that there was not sufficient evidence to judge him incompetent, his request was honored and the report of the findings was given only to him (despite his parents' request for a copy). Mr. B was encouraged to stay in regular contact with his family, and he was given the name of a local psychologist who could see him in therapy if he so desired. He was also given the name and number of a psychiatrist specializing in bipolar disorder, in case his symptoms became distressing or problematic in the future. In referring back to the definition of competence given by Appelbaum and Grisso (1988) at the beginning of the section, Mr. B demonstrated the ability to (1) communicate a choice, (2) understand relevant information, and, at least partially, (3) manipulate information rationally. The component of this process most problematic for Mr. B was the ability to appreciate the situation and its consequences. His clinical symptoms prevented him from seeing his current clinical state clearly, and his awareness of his illness and its consequences was poor. While it could be debated that his untreated bipolar disorder was a threat to his well being, he had functioned at this level for an extended period of time, and there was no strong evidence that he was in the process of decompensating. Therefore, no action was taken to try to compel him into treatment or to disclose the results of this evaluation to treating health care professionals. The neuropsychologist provided the patient with the necessary contact information should he begin to decompensate and encouraged him to engage in therapy so his clinical course could be monitored. Mr. B did begin attending therapy on a biweekly basis, and at the time of this writing he is still involved in treatment with the same psychologist.

Case 2

Mr. D was a 27-year-old Filippino male referred by the attending neuropsychiatrist from the inpatient psychiatry unit for assessment of judgment, problem solving, and decision making, as well as the nature and etiology of any cognitive deficits. According to records, Mr. D had a longstanding history of impulsive and aggressive behavior and several psychotic episodes dating back to the age of 18. His history was also significant for a prior injury to his legs and head. One year prior to the current hospitalization Mr. D had become psychotic and physically aggressive toward his sister. During this episode, he climbed to the roof of a three-story building and subsequently jumped (thinking he would be able to fly to the next building). He suffered two compound fractures of the right and left legs and sustained a mild head trauma, based on a 3–5 minute loss of consciousness noted at the scene. While his right leg healed with the use of a cast, his left leg required the placement of three bone screws to stabilize the fracture. However, the bone had not healed well and two of the screws were noted to be broken on X-ray. MRI of the head revealed asymmetry of the ventricles (R>L) and an ependymal cyst on the right. Other diagnostic studies (i.e., EEG, blood work) were negative. When discussing the case with the orthopedic surgeon and the psychiatrist, Mr. D acknowledged that two of the three screws had broken, although he appeared to be unconcerned about the last screw and the possible consequences of refusing further treatment. Despite repeated warnings and statements to the contrary, Mr. D insisted that the final screw would hold indefinitely. As such, he flatly refused any surgery and continued to walk about the unit despite being specifically instructed to stay off of his legs. Mr. D's parents and older sister were quite involved in his treatment and were supportive of surgery to repair his leg. Despite their efforts, Mr. D was still resistant to having surgery.

At the time of his assessment, Mr. D was living with his parents and older sister. Mr. D had 12 years of education and was described as a C-D student throughout his academic experiences. He worked at odd jobs during school but was never gainfully employed full-time. Following his first onset of psychosis at age 18, Mr. D was unable to live independently. His mother took care of all financial tasks and helped Mr. D in his basic activities of daily living, such as laundry and cooking. Mr. D was reported to be quite isolated, with no immediate friends outside of his family. He had never dated. With the exception of the injuries noted previously, Mr. D's medical history was generally unremarkable. There was no report of significant drug or alcohol use. A family history of schizophrenia was noted in Mr. D's maternal grandfather and paternal uncle. No report of familial neurologic disease was revealed. Medications at time of testing included Risperdal.

When queried about his understanding of his condition, Mr. D stated that his leg was "fine," and that "it would heal on its own." He subsequently proceeded to show the examiner his belief by springing up and down on his legs on the floor. He stated that the "doctors were wrong" about his leg and that he was a "good healer." Even when the examiner pointed out the discoloration in his left leg due to impairment in blood flow, Mr. D stated that his leg "was always darker on that side." In general, Mr. D was able to express how he had ended up in the hospital but seemed unable to reconstruct what had happened to him in his injury. He did not recall his fall one year ago but was able to generally state what had been told to him. After getting a detailed explanation of his injury (~ two hours), complete with graphs and a model of the bone affected, Mr. D was unable to explain what was wrong with his leg or any of the treatments or interventions to take place. Despite frequent repetitions of the treatment plan and risks and benefits, Mr. D showed no improvement in his comprehension or understanding of his status. When asked to formulate a treatment plan of his own, Mr. D was unable to do so without a staff member's help.

Mr. D was oriented to self, place, and time. He presented as alert, cooperative, and motivated to perform his best. Affect was slightly restricted but was stable and congruent to conversation. Thought processes appeared relevant and goal-directed. However, responses were generally very slow, concrete and suggested poor insight regarding future consequences of behavior. Moreover, several responses included violent themes. For example, when asked to define 'terminate' he responded, "to kill like the Terminator, injection death." He also showed a tendency to perseverate on verbal stimuli, which produced additional irrelevant verbalizations. He appeared amused by his verbalizations and would often laugh out loud. He endorsed daily auditory hallucinations that were fully formed and localized outside of his head. He stated that he had experienced these voices since age 19 or 20. Mr. D demonstrated significant impulsivity and socially inappropriate behaviors. Some repetition of instructions was necessary for comprehension. Spontaneous speech was within normal limits in terms of rate, range, and intensity. Comprehension seemed marginal.

Results of intellectual assessment revealed abilities in the Borderline range of intellectual functioning, with non-verbal abilities significantly lower than verbal skills (VIQ>PIQ). Verbal and non-verbal reasoning skills were among his poorest performances on intellectual assessment. Basic academic skills were in line with obtained IQ, with very limited reading comprehension skills. Neuropsychological testing revealed marked impairments in verbal and non-verbal problem-solving skills. Mr. D was impaired in cognitive flexibility and in higher level categorical reasoning, and he showed significant impulsivity. Deficits in response inhibition were seen throughout the testing. Memory for structured verbal and non-verbal information was marginal, whereas memory for information requiring organization on his part (e.g., California Verbal Learning Test; Delis et al., 1987) was severely impaired. Mr. D had a significant degree of perseverative responding, as well as a high number of intrusions. Visual-perceptual skills were moderately impaired, with distortions of basic perception being noted. Basic auditory verbal comprehension was poor, while expressive abilities were generally intact. Left-sided tactile suppressions were noted on sensory examination, and mild lateralized deficits were seen on tests of fine motor speed and coordination. Examination of the MMPI-2 validity scales indicated a highly invalid pattern of responses. Specifically, his response profile was consistent with confusion and poor understanding of questions (questions were presented via tape recorder due to his poor reading skills). He denied any frank depression or anxiety on clinical measures.

Outcome

The ethics of informed consent require that a patient be able to communicate a choice, understand relevant information, appreciate the situation and its consequences, and manipulate information rationally. Analysis of Mr. D's case indicated that while he was able to communicate a choice, he had deficits in comprehending information accurately and possessed poor insight into his illness and the consequences posed by not treating his leg. Furthermore, he was unable to take the information available to him and formulate why he made this decision. Thus, he could not logically plan an alternative course of treatment nor explain his reasoning leading to his choice. His deficits in these areas were also supported by the neuropsychological evaluation, which documented Borderline intellectual ability and specific deficits in frontal system functioning, memory, auditory-verbal comprehension, and visual-spatial abilities. Notably, deficits in frontal system function have implications for patient autonomy. These systems are implicated in executive functions, ranging from coordination of simple ideas and movements to complex goal-directed action and long-range planning. As recently noted by Workman and associates (2000), deficits in executive control can significantly impact two of the three major aspects of patient autonomy, specifically intentionality and voluntariness (the third being comprehension). Mr. D showed impairment in

[handwritten annotation: n psych scores are not necessarily essential to determine this]

all of these aspects, and, based on the immediate risk to his well being and the potential loss of his leg, surrogate decision making was sought from his parents and older sister. The treatment team again reviewed the procedure with Mr. D, sought assent to the intervention, and reconsidered the treatments in Mr. D's best interests. Following this course, Mr. D was judged to be incompetent to make this treatment decision by the neuropsychologist and the attending psychiatrist, and court approval for a substituted consent was obtained, consistent with the APA Ethical Standard 4.02(b) when persons are legally incapable of giving informed consent, psychologists obtain informed permission from a legally authorized person, if such substitute consent is permitted by law; (c) in addition, psychologists (1) inform those persons who are legally incapable of giving informed consent about the proposed interventions in a manner commensurate with the person's psychological capacities, (2) seek their assent to those interventions, and (3) consider such persons' preferences and best interests.

As noted in the vignette, the clinicians tried repeatedly to provide information to the patient so that he could best understand his treatment options (including graphs and models). They also attempted to gain his assent to treatment, which he declined. Despite these attempts and his subsequent refusal, the treatment team considered the course of action in Mr. D's best interests, and a court order sought to proceed with the surgical intervention. Mr. D's family provided consent to proceed with the surgery, and Mr. D's leg was repaired. In follow-up, Mr. D still felt that the surgery was not necessary, but seemed pleased that his leg felt "better" and that it was "the same color as the other leg."

These vignettes aim to illustrate the diversity of patients with different capacities that may present themselves to the neuropsychologist when dealing with people suffering from neuropsychiatric disorders. In each case, both clinical variables and neuropsychological factors had an impact on judgment of decisional capacity and, eventually, outcome. The challenge for neuropsychology lies in the development of standardized and *quantitative* measures to begin to address the ethical issues daily faced by the clinician. Such measures can help document which neuropsychological functions are most related to different components of decision-making skills and which aspects of these decision-making abilities are most relevant to research and clinical decisions.

References

Amador, X.F., Strauss, D.H., Yale, S.A., & Gorman, J.M. (1991). Awareness of illness and schizophrenia. *Schizophrenia Bulletin, 17*, 113-132.

American Psychological Association. (1992a). Ethical principles of psychologists and code of conduct. *American Psychologist, 47*, 1597-1611.

American Psychological Association, Ethics Committee. (1992b). Rules and procedures. *American Psychologist, 47*, 1612-1628.

Appelbaum, P.S. (1998). Missing the boat: Competence and consent in psychiatric research. *American Journal of Psychiatry, 155,* 1486-1488.

Appelbaum, P.S., & Grisso, T. (1988). Assessing patients' capacity to consent to treatment. *New England Journal of Medicine, 319,* 1635-1638.

Appelbaum, P.S., & Grisso, T. (1995). The MacArthur Treatment Competence Study, I, II, III. *Law and Human Behavior, 19,* 105-174.

Appelbaum, P.S., & Grisso, T. (1996). *The MacArthur Competence Assessment Tool–Clinical research.* Sarasota, FL: Professional Resource Press.

Appelbaum, P.S., Roth, L.H., & Lidz, C.W. (1982). The therapeutic misconception: Informed consent in psychiatric research. *International Journal of Law and Psychiatry, 5,* 319-329.

Benson, P.R., Roth, L.H., Winslade, W.J. (1985). Informed consent in psychiatric research: Preliminary findings from an ongoing investigation. *Social Science & Medicine, 20,* 1331-1341.

Bilder, R.M., Mukherjee, S., Rieder, R.O., & Pandurangi, A.K. (1985). Symptomatic and neuropsychological components of defect states. *Schizophrenia Bulletin, 11,* 409-414.

Carpenter, W.T., Gold, J.M., Lahti, A.C., Queern, C.A., Conley, R.R., Bartko, J.J., Kovnick, J., & Appelbaum, P.S. (2000). Decisional capacity for informed consent in schizophrenia research. *Archives of General Psychiatry, 57,* 533-538.

Censits, D.M., Ragland, J.D., Gur, R.C., & Gur, R.E. (1997). Neuropsychological evidence supporting a neurodevelopmental model of schizophrenia: A longitudinal study. *Schizophrenia Research, 24,* 289-298.

Charland, L.C. (1999). Appreciation and emotion: Theoretical reflections on the MacArthur Treatment Competence Study. *Kennedy Institute for Ethics Journal, 8,* 359-376.

Delis, D.C., Kramer, J.H., Kaplan, E., & Ober, B.A. (1987). *California Verbal Learning Test, Manual.* San Antonio: Harcourt Brace Jovanovich.

DeRenzo, E.G., Conley, R.R., & Love, R. (1998). Assessment of capacity to give consent to research participation: State-of-the-art and beyond. *Journal of Health Care, Law & Policy, 1,* 66-87.

Dresser, R. (1996). Mentally disabled research subjects: The enduring policy issues. *Journal of the American Medical Association, 276,* 67-72.

Elliot, C. (1997). Caring about risks: Are severely depressed patients competent to consent to research? *Archives of General Psychiatry, 54,* 113-116.

Flashman, L.A., McAllister, T.W., Andreasen, N.C., & Saykin, A.J. (2000). Smaller brain size associated with unawareness in patients with schizophrenia. *American Journal of Psychiatry, 157,* 1167-1169.

Flashman, L.A., McAllister, T.W., Saykin, A.J., Johnson, S.C., Rick, J.H., & Green, R.L. (2001). Specific frontal lobe regions correlated with unawareness of illness in schizophrenia: A preliminary study. *Journal of Neuropsychiatry and Clinical Neuroscience, 13,* 255–257.

Freedman, B. (1981). Competence, marginal and otherwise: Concepts and ethics. *International Journal of Law and Psychiatry, 4,* 53-72.

Gibson, J.M. (1990). Values history focuses on life and death decisions. *Medical Ethics Physician, 17,* 1-2.

Goldberg, T.E., Hyde, T.M., Kleinman, J.E., & Weinberger, D.R. (1993). Course of schizophrenia: Neuropsychological evidence for a static encephalopathy. *Schizophrenia Bulletin, 19,* 797-804.

Grant, I., & Adams, K.M. (1986). *Neuropsychological assessment of neuropsychiatric disorders.* New York: Oxford University Press.

Grisso, T., & Appelbaum, P.S. (1995). The MacArthur Treatment Competence Study, III: Abilities of patients to consent to psychiatric and medical treatments. *Law and Human Behavior,19,* 149-174.

Grisso, T., Appelbaum, P.S., & Hill-Fotouhi, C. (1997). The MacCAT-T: A clinical tool to assess patients' capacities to make treatment decisions. *Psychiatric Services, 48*, 1415-1419.

Grossman, L., & Summers, F. (1980). A study of the capacity of schizophrenic patients to give informed consent. *Hospital & Community Psychiatry, 31*, 205-206.

Gur, R.E., & Gur, R.C. (2000). Schizophrenia: Brain structure and function. In H.I. Kaplan & B.J. Sadock (Eds.), *Comprehensive textbook of psychiatry/VII* (pp. 1117–1129), Philadelphia: Lippincott Williams & Wilkins.

Gur, R.C., Ragland, J.D., & Gur, R.E. (1997). Cognitive changes in schizophrenia: A critical look. *International Review of Psychiatry, 9*, 449-457.

Hilts, P.J. (1998). Psychiatric researchers under fire. *New York Times*, May 14, p. F1.

Kleinman, I., Schacter, D., Jeffries, J., & Goldhamer, P. (1993). Effectiveness of two methods for informing schizophrenic patients about neuroleptic medications. *Hospital and Community Psychiatry, 44*,1189-1191.

Lidz, C.W., Meisel, A., Zerubavel, E., Carter, M., Sestak, R.M., & Roth, L.H. (1984). *Informed consent: A study of decision making in psychiatry*. New York: Guiliford Press.

Lucassen, A. (1998). Ethical issues in genetics of mental disorders. *Lancet, 352*, 1004-1005.

Marson, D.C., Cody, H.A., Ingram, K.K., & Harre1, L.E. (1995). Neuropsychologic predictors of competency in Alzheimer's disease using a rational reasons legal standard. *Archives of Neurology, 52*, 955-959.

Marson, D.C., Ingram, K.K., Cody, H.A., & Harrell, E. (1995). Assessing the competency of patients with Alzheimer's disease under different legal standards: A prototype instrument. *Archives of Neurology, 52*, 949-954.

Meisel, A., & Roth, L.H. (1981). What we do and do not know about informed consent. *Journal of the American Medical Association, 246*, 2473-2477.

Overall, J.E., & Gorham, D.E. (1961). The Brief Psychiatric Rating Scale. *Psychological Reports, 10*, 799-812.

President's Commission for the Study of Ethical Problems in Medicine and Biomedical and Behavioral Research (1982). *Making health care decisions: A report on the ethical and legal implications of informed consent in the patient–practitioner relationship, Vol 1*. Washington, DC: Government Printing Office.

Randolph, C. (1998). *The repeatable battery for the assessment of neuropsychological status*. San Antonio, TX: The Psychological Corporation.

Roberts, L.W. (1998). The ethical basis of psychiatric research: Conceptual issues and empirical findings. *Comprehensive Psychiatry, 39*, 99-110.

Roberts, L.W., & Roberts, B.R. (1999). Psychiatric research ethics: An overview of evolving guidelines and current ethical dilemmas in the study of mental illness. *Biological Psychiatry, 46*, 1025-1038.

Roberts, L.W., Warner, T.D., & Brody, J.L. (2000). Perspectives of patients with schizophrenia and psychiatrists regarding ethically important aspects of research participation. *American Journal of Psychiatry, 157*, 67-74.

Roth, L.H., Appelbaum, P.S., Lidz, C.W., Benson, P., & Winslade, W.J. (1987). Informed consent in psychiatric research. *Rutgers Law Review, 39*, 425-441.

Saykin, A.J., Gur, R.C., Gur, R.E., Mozley, D., Mozley, L.H., Resnick, S.M., Kester, D.B., & Stafiniak, P. (1991). Neuropsychological function in schizophrenia: Selective impairment in memory and learning. *Archives of General Psychiatry, 48*, 618-624.

Saykin, A.J., Shtasel, D.L., Gur, R.E., Kester, D.B., Mozley, L.H., Stafiniak, P., & Gur, R.C. (1994). Neuropsychological deficits in neuroleptic naive, first episode schizophrenia patients. *Archives of General Psychiatry, 51*, 124-131.

Schachter, D., Kleinman, I., Prendergast, P., Remington, G., & Schertzer, S. (1994). The effect of psychopathology on the ability of schizophrenic patients to give informed consent. *Journal of Nervous and Mental Disease, 182,* 360-362.

Schaeffer, M.H., Krantz, D.S., Wichman, A., Masur, H., Reed, E., & Vinicky, J.K. (1996). The impact of disease severity on the informed consent process in clinical research. *American Journal of Medicine, 100,* 261-268.

Shamoo, A.E. (1997). *Ethics in neurobiological research with human subjects: The Baltimore Conference in Ethics.* New York: Gordon & Breach.

Shore, D. (1996). Ethical principles and informed consent: An NIMH perspective. *Psychopharmacology Bulletin, 32,* 7-10.

Soskis, D.A. (1978). Schizophrenic and medical inpatients as informed drug consumers. *Archives of General Psychiatry, 35,* 645-647.

Stanley, B., Sieber, J.E., & Melton, G.B. (1987). Empirical studies of ethical issues in research. *American Psychologist, 42,* 735-741.

Stanley, B., Stanley, M., Guido, J., & Garvin, L. (1988). The functional competency of elderly at risk. *Gerontologist, 28,* 53-58.

Stanley, B., Stanley, M., Lautin, A., Kanw, J., & Schwartz, N. (1981). Preliminary findings on psychiatric patients as research subjects: A population at risk? *American Journal of Psychiatry, 38,* 669-671.

Sugarman, J. (1999). Empirical research on informed consent: An annotated bibliography. *Hastings Center Report (Special Supplement* January-February).

Szasz, T. (1996). *The meaning of mind: Language, morality, and neuroscience.* Westport, CT: Praeger.

Wechsler, D. (1997). *Wechsler Adult Intelligence Scale-3rd Edition: Administration and Scoring Manual.* San Antonio, TX: The Psychological Corporation.

Weiderholt, J.L., & Bryant, B.R. (1992). *Gray Oral Reading Tests,* (3rd ed.). Austin, TX: Pro-Ed.

Wilkinson, G.S. (1993). *Wide Range Achievement Test-3rd Edition: Administration Manual.* Wilmington, DE: Wide Range Inc.

Workman, R.H., McCullough, L.B., Molinari, V., Kunik, M.E., Orengo, C., Khalsa, D.K., & Rezabek, P. (2000). Clinical and ethical implications of impaired executive control functions for patient autonomy. *Psychiatric Services, 51,* 359-363.

Chapter 10

ETHICAL NEUROPSYCHOLOGICAL PRACTICE IN MEDICAL SETTINGS

Elisabeth Wilde, Shane Bush, and Penelope Zeifert

Introduction

The roles of neuropsychologists in medical settings are many and varied, and the potential reasons for ethical misconduct are equally diverse. However, it seems likely that most ethical misconduct in medical settings is not intentional but rather is the result of unfamiliarity with general medical ethics, relevant ethics codes, and laws. Even for neuropsychologists who are sensitive to ethical issues and follow accepted standards of practice, situations may arise in which two or more ethical principles conflict with each other. In such situations the neuropsychologist must choose a course of action that favors one principle over the other.

While the neuropsychologist in a medical setting may function as a clinician, teacher, researcher, administrator or a combination of these, the focus of this chapter is on the provision of clinical services. Within the clinical realm, roles may vary based on whether neuropsychological service is provided throughout the medical center or to a specific unit, the type of unit, whether the neuropsychologist is a consultant or member of the medical team, the expertise and interests of the neuropsychologist, and the relationship between neuropsychology and other specialists. Each of these factors contributes to the types of potential ethical challenges that the neuropsychologist may face.

Ethical conflicts may be resolved in a variety of ways depending upon the context. Laws, institutional regulations, general biomedical ethics (beneficence, non-maleficence, justice, autonomy; Beauchamp & Childress, 1989), and specific ethics codes exist to guide the neuropsychologist in the identification and resolution of ethical conflicts. In addition, experienced colleagues with ethical expertise often prove to be a most valuable resource. By increasing familiarity with the APA Ethical Standards, aspiring to practice in a manner consistent with the Ethical Principles, and utilizing the above resources, the neuropsychologist can meet the ethical challenges confronted in medical settings and be of service to colleagues practicing with less awareness of, or investment in, ethical neuropsychological practice.

The purpose of this chapter is to highlight some of the ethical challenges that neuropsychologists commonly face in medical settings. Each section begins with a clinical vignette that illustrates select ethical issues; the ethical issues are then each examined in detail. Each section concludes with recommendations for negotiating such challenges when confronted in the course of neuropsychological practice.

Vignette 1

An 80-year-old gentleman is referred to Dr. Young for a neuropsychological evaluation to aid with differential diagnosis and to determine his current cognitive abilities. The patient was admitted to the hospital five days earlier due to progressive mental status changes during the previous 4–6 weeks, visual hallucinations involving his deceased relatives, and increased stiffness and slowness when he walks. The referral also indicates the staff's concern that the patient repeatedly voices his concern about his son's involvement in his financial affairs.

The patient's medical history is complex and includes multiple aspects of cardiovascular (congestive heart failure, coronary artery disease, abdominal aortic aneurysm, peripheral vascular disease, hypertension), pulmonary (severe chronic obstructive pulmonary disease), renal disease, and diabetes. He takes a number of medications associated with these disease processes as well as analgesics. Recent repeat CT compared to previous studies four years prior and two years prior reveals no interval change and is suggestive of chronic ischemic small vessel disease. However, recent PET scan was noted to reveal mild hypometabolism in the temporal-parietal lobes bilaterally.

During the course of the assessment, the patient's attending physician approaches Dr. Young and reports that following further medical testing and work-up, consulting physicians have determined that the patient's abdominal aortic aneurysm has substantially increased in size, and they are recommending surgical repair. The physician also notes that the patient has obviously not been adhering to previous medical treatment plans regarding the management of his diabetes. Furthermore, he reports that the patient's family has contacted him with concerns about the patient's ability to live independently, to monitor his finances, and to drive. However, the patient has flatly refused

*to consider placement in an assisted care facility and complains that his fam-
ily is "just after the money." He has also told his attending physician that
he will "probably not" elect to have his aneurysm surgically repaired. This
physician requests that Dr. Young now also assess the patient's competence.*

*During clinical interview, the patient reports that he resides in his own
home with a younger, unrelated roommate. He reports that he retains control
of his finances. He appears very concerned about the fact that his estranged
son suddenly has an interest in his well being and wants him to sell his home
and grant him power of attorney over his financial affairs. He states that he
is comfortable in his own home and manages well unless he "gets sick." He
reports that he is still driving and is not having any difficulties.*

*Dr. Young interviews the patient's son who states that due to personal
differences and the fact that the patient lives in another state, they have had
limited contact over the past 10 years. However, he reports that the patient's
roommate has contacted him on several occasions because the patient "didn't
seem himself" and also following three minor fender-bender accidents. The
patient's son reports that he does not know if the patient is able to correctly
monitor his medications.*

Discussion

This vignette presents a conflict between a wish to respect the patient's ability
to make decisions independently (autonomy) and the desire to do something
that may be in the patient's best interest, to ensure his safety and well being
(beneficence). Determining which of these two general biomedical ethical
principles to endorse for this patient is of primary concern. The neuropsychologist's task is to determine how best to serve the needs of this patient
and the referral source.

Questions regarding a patient's cognitive functioning may be common
in many areas of the medical setting, including floors or units other than
those where neuropsychologists typically spend most of their time. In some
instances, an unexpected injury, disease process, or medication effect is
severe enough to temporarily impact the patient's ability to reason. In other
instances, a patient may be brought to the hospital for reasons relating to a
chronically progressive deterioration or a subacute exacerbation of a long-
standing illness that impacts mental functioning. Other patients may be hospitalized for increased disability presumably secondary to a severe psychiatric
disturbance. Therefore, the neuropsychologist may encounter consults for
recommendations surrounding competence and decision-making in a range
of contexts for various reasons. For example, since the medical community
requires that a patient possess adequate decision-making capacity as a basis
for informed consent before undergoing many medical procedures or treatments, a neuropsychology consult may be requested when there is concern
about a patient's decision-making capacity. Second, there is often concern
about the patient's safety following disposition from the medical setting (e.g.,
ability to live independently). Third, the physician may be under legal or ethi-

cal obligation to intervene when a patient refuses to comply with a treatment recommendation in the interest of the safety of the patient or the public (e.g., impaired capacity to drive, impaired capacity to practice as a professional).

While competency in the strictest sense is ultimately a legal issue, the reality is that clinicians often make decisions informally (Fowles & Fox, 1995), and physicians and other members of a multidisciplinary team are frequently called upon to provide the information that is used in a formal competency evaluation. In many respects, the neuropsychologist is an ideal member of a team of professionals who contributes to a competency evaluation. The most obvious reason is that competency in large part involves or is dependent upon cognitive functioning. The experienced neuropsychologist may be an invaluable resource in providing information about the nature and extent of deficits in different domains of cognition. Furthermore, he or she may be able to contribute substantially to difficult distinctions that the team must make between possible sources of cognitive impairment, including primary dementing processes, toxic/metabolic disturbances, adverse effects of medications, psychiatric disorders, etc. No less important, though perhaps less visible, is the armamentarium of skills that a neuropsychologist may draw upon as a result of his or her primary identity as psychologist. In what may become very emotionally charged and difficult decisions, such skills may include a sensitivity to group and family dynamics which may be contributing to the conflict, an awareness of psychological variables which may be influencing the patient's decision (e.g., unverbalized or less observable fear and anxiety aroused by the proposed treatment), and a keen ability to monitor the impact of a patient's decision or inability to make an informed decision upon the patient, the patient's family members, and members of the medical staff. However, precisely because such situations may be complex and demanding and because the consequences may be substantial, special consideration should be given to issues such as informed consent, boundaries of professional competency, assessment with special populations, and respect for a patient's values or beliefs when they differ from those of the medical staff or the neuropsychologist.

Informed Consent

> *APA Ethical Standard 1.07: "When psychologists provide assessment, evaluation...or other psychological services to an individual, they provide, using language that is reasonably understandable to the recipient of those services, appropriate information beforehand about the nature of such services and appropriate information later about results and conclusions."*

The issue of obtaining informed consent prior to assessment has recently emerged as a topic of interest and debate among neuropsychologists. In their commentary on the applications of the Ethics Code to neuropsychological

This has changed

assessment, Binder and Thompson (1995) report that "the current Ethics Code...does not require the patient to give informed consent for assessment." This is consistent with some literature in the medical arena where a 'sliding scale' approach is utilized; that is, non-invasive interventions or treatment procedures with limited probable risk and obvious benefit require less stringent application of consent, and assent alone is sufficient (Drane, 1984; Fellows, 1998; Venesy, 1994). However, other authors have reasoned that in any situation where psychological assessment or intervention is performed, some degree of informed consent is required. Although the APA ethical standard is somewhat non-specific about obtaining formal consent, the APA Standards for Educational and Psychological Testing 7.4 dictate that "informed consent should be obtained from test takers or their legal representatives before testing is done...When testing is not required, test takers should be informed concerning the testing process" (AERA, APA & NCME, 1999). In fact, the Canadian Code of Ethics for Psychologists (Canadian Psychological Association, 1991) specifies that the psychologist should "obtain informed consent from all independent and partially dependent persons for any psychological services provided to them" (Standard 1.13). From an ethical point of view, this recommendation is derived from concern for basic rights such as privacy, autonomy and self-determination. From an institutional point of view, documentation of formal informed consent for any procedure may be encouraged as a legal safeguard. From a practical point of view, a valid neuropsychological assessment demands willing participation and adequate effort.

Obtaining informed consent prior to performing an assessment on a patient who is questionably competent to make decisions about treatment interventions may seem ironic, and the process itself may be complex. Johnson-Greene et al. (1997) highlight some potential dilemmas surrounding the process of obtaining informed consent for neuropsychological testing which include a patient being less disclosing about psychosocial variables, premorbid history, and perceived cognitive deficits or, alternatively, refusing to participate in an assessment which may limit their decision or ability to participate in certain activities (see also Binder & Thompson, 1995). Furthermore, concern for the patient's understanding of the limits of confidentiality may arise when there is an increased likelihood of a formal competency evaluation where the information may be used by the courts against the wishes of the patient.

Examiner Boundaries of Competence

APA Ethical Standard 1.04a: "Psychologists provide services...only within the boundaries of their competence, based on their education, training, supervised experience, or appropriate professional service."
Standards for Educational and Psychological Testing 7.4: "Test users should determine from the manual or other reported evidence whether the construct being measured corresponds to the nature of the assessment that is intended."

The competency evaluation may be considered an activity that requires specific and supervised experience. Participating in a competency evaluation as a neuropsychologist not only requires experience in the formal administration of neuropsychological tests, but also may require the clinician to have specialized experience in the assessment of a particular age group (e.g., elderly patients), as well as adequate knowledge to anticipate and evaluate likely areas of impairment resulting from the patient's presumed medical or psychiatric condition. For example, in some situations, particularly involving elderly patients with multiple medical issues, disentangling acute or sub-acute delirium versus a dementia versus a delirium superimposed upon a progressive neurodegenerative condition may, on its own, be an extremely difficult process with a limited degree of certainty. In the above vignette, it may be entirely possible that the hallucinations and reported motor slowing that the patient experiences are a result of toxic/metabolic or medication-induced processes. Alternatively, it is also possible that the patient's hallucinations and motor symptoms are associated with a progressive long-standing process such as Lewy Body Dementia, which has gone undiagnosed due to lack of contact with family members who might otherwise report a decline in cognitive functioning.

Finally, the psychologist should be aware of the legal criteria that courts apply in competency judgments, relevant statutory definitions of competency, and a general knowledge of the legal procedures involved in a formal determination of competency. In the past, legal competency was considered to be an all-or-none capacity where an individual was either deemed competent or incompetent to make all types of decisions. Although modern law now favors increased patient involvement and the optimization of decision-making autonomy where possible, clinicians may still fail to recognize the need for situation-specific or capacity-specific abilities (Moye, 2000; Rosenthal, 1996). In the above scenario, the neuropsychologist must bear in mind that several aspects of competency are at issue and that each should be assessed as a separate domain of functioning. In addition to an assessment of the capacity to make medical treatment decisions, a number of possible other aspects of competence arise in the patient who is mentally ill or cognitively compromised. These may include, but are not limited to, capacities relating to driving, managing finances, living independently (including the ability to maintain adequate nutrition and self-care), managing administration of medication, caring for children, controlling a firearm, and continuing to function in an occupational capacity.

In addition to having a solid understanding of, and experience with, the intricacies of competency evaluations, the neuropsychologist should acknowledge that literature in this area is constantly evolving as more research is performed and as case law is created. The neuropsychologist should strive to stay abreast of empirically-based advances in the area, including a knowledge of the ecological validity and the limitations of different neuropsychological measures used for this assessment purpose. Section 2.02 of the APA Ethics

Code mandates that assessment techniques will be utilized "for purposes that are appropriate in light of the research on or evidence of the usefulness and proper application of the techniques."

Use of Assessment with Special Populations and In Special Contexts

Testing patients with sensory deficits or functional limitations associated with their medical conditions may pose some unique challenges for standardized administration and scoring as well as interpretation. For some tests, certain sensory abilities (e.g., eyesight or hearing) are prerequisite to a patient's ability to apprehend the stimuli. In other cases, motor limitations resulting from any number of causes (e.g., hemiparesis, movement disorder, arthritis, carpal tunnel syndrome, orthopedic injury) may preclude a patient from performing well on a standardized test. Furthermore, a number of situational variables may require further consideration, including time constraints of the patient and the clinician.

For example, delirium is, by definition, "a change in cognition... [that] develops over a short period of time (usually hours to days) and tends to fluctuate during the course of the day" (DSM-IV, American Psychiatric Association, 1994). Therefore, it is also likely that competence, which is dependent upon cognition, may fluctuate during the course of hospitalization, or even during the course of the evaluation. Numerous factors, such as the time of the day, medication effects, and metabolic changes, may be directly associated with these fluctuations. Even in cases where there is a dementing illness present, such physiological factors may be influential. Confusion may be further exacerbated at certain times of the day as a result of being in an unfamiliar or overstimulating environment. Finally, regardless of the presence or absence of delirium and/or dementia, dynamic factors such as pain and mood disturbance may exert a subtle influence and contribute to fluctuations in ability.

Respecting Others

> *APA Ethical Standard 1.09: "In their work-related activities, psychologists respect the rights of others to hold values, attitudes, and opinions that differ from their own."*
> *Canadian Code of Ethics for Psychologists II.10: Psychologists "evaluate how their own experiences, attitudes, culture, beliefs, values, social context, individual differences, and stresses influence their interactions with others, and integrate this awareness into all efforts to benefit and not harm others."*

Questions involving competency or decision-making capacity are most likely to arise when a patient refuses a medical intervention or aspects of a physician's treatment plan. Often in situations where decision-making capacity for an emergent or higher risk medical procedure or treatment is at stake, medical staff may become caught in a dual responsibility to the patient: they must use their knowledge and expertise to promote the well-being of the patient through advocating interventions with known or possible benefit, and they must also respect the patient's autonomy and right to govern what interventions will occur.

Given that the patient has adequate cognitive abilities to make an informed decision, the explanation of a patient's decision may be illuminating. For example, in the above vignette, the patient may have been able to accurately report the advice of the treatment team, the presumed risks and benefits of the surgery or the risks of not having the surgery, and the available treatment alternatives. He may have responded, "You know, I'm eighty years old and I'm pretty fragile at this point. They've told me that there is a chance that I may have complications during the surgery, including a stroke. I'm just not sure I'd survive it or that I'd want to spend the little time I've probably got left trying to recuperate. My time is coming soon anyway and I'd rather spend whatever time I've got left doing the few things that I look forward to anymore — not in some hospital. I'd rather have the aneurysm take me by surprise than worry about the surgery." Such a response may seem reasonable to many people from a quality of life perspective, particularly those who have worked extensively with older patients in a long-term care setting.

Situations may also arise where a competent patient refuses a treatment decision that may have imminent and serious or life-threatening consequences for that patient. Such examples may include patients who refuse treatment due to perceived decrements in quality of life (e.g., a diabetic patient who refuses an amputation or a cancer patient who refuses additional surgery or chemotherapy) or patients who refuse medical treatments that are at odds with religious beliefs or cultural practices (e.g., a Jehovah's witness who refuses a blood transfusion, a patient who elects 'spiritual healing' over antibiotics, or a patient who refuses to abort a child whose existence threatens her own life).

Recommendations

1. *Conduct a competency evaluation only if qualified to do so.* Determination of competency can potentially be a very complex process with life-altering ramifications. The neuropsychologist who agrees to address such a referral should be knowledgeable about the patient's medical and/or psychiatric illness as well as state laws and regulations pertaining to the areas of competency in question. The clinician should have an up-to-date knowledge of ecologically valid instruments that may be useful in determining competence in different areas. Recent publications may serve as useful guides for clinicians in medical settings who elect to become involved in competency decisions, including the Department of Veterans Affairs' *Assessment of Competency and Capacity of the Older Adult: A Practice Guide for Psychologists* (1997), Grisso and Appelbaum's *Assessing Competence to Consent to Treatment* (1998), and Sugarman's *20 Common Problems — Ethics in Primary Care (2000).*

2. *Develop a thorough understanding of the context of the evaluation.* The neuropsychologist must work closely with the health care team and, where applicable, the patient's family, to determine any critical events or mitigating circumstances which may have precipitated the referral. The neuropsychologist should have a good understanding of specific areas of skill and function that are at issue, the nature of the patient's current responsibilities, and the social context in which he or she operates. The initial stages of the assessment should include gathering and reviewing multiple sources of data, including relevant information pertaining to ethnic background, religious beliefs, family values, etc. In addition, past, recurrent, or present psychiatric conditions should be taken into consideration.

3. *Obtain appropriate informed consent prior to the evaluation.* It may be advisable to begin any interview with appropriate probes about the purpose of the evaluation and the patient's expectations about the assessment process and consequences (Tuokko & Hadjistavropoulos, 1998). However, particularly in situations such as the above, adequate explanation should be given regarding the purpose of the evaluation and limits of confidentiality, including the possibility that the records may be used for legal purposes, treatment decisions, or disposition planning (APA, 1998). Obtain written documentation of informed consent from the patient or the patient's legal guardian or proxy decision-maker. If this is not possible, assess the patient's assent and note the process in the report. Ultimately, however, the clinician should consider the underlying ethical principles reflected in the Canadian Code of Ethics for Psychologists, such as the need to "seek as full and active participation as possible from others in decisions which affect them" (1.11) and "recognize that informed consent is the result of a process of reaching an agreement to work collaboratively, rather than simply having a consent form signed" (1.16).

4. *Conduct an evaluation that is appropriately thorough but realistic given the constraints of the situation.* Neuropsychologists working with inpatients in medical settings are frequently expected to operate within a context that is, by nature, not conducive to eliciting a patient's optimal performance. Numerous factors make a standard assessment difficult or unrealistic, including the physiological and psychological impact of the patient's illness, adverse effects of medication, mobility constraints, competition with other staff for time with the patient, or the need for immediate information so that the treatment team can proceed. Nevertheless, if the neuropsychologist can work with the treatment team to reduce the impact of these variables, adequate assessment may be possible. Although most assessments will require evaluation of cognitive domains such as attention, memory, reasoning and problem-solving, language, visuospatial functioning and executive functioning, some areas may require more or less emphasis based upon the patient's environment and the specific area of competency in question.

5. *Recognize that competence is not a unitary concept.* Each ability being questioned must be addressed separately since a lack of competency in one

domain does not necessarily preclude other capacities. In addition to decision-making capacity for medical decisions or legal decisions which may require a formal competency evaluation, a physician may ask for 'routine' recommendations regarding other capacities such as driving, managing medications, continuing to live independently, executing an advanced directive, or consenting to research.

6. *Competence is not an all-or-nothing phenomenon.* Since the legal definition of competency involves an individual's general ability to function within and manage an environment (Venesy, 1994), formal neuropsychological testing should be supplemented with information about the patient's history of previous mistakes in certain areas as well as any evidence that a patient may be able to function in an adapted environment. The individual's awareness of his or her deficits may be an important determining factor in the ability to compensate for the deficits and reduce the degree to which safety is at risk. Educating the patient and the patient's family members about specific cognitive strengths and weaknesses may be crucial in recruiting their support and understanding. Encourage the family and the patient to strive for a balance between activity and safety, and help the system construct specific ways in which this can be done. For example, although a patient may not be capable of driving in all contexts (darkness, high-traffic areas, freeways, unfamiliar routes, long-distances, unaccompanied), there may be situations where more limited driving is appropriate (Green, 2000).

7. *Competence is not a static determination.* The patient should be medically stable at the time of each assessment. Careful attention should be paid to factors that may impede test performance on standardized tests but may not necessarily impair decision-making capacity. Reassessment of competency may be warranted in patients where there is an expected recovery curve or decline in functioning. In patients where decision-making capacity is at issue for an imminent invasive medical procedure, the competence assessment should include at least two periods of contact on two different days to ensure stability of the decision over time (Venesy, 1994).

8. *Respect human differences.* The values of the patient making the decision of whether or not to undergo a medical procedure may differ from the perspectives and perceived obligations held by other family members or members of the treatment team. The patient's own value system remains an important aspect of the assessment process and may require explicit discussion of issues such as autonomy, privacy, quality of life, etc. Determine whether a patient's decision is consistent with the patient's personal beliefs and goals. If a patient that appears otherwise competent from a cognitive point of view refuses a medical treatment with known benefit, attempt to determine whether this is consistent with the patient's long-held values. Carefully determine other psychological pressures that may be contributing to a patient's decision (e.g., financial concerns, not wanting to be perceived as a burden by the family, depression). Consider cul-

tural, religious, and ethnic differences and "respect and integrate as much as possible the opinions and wishes of others regarding decisions which affect them" (CCEP 1.12)
9. *Carefully document all aspects of the competency evaluation.* Particularly in evaluations of a patient's decision-making capacity for medical decisions, documentation may include the following: (a) the extent of the disclosure given to the patient regarding risks and benefits of the proposed medical procedure or treatment, (b) evidence of their understanding of that information, (c) other persons present for the discussion, and (d) any materials used to help address the issue (Venesy, 1994). Detailed documentation regarding specific recommendations and conclusions should be made.

Vignette 2

As a neuropsychologist in a large training hospital, Dr. Smith's responsibilities include teaching and supervising aspects of training for the interns and post-doctoral fellows in her program. After spending years building a collegial relationship with members of the neurology department, she finally arranges to provide each of her interns and fellows with the opportunity of rotating with the neurology residents and the attending neurologists on the inpatient units and specialty clinics. She believes this will be a very useful and dynamic exposure to the neurological examination, synthesis of neurodiagnostic test data, diagnosis, and treatment of a wide range of diseases with neurologic manifestations. Following each patient's consent, her trainees are allowed to observe all aspects of interview and history taking, medical chart review, physical and mental status examination, as well as participate in supervisory rounding and discussion of the cases. Her trainees uniformly agree that this is an invaluable experience not only in terms of learning about brain–behavior relationships, but also in their exposure to and respect for particular areas of expertise in their medical colleagues. After several months, a neurologist who has been working with Dr. Smith's trainees approaches Dr. Smith and states that she has several residents who are particularly interested in pursuing behavioral neurology or geriatric medicine following residency. She requests that her residents be granted an opportunity to observe neuropsychological examinations with patients so that they may learn more about the measures used in cognitive testing and how different score profiles relate to different neurological disorders.

Discussion

Initially, such a scenario may seem a welcome opportunity to enhance collaborative training and research possibilities as well as to foster a network of mutual respect among specialty areas treating patients with cognitive difficulties. In many neuropsychology training programs based in medical centers, trainees are required to develop an understanding of central nervous system-based compromise and neurodiagnostic data which may include, among other things, direct exposure to the neurologic examination, neuroradiologic

techniques, EEG, and basic laboratory findings. Presumably, such experience is intended to help training neuropsychologists synthesize patient data,
adequately consider diagnostic possibilities, and identify possible pathologic
behaviors that may require referral to neurology or another medical specialty. Indeed, such experience may be required to establish competence as
a neuropsychologist and to promote the welfare of patients. Furthermore,
such experience exemplifies the spirit of ethical principles and standards.
For example, the Canadian Code of Ethics for Psychologists requires that
psychologists "demonstrate appropriate respect for the knowledge, insight,
experience, and expertise of others" (1.1) and emphasizes the need to "make
[psychologists] aware of the knowledge and skills of other disciplines (e.g.,
law, medicine) and advise the use of such knowledge and skills, where relevant to the benefit of others" (II.19).

Similarly, the above scenario could be viewed as an opportunity to educate
resident physicians about the potential benefit of obtaining neuropsychological testing on future patients. Such education may enable physicians to better
determine appropriate neuropsychology referral and to more clearly define
referral questions. This education is consistent with recent APA guidelines
that direct psychologists to "educate health care professionals who may be
administering mental status examinations or psychological screening tools
regarding the psychometric properties of these instruments and their clinical
utility for particular applications" (APA, 1998). The neurologist's request
seemingly yields potential benefit for the institution, the physician, the neuropsychologist, and ultimately, a number of future patients. However, in
anticipating other possible consequences of such a scenario, there are several
ethical issues that deserve thoughtful consideration, including test security,
user competence, and third-party observation.

Test Security

> APA Ethical Standard 2.10: "Psychologists make reasonable efforts
> to maintain the integrity and security of tests and other assessment
> techniques."
> Standards for Educational and Psychological Testing 15.7: "Test users
> should protect the security of test materials. Those who have test mate-
> rials under their control should take all steps necessary to assure that
> only individuals with a legitimate need for access to test materials are
> able to attain such access."
> Canadian Code of Ethics for Psychologists IV.9: Psychologists "pro-
> tect the skills, knowledge, and interpretations of psychology from
> being misused, used incompetently, or made useless (e.g., loss of secu-
> rity of assessment techniques) by others."

The issue of test security has been the subject of some concern for neuropsychologists, arising predominantly from experience in the forensic setting. One

of the primary issues at stake is the potential distortion of a patient's test scores through prior knowledge of, or exposure to, the testing material or by coaching from an attorney. Admittedly, it is not likely that other health professionals within a medical setting would intentionally attempt to coach patients or give them information about the testing with the intent to artificially impact an evaluation. However, it is conceivable that health professionals that are not well familiarized with the testing process and standardization techniques may inadvertently give information about a testing procedure which relies heavily upon novelty and lack of familiarity (e.g., "they'll show you some cards that you have to sort according to color, shape, or amount and then see if you can switch the concept to see if you possess the mental flexibility necessary for driving") or begin to incorporate standardized test questions in their own examinations (e.g., using questions from the Information, Comprehension or Similarities subtests of the Wechsler intelligence scales). It is also possible that well-meaning non-psychologist members of a cognitive rehabilitation team may attempt to utilize unsecured test materials to 'practice' or 'improve' cognitive skills. While absent of any ill intent, such instances may also unfortunately jeopardize the validity and integrity of standardized tests (The National Academy of Neuropsychology Policy and Planning Committee, 2000a).

User Competence

> APA Ethical Standard 2.02b: "Psychologists refrain from misuse of assessment techniques, interventions, results, and interpretations and take reasonable steps to prevent others from misusing the information these techniques provide."
> APA Ethical Standard 2.06: "Psychologists do not promote the use of psychological assessment techniques by unqualified persons."

Also germane to the above scenario are concerns for restricting the use of test material by unqualified persons and, by extension, reducing the potential for misinterpretation of test data. A primary issue for the neuropsychologist relates to user competence, namely, that after limited exposure to testing methods and expected patterns of difficulty in different neurological or psychiatric disorders, another health professional may believe that he or she is qualified to understand and interpret individual test scores or patterns of deficits. An example of such might include the psychiatry resident that hastily concludes that a patient "must be schizophrenic" after viewing an MMPI-2 profile sheet in the patient's file with an elevated scale 8. Of similar concern is the neurologist who concludes that his 56-year-old patient who is a zoology professor demonstrates "no impairment" with respect to verbal fluency since the patient is "easily able to name about 10 animals within a minute's time." Lack of understanding regarding standardization, measurement theory, and normative data as well as lack of experience with the assessment tools and their specific application to patients in special populations may prove fertile ground for misuse of neuropsychology's psychometric assessment techniques.

Third-party observation

The issue of third-party observation has been a topic of some controversy in recent years. While much of the literature on third-party observation in neuropsychological assessment specifically targets concerns arising during examination for forensic purposes, the principle issues that have been raised may again extend to a more general arena. These may be applicable not only to non-psychologist trainees, as in the above vignette, but may also apply to other situations often encountered in the medical setting involving 'benign' third-parties, such as family members, hospital roommates, and other hospital staff. Limited empirical data exist pertaining to the presence of such parties, so the effects of these observers is not well understood (McSweeny et al., 1998). While there are certainly instances where the presence of such individuals is warranted or unavoidable, there are three reasons why this matter may deserve deliberate clinical judgment on a case-by-case basis.

The first concern is that the introduction of an additional person may increase the potential for distraction, particularly in individuals that already possess a compromised ability to selectively focus or sustain attention. The Standards for Educational and Psychological Testing (AERA, APA, & NCME, 1999) clearly call for a testing environment "of reasonable comfort and with minimal distractions." Second, there is the possibility of misleading assessment results secondary to a "social facilitation effect" or the potential impact of performing differently as a result of being observed by others (McCaffrey et al., 1996; The National Academy of Neuropsychology Policy and Planning Committee, 2000b). The implication of social facilitation originates from a series of observations that subjects typically exhibit better performance on tasks that are easy or well-learned and decreased performance on tasks that are difficult or novel. McCaffrey et al. (1996) caution that neither cognitive compromise nor immaturity make one immune from the impact of social facilitation, and that the use of one-way mirrors and videotaping may also elicit the effect. Finally, the presence of a third party may represent a 'non-standardized' aspect of the test administration that may also jeopardize the validity of the assessment techniques (McCaffrey et al., 1996). Standards for Educational and Psychological Testing direct that in usual applications examiners should carefully follow the standardized administration and scoring procedures established by the test publisher. This issue is specifically addressed in recent manuals of the Wechsler tests, such as the WAIS-III, which specifies that "as a rule, no one other than you and the examinee should be in the room during the testing" (Wechsler, 1997, p. 29).

For those who might argue that the above issues regarding third party presence should extend to neuropsychology trainees, results of a recent survey of NAN members suggest that many neuropsychologists (70% of 817 respondents) believe that it is acceptable to have a trained observer present during neuropsychological examinations (Sewick et al., 1999). By having such a trained observer, such as a neuropsychologist, neuropsychology trainee, or trained technician as an observer, test security would remain intact. However, there exists a need for further studies to determine if the presence of such an observer would have a substantial effect on the performance of the patient. While this study supports the presence of neuropsychology trainees in the examination room with their supervisors, an astute neuropsychologist will likely be able to utilize a number of opportunities to both formally and informally educate his or her non-psychology colleagues and patients' family members about neuropsychological testing without compromising the welfare of any individual patient or violating principles such as test security and user competence.

Recommendations

1. *Make reasonable efforts to minimize influences that may adversely affect the validity of a patient's assessment.* The psychologist's primary obligation is to the patient being evaluated. He or she should strive to provide accurate and standardized administration of the assessment tools in order to achieve valid conclusions about cognitive functioning. Thoughtful consideration should be given to the potential for increased distraction and social facilitation effects, regardless of whether the observer is a non-psychologist trainee, interpreter, family member, hospital roommate, or other health care professional. Obviously, situations where patients may be particularly prone to the distracting influence of the observer should be avoided. The National Academy of Neuropsychology (NAN) Policy and Planning Committee concedes that there may be non-forensic training situations where a neutral third party observer is entirely appropriate (i.e., when students or other professionals in psychology observe testing as part of their formal education or a parent remains in the testing room during a child's evaluation to act as a calming influence). The NAN Policy and Planning Committee has recommended that neuropsychologists "strive to minimize all influences that may compromise accuracy of assessment and should make every effort to exclude observers from the evaluation" (The National Academy of Neuropsychology Policy and Planning Committee, 2000b).

2. *Consider and explicitly address important training differences before instructing non-psychologists about neuropsychological testing.* Just as difficulties may arise for psychologists who are new to the adversarial approach of attorneys, differences in training or diagnostic/treatment approaches between other health professionals (physicians, nurses, speech therapists, occupational therapists, etc.) and psychologists may also give rise to unanticipated difficulties. The neuropsychologist may need to explain that neuropsychological testing may be more prone to influence

of psychological or social effects than many aspects of physical examination. An explicit discussion involving issues of standardization procedures, user competence, test security, and confidentiality is also advisable. The neuropsychologist may offer other teaching alternatives in lieu of observing an actual patient examination and may consider using simulated test questions or general explanation on concepts rather than the actual test items.

3. *When the neuropsychologist elects to train others about neuropsychological assessment, the importance of expertise and appropriate referral should be reinforced.* Recent APA guidelines suggest that although education of health care professionals regarding simple psychometric screening instruments is encouraged, "education is also provided about the differences between brief screening examinations and more comprehensive psychological or neuropsychological evaluations" (APA, 1998).

4. *Include a section in the report where potentially confounding factors affecting the test performance are identified and their presumed impact is explained.* If there is a third party present for any aspect of the evaluation, it has been recommended that both the behavior of the third party and the presumed impact of the third party upon the patient be noted (McCaffrey et al., 1996). In addition, neuropsychologists working on medical units will likely be familiar with the challenges that such environments pose in terms of bedside testing and unavoidable interruptions by hospital staff, and the potential impact of such interruptions should also be reported.

Vignette 3

Mrs. Jones, a 67-year-old divorced woman, is referred for a neuropsychological evaluation in the context of an 18-month history of cognitive decline of insidious onset. The patient comes to the appointment accompanied by her daughter. The patient reports that she was referred for the testing by her primary care physician "to find out what's wrong." The patient reports that she has had great difficulty with her spelling and handwriting and notes that "her hand moves a lot." She also reports some memory problems, word-finding difficulties, and difficulties performing some more complex household chores. Her medical history is significant only for osteoporosis, and she takes Fosamax and vitamin supplements. Recent MRI indicates mild generalized atrophy in relation to her age, more so on the left hemisphere than on the right. She reports a history of depressive episodes although she has never been formally treated for depression. She is clearly very distressed by her difficulties and tells you that she "would rather die" than be diagnosed with "dementia." Although her daughter recognizes that her mother has significant cognitive problems, she asks that you not tell her mother that she has 'dementia' because it generates enormous anxiety for the patient.

During the course of the evaluation, the patient evidences a mild alien limb syndrome and intermittent myoclonic jerking in her right arm. In addition, the patient appears notably dyspraxic with her dominant (right) hand. Her neuropsychological examination reveals severe difficulties with verbal memory, sustained attention, confrontation naming, verbal fluency, and executive functioning. In addition, she evidences decreased reaction time and motor functioning, particularly with her right hand. The neuropsychologist suspects that she may have corticobasal ganglionic degeneration (CBGD) and recommends that she be referred to neurology for further evaluation.

Immediately following the patient's neurological evaluation, the neurologist tells the patient that her diagnosis is CBGD — a form of progressive dementia for which there is no treatment, and that based on the results of neuropsychological testing, she is already severely cognitively impaired. The following week the patient's daughter calls, and angrily accuses the neuropsychologist of "making her mother so depressed that she won't do anything at all." She states that she is upset since she specifically told the neuropsychologist that the term 'dementia' would create further difficulties for her mother. She explains that the neurologist appeared very hurried in the examination and recommended that her mother look up information about the disease on the Internet. The patient's daughter further explains that she went to the website herself, and the condition was described as one that is "relentlessly progresses, with probable involvement of all extremities and increasingly severe cognitive deterioration until death ensues."

Discussion

Disclosure and communicating assessment results

> *APA Ethical Standard 2.09: "Psychologists ensure that an explanation of the results is provided using language that is reasonably understandable to the person assessed or to another legally authorized person on behalf of the client."*

The ethics code does not explicitly address the issue of disclosure of diagnosis and prognosis per se, although neuropsychological testing is often utilized to contribute information in answering these questions. There are many psychologists who might argue that there may be situations where informing a patient of his or her diagnosis is neither necessary nor particularly beneficial for the patient (e.g., diagnosis of Borderline Personality Disorder) as long as the patient is given appropriate general information about the evaluation results. Similarly, there may be good reasons to avoid using diagnostic labels in communicating assessment results to a child or any patient with a limited ability to appreciate the diagnostic term. It has been argued that potentially stigmatizing diagnoses (e.g., brain dysfunction or dementia) may result in loss of self-esteem and/or an altered perception and treatment of an individual by family, friends, and employers to the detriment of the patient (Binder & Thompson, 1995). However, in most situations it would be clearly unethical not to provide a competent adult patient both with information relating to the presumed etiology of their cognitive deficits as well as any treatment recommendations; in most cases, the patient and family members clearly benefit from such information. Difficulties may arise, however, when the clinician must deliver particularly upsetting information to an ill-prepared audience. Medicine approaches the issue by stating, "In general, disclosure to patients is a fundamental ethical requirement. However, society recognizes the 'therapeutic privilege,' which is an exemption from *detailed* [emphasis added] disclosure when such disclosure has a high likelihood of causing serious and irreversible harm to the patient. On balance, this privilege should be interpreted narrowly; invoking it too broadly can undermine the entire concept of informed consent" (American College of Physicians, 1992). Providing patients and their family members with enough information to adequately understand and cope with present cognitive and behavioral difficulties, as well as anticipate future decline or residual cognitive difficulties, is perhaps the most important aspect of the evaluation from the neuropsychologist's point of view. However, the neuropsychological examination may be part of a series of tests required for diagnosis, and providing feedback to a patient in the middle of this process may not always be an easy task (Green 2000; Tuokko & Hadjistavropoulos, 1998).

In some situations, results from the neuropsychological examination are provided by the professional who requested the evaluation (e.g., neurologist, geriatric internal medicine doctor) in the context of other information that is used to make a diagnosis. Although the physician ideally gives the patient adequate information in terms that he or she can understand and remains sensitive to the patient's responses, the reality is that this may be difficult for some physicians to do for various reasons. This may be particularly true in communicating about neuropsychological test results when the physician's own familiarity with testing is rather limited. The Ethics Code implies that the psychologist is ultimately responsible for ensuring that the patient receives adequate feedback about the results of psychological testing; however, it appears that the clinician must use his or her own judgment in determining exactly what that "explanation" entails and the setting in which that information is communicated.

Recommendations
1. *Discuss the setting in which results will be communicated.* Consider the relative advantages or disadvantages to having other family members present for the feedback session. If someone other than the neuropsychologist will be communicating the results, identify for the patient (or the appropriate caregiver) the name and role of that professional. Offer the patient or caregiver the opportunity to contact the neuropsychologist directly if there are further questions or if clarification is needed.
2. *Consider the benefits of a formal feedback session*, particularly when a patient or caregiver will be given information that is potentially upsetting. Aspects of the feedback session may include a review of the purpose of

testing, a basic explanation that the tests assess cognitive and behavioral skills that are associated with different brain areas and measure the functionality and integrity of the brain, and an explanation of strengths and weaknesses. If appropriate, information regarding diagnosis or etiology may follow. Finally, recommendations intended to help the patient and family members manage the present and prepare for the future should be considered. However, the clinician should remain sensitive to both verbal and non-verbal information that indicates distress or confusion and should carefully track the impact of the information upon the patient.

3. *Consider whether or not it may be appropriate to provide the patient with a copy of the written report.* Some neuropsychologists perceive several distinct practical advantages in providing the patient (or the patient's guardian) with a copy of the written report and encouraging him or her to keep the information in a file with other medical information. This practice may make sense in situations where a large number of subsequent treatment providers outside the neuropsychologist's institution may benefit from the information and treatment recommendations contained in a report which the patient can readily provide at the time he or she is seen in the future. However, other neuropsychologists raise concern about the potential for information contained in written reports to be confusing or disturbing to patients. It is, of course, always advisable to construct written reports carefully and in a manner that decreases the potential for confusion or stigmatization by any potential audience. It may also be wise to discuss information contained in the report prior to releasing it to the patient in an attempt to minimize confusion. Providing a non-technical summary of the findings and recommendations has also been recommended by other neuropsychologists (Binder & Thompson, 1995).

Vignette 4

A 48-year-old male patient is referred for neuropsychological evaluation as part of his neurologic work-up to characterize the nature and extent of his reported cognitive difficulties. The patient reports a two-year history of headaches, fatigue, short-term memory loss, and difficulty with concentration. In a collateral interview with the patient's wife, she reports that she noticed some cognitive changes and personality changes that corresponded to three very stressful events that occurred at about the same time. The first was a brief exposure to a toxic agent at his place of work after which the patient became intensely dissatisfied with the way the situation was handled and left his job. His wife further indicates that just prior to this incident, she discovered that she was pregnant. Since the couple never planned on having children, this was not only unexpected, but also unwelcome. Finally, she reports that the patient's mother died suddenly and that the patient "seemed to have a lot of unfinished business from his childhood."

When you ask the patient how old his daughter is, he begins to cry and states, "I love her and we just couldn't have had an abortion, but I wish that we'd never had children." His wife notes that he continues to have difficulty adjusting to the presence of the baby and frequently becomes agitated and "verbally abusive" toward the child. She also reports that they have had some relationship difficulties since she reported an episode of domestic violence eight months ago.

When you ask if the patient is intending to pursue worker's compensation or any litigation against his former employer, the patient reports that he has not decided. The patient's personality testing reveals substantial depression and cognitive testing is significant only for mild difficulties with attention/ concentration and immediate recall. The neuropsychologist concludes that the cognitive deficits are relatively mild and likely related to severe depression, particularly since the patient's exposure to the toxic agent is not likely to produce the patient's reported difficulties.

Discussion

Assuming that the neuropsychologist is certain that the child is not in immediate danger of being physically harmed, he or she is left to decide how much of the information obtained in the interview is appropriate to include in a report that will be accessible not only to the referring physician, but also to his insurance company and, in this case, to any health professional with access to the patient's computerized record. In addition, information contained in the interview notes and formal report may be discoverable to a potential attorney for use to the detriment of the patient at a later point in time. One could argue that specific information may substantiate a claim that mood-related influences are causing or exacerbating the patient's difficulties with memory and concentration. Furthermore, one could argue that documenting certain aspects of the above information is also likely to result in timely referral and reinforcement for much needed psychiatric/psychological services. However, one can also imagine destructive consequences resulting from the inclusion of detailed information about issues that are deemed sensitive by the patient, the patient's family members, or other individuals within a patient's social context.

Privacy and Confidentiality

APA Ethical Standard 5.03(a): "In order to minimize intrusions on privacy, psychologists include in written and oral reports, consultations, and the like, only information which is germane to the purpose for which the communication is made."
CCEP Ethical Standard 1.32: Psychologists "explore and collect only that information which is germane to the purpose(s) for which consent has been obtained."
APA Ethical Standard 5.05(a): "Psychologists disclose confidential information without the consent of the individual only as mandated by law, or where permitted by law for a valid purpose, such as (1)

to provide needed professional services to the patient..., (2) to obtain appropriate professional consultations,(3) to protect the patient or client or others from harm..."

In most situations, it is relatively easy to omit detailed information that is not relevant to the purpose of the consult. However, there are occasionally more complex situations where the neuropsychologist may believe that sensitive information is potentially important to the immediate well being or continuing care of the patient, whether it relates directly to the initial referral question or not. Furthermore, there may be situations in which cognitive difficulties could be attributable to sensitive factors that were not identified by the referral source, such as repeated severe domestic violence, an inherited genetic disorder, HIV/AIDS, or illicit substance abuse.

Computerized Records

APA Ethical Standard 5.04: "Psychologists maintain appropriate confidentiality in creating, storing, accessing, transferring, and disposing of records under their control, whether these are written, automated, or in any other medium."

Maintaining confidentiality has become increasingly difficult in medical settings where records are computerized and electronically processed. New advances in technology have brought enormous benefits in being able to access patient information, particularly in situations where evaluation and treatment of a patient is shared between numerous medical professionals and institutions. However, it also brings increased risks and may make it difficult to ensure that certain information be provided only to the referral source or on the basis of 'need to know.' While it is unlikely that any health professional with appropriate access to a patient's record would intentionally disclose or distort sensitive information, situations may arise where information contained in a report is more prone to misinterpretation when viewed by a professional treating a patient for an unrelated issue (and without an understanding of the referral context) or by a professional who briefly read only a portion of the report.

Recommendations
1. *Keep patients informed.* Routinely inform all patients of the limits of confidentiality, remind them of the referral source, and alert them that others within the medical system will likely have access to the information. Discuss any concerns that they may have about this.
2. *Be aware of the potential for litigation.* Attempt to anticipate instances where there is an increased likelihood that the report may be used for worker's compensation, disability, or litigation purposes and inform the patient of any further limits of confidentiality associated with these processes.

3. *Minimize intrusions on privacy.* Include in reports only information that is pertinent to the referral question or ongoing treatment, particularly when information is sensitive. "Be acutely aware of the need for discretion in the recording and communication of information, in order that the information not be interpreted or used to the detriment of others" (CCEP II.28).
4. *Keep in mind the audience that you are writing for.* When the audience is likely to be a physician who reads only the concluding paragraph of your report three minutes before seeing the patient, write in a manner that is likely to decrease the possibility of misinterpretation.
5. *Recognize differences in reporting guidelines for psychologists and physicians.* Recognize that although reporting laws for physicians and psychologists may have several common areas of overlap (i.e., abuse of a child or vulnerable person, risk of self-harm, risk of harm to another specific, identifiable person, etc.) there may be areas where physicians have different legal or institutional obligations than psychologists to respond to reported information. For example, state laws may require a physician to report some situations involving suspected domestic violence, habitual narcotic use (Rutberg, 1999), or medical conditions which preclude driving.
6. *Safeguard records.* Take appropriate steps to ensure that information is appropriately transferred, stored, and disposed of, particularly in electronic systems where the difference between one patient's file and another patient's file is a single keystroke.

Vignette 5

A neuropsychologist receives a referral from a geriatrics specialist to evaluate a 60-year-old man with a long history of alcohol abuse and declining general health. In addition, there is a question of possible dementia. The referral requests that the neuropsychologist make a determination about the etiology and extent of the cognitive disturbance. The patient's first and dominant language is Chinese, although the patient has lived in the United States for 30 years. He reports some formal schooling in his childhood, although he does not remember at exactly what age he left school. The medical examination and laboratory testing that was done upon admission indicated that the patient had very poorly controlled diabetes and possible liver disease; however, because the patient reports that he "just didn't go to doctors," little else is known about his medical history. The patient's wife has passed away. He has recently moved in with a daughter in the area who reports that her father has been exhibiting mood lability and periods of confusion in addition to difficulties with his vision and balance. She states that she believes her father's command of the English language has never been very good. She cannot say whether his receptive and expressive faculties have decreased in English or Chinese since she does not speak Chinese and has not had contact with him for many years.

Discussion

Scores generated by formal neuropsychological testing can never be diagnostic in isolation. Rather, the ability to interpret those scores within the individual's context is the very reason that neuropsychological testing is useful at all in the process of delineating diagnostic possibilities. In fact, establishing the context of the individual's performance on neuropsychological testing is required in order to say anything at all about the nature of the patient's deficits, the extent of the difficulties, the possible causes of those difficulties, or ways in which those difficulties can be remedied. Therefore, establishing an accurate context is fundamental before proceeding toward any interpretation.

In addition to variables which are always essential to the interpretation of test data (e.g., age, gender, level of education, fluency in the testing language, previous level of functioning), the neuropsychologist must attempt to ascertain the timing and nature of initial symptoms, the progression of cognitive difficulties, and any other variables in the medical history which could contribute to a patient's cognitive decline. The neuropsychologist should also attempt to gather information from the medical records, the patient, and collateral sources about any alterations in a patient's personality, behavior, or ability to function in his or her environment.

It is not uncommon to encounter situations in the medical setting where one or more of these contextual variables is obscured to varying degrees. The above situation presents numerous difficulties since the neuropsychologist is not able to obtain reliable background information relating to the course of the cognitive difficulties or the patient's premorbid level of functioning. Furthermore, there is limited data on past and current medical conditions that may potentially impact the patient's functioning. For example, without further information, it is difficult to establish where the vision and balance difficulties are attributable to possible complications of diabetes (i.e., retinopathy, diabetic neuropathy) versus another etiology impacting the central nervous system. Perhaps most worthy of consideration, however, are the potential issues raised by age, language, and cultural variables.

Use of Tests with Special Populations

APA Ethical Standard 2.04: "Psychologists who perform interventions or administer, score, interpret, or use assessment techniques are familiar with the reliability, validation, and related standardization or outcome studies of, and proper applications and uses of the techniques they use... Psychologists attempt to identify situations in which particular interventions or assessment techniques or norms may not be applicable or may require adjustment in the interpretation because of factors such as individuals' gender, age, race, ethnicity, national origin, religion, sexual orientation, disability, language or socioeconomic status."

There are obvious difficulties posed by administering language-dependent tests to non-English speaking patients or patients with very visible "handicaps". However, Artiola i Fortuny and Mullaney (1998) have also questioned the quality of neuropsychological testing with patients who have an incomplete command of the English language. Furthermore, they advocate caution in the interpretation of the test scores of a patient with limited formal education.

Using valid norms

> *Standards for Educational and Psychological Testing 13.1: "For non-native English speakers or for speakers of some dialects of English, testing should be designed to minimize threats to test reliability and validity that may arise from English differences."*

Normative data is a fundamental piece of the context within which the data must be interpreted. In keeping with the ethical obligation to understand the psychometric properties of the assessment tools that they utilize, psychologists should be aware of the standardization sample and the reliability and validity of the measure being employed. Serious errors may occur when a clinician makes assumptions about aspects of cognitive functioning for an individual who is not fairly equipped from a linguistic perspective. In addition, errors can also result from comparing non-linguistic aspects of cognition in those with little or no formal education to a standardization sample comprised of the more mainstream U.S. population (Artiola i Fortuny & Mullaney, 1998). Furthermore, there are many known cognitive changes that occur with aging, and the clinician should be aware of suitable norms when administering neuropsychological tests to older adults (APA, 1998; Tuokko & Hadjistavropoulos, 1998).

Limitations of Testing Results

> *APA Ethical Standard 2.05: "When interpreting assessment results, including automated interpretations, psychologists take into account the various test factors and characteristics of the person being assessed that might affect the psychologist's judgments or reduce the accuracy of their interpretations. They indicate any significant reservations that they have about the accuracy or limitations of their interpretations."*

Since it may be easy for a clinician with limited experience in working with non-English-speaking patients, the elderly, or individuals with little formal education to over- or under-attribute pathology, the neuropsychologist must consider and utilize all appropriate avenues to provide an accurate assessment. This optimally includes referral to a qualified neuropsychologist with specialized training in these areas. Introducing any potential confounds through the use of interpreters, unpublished or non-standardized alternate versions of tests, or norms that are not compatible with the age, education, and language characteristics of the patient should be avoided if possible or utilized only with appropriate caution and explicit caveats. Furthermore, it is advisable to determine whether doing so allows the clinician to remain within the appropriate boundaries of personal professional competence and the standards of practice set by the field. In cases where there are conceivable limitations on the neuropsychological findings, diagnosis and treatment recommendations are best made through a convergence of multiple sources of data, with increased reliance upon more objective medical findings. Artiola i Fortuny and Mullaney (1998) conclude that if the existence or severity of an insult cannot be based on 'verifiable evidence,' neuropsychologists should avoid making diagnostic statements altogether.

Recommendations

1. *Develop and maintain competency.* Establish a competency in general information that is relevant to patient populations that you work with.
2. *Practice only within your competencies.* Decline or refer out if you are not well trained with a certain population.
3. *Know the patient.* Balance information and assumptions relevant to a group or population with information specific to the individual. Conduct thorough interviews with patients and/or family members who are accurate historians. Attempt to obtain information that is necessary in creating an appropriate context specific to the patient.
4. *Acknowledge limitations of the evaluation or results.* Factors that limit the clinician's ability to establish a context will ultimately limit the certainty with which conclusions can be drawn. This is particularly true in situations where the neuropsychologist is asked to provide or assist with diagnosis or prognosis. The neuropsychologist is admonished to "acknowledge the limitations of [the neuropsychologist's] knowledge, methods, findings, interventions, and views" (CCEP III.8). Document factors that limit findings from neuropsychological testing and explicitly state areas where conclusions are to be considered tentative.

Conclusions

Clinical neuropsychologists provide medical facilities with a critical service through their ability to evaluate and treat patients with known or suspected neurological disorders. However, numerous situations may arise in medical settings that challenge the neuropsychologist's ability to practice within ethical parameters. Some of the conditions that provide richness in clinical practice, such as interdisciplinary interaction, training opportunities, and the potential to work with an array of interesting patients, also serve as potential ethical pitfalls. Awareness of these pitfalls and ways to avoid or resolve them is the key to sustaining an ethical practice.

The purpose of this chapter was to present some of the common ethical challenges encountered in medical settings and ways to successfully resolve them. Through exposure to vignettes and the ethical issues they raise, the neuropsychologist is better able to anticipate ethical dilemmas, identify them when they occur, and follow an established sequence of steps to resolve them. While situations will inevitably arise that are unique and challenge even seasoned, ethically-informed clinicians to arrive at a consensus regarding the optimal course of action, familiarity with the collective experiences found in writings such as this may increase the confidence with which one pursues the best course of action for the patient and the profession.

References

American College of Physicians (1992). American College of Physicians ethics manual — third edition. *Annals of Internal Medicine, 117,* 947-960.

American Educational Research Association, American Psychological Association, National Council on Measurement in Education (1999). *Standards for educational and psychological testing.* Washington, DC: American Educational Research Association.

American Psychiatric Association (1994). *Diagnostic and statistical manual of mental disorders (DSM-IV).* Washington, DC: American Psychiatric Association.

American Psychological Association (1992). *Ethical principles of psychologists and code of conduct.* Washington, DC: American Psychological Association.

American Psychological Association (1998). Guidelines for the evaluation of dementia and age-related cognitive decline. *American Psychologist, 53,* 1298-1303.

Artiola i Fortuny, L., & Mullaney, H. A. (1998). Assessing patients whose language you do not know: Can the absurd be ethical? *The Clinical Neuropsychologist, 12,* 113-126.

Beauchamp, T. L., & Childress, J. F. (1989). *Principles of biomedical ethics, 3 ed.* New York: Oxford University Press.

Binder, L. M., & Thompson, L. L. (1995). The ethics code and neuropsychological assessment practices. *Archives of Clinical Neuropsychology, 10,* 27-46.

Canadian Psychological Association (1991). *The Canadian code of ethics for psychologists, Revised.* Old Chelsea, Quebec: Canadian Psychological Association.

Department of Veterans Affairs (1997). *Assessment of competency and capacity of the older adult: A practice guideline for psychologists* (Publication No. PB97-147904). Milwaukee, WI: National Center for Cost Containment.

Drane, J. F. (1984). Competency to give an informed consent: A model for making clinical assessment. *Journal of the American Medical Association, 252,* 925-927.

Fellows, L. K. (1998). Competency and consent in dementia. *Journal of the American Geriatric Society, 46,* 922-926.

Fowles, G. P., & Fox, B. A. (1995). Competency to consent to treatment and informed consent in neurobehavioral rehabilitation. *The Clinical Neuropsychologist, 9,* 251-257.

Green, J. (2000). *Neuropsychological evaluation of the older adult: A clinician's guidebook.* New York: Academic Press.

Grisso, T., & Appelbaum, P. (1998). *Assessing competence to consent to treatment: A guide for physicians and other health professionals.* New York: Oxford University Press.

Johnson-Greene, D., Hardy-Morais, C., Adams, K. M., Hardy, C., & Bergloff, P. (1997). Informed consent and neuropsychological assessment: Ethical considerations and proposed guidelines. *The Clinical Neuropsychologist, 11,* 454-460.

McCaffrey, R. J., Fisher, J. M., Gold, B. A., & Lynch, J. K. (1996). Presence of third parties during neuropsychological evaluation: Who is evaluating whom? *The Clinical Neuropsychologist, 10*(4), 435-449.

McSweeny, A. J., Becker, B., Naugle, R. I., Snow, W. G., Binder, L. M., & Thompson, L. L. (1998). Ethical issues related to the presence of third party observers in clinical neuropsychological evaluations. *The Clinical Neuropsychologist, 12,* 552-559.

Moye, J. (2000). Ethical issues. In V. Molinari (Ed.), *Professional psychology in long term care* (pp. 329-248). Long Island City, NY: Hatherleigh Press.

National Academy of Neuropsychology Policy and Planning Committee (2000a). Test security: Official position statement of the National Academy of Neuropsychology. *Archives of Clinical Neuropsychology, 15,* 383-386.

National Academy of Neuropsychology Policy and Planning Committee (2000b). Presence of third party observers during neuropsychological testing: Official statement of the National Academy of Neuropsychology. *Archives of Clinical Neuropsychology, 15,* 379-380.

Rosenthal, M. (1996). Ethical issues in the evaluation of competence in persons with acquired brain injuries. *NeuroRehabilitation, 6,* 113-212.

Rutberg, M. P. (1999). Medical-legal issues facing neurologists. *Neurologic Clinics, 17,* 307-313.

Sewick, B.G., Blase, J.J., & Besecker, T. (1999). Third party observers in neuropsychological testing: A 1999 survey of NAN members [abstract]. *Archives of Clinical Neuropsychology, 14,* 753-754.

Sugarman, J. (2000). *20 common problems — Ethics in primary care.* New York: McGraw Hill.

Tuokko, H., & Hadjistavropoulos, T. (1998). *An assessment guide to geriatric neuropsychology.* Mahwah, NJ: Lawrence Erlbaum Associates.

Venesy, B. A. (1994). A clinician's guide to decision-making and ethically sound medical decisions. *American Journal of Physical Medicine and Rehabilitation, 73,* 219-226.

Wechsler, D. (1997). *WAIS-III administration and scoring manual.* San Antonio: The Psychological Corporation.

Chapter 11

ETHICAL DECISION MAKING WITH INDIVIDUALS OF DIVERSE ETHNIC, CULTURAL, AND LINGUISTIC BACKGROUNDS

Josette G. Harris

Introduction

Neuropsychologists are increasingly becoming sensitized to the unique considerations that should attend assessment, treatment, and research with individuals from diverse ethnic, cultural, and linguistic backgrounds. Yet, many professionals remain uncertain about whether or how to provide services to diverse individuals in a manner that will be beneficial and ethical. One way in which neuropsychologists attempt to guide their decision making is by consulting professional guidelines or rules regarding what they ought to do when confronted with the complex dilemmas of providing services to and conducting research with individuals whose culture or language they do not share. The American Psychological Association (APA) Ethical Principles of Psychologists and Code of Conduct (APA, 1992), hereinafter referred to as the Ethics Code, is one such resource that neuropsychologists utilize. However, some professionals attempt to rely upon the Ethics Code as a source for *definitive* direction. This unnecessarily narrow and restrictive approach may inadvertently result in the very type of unethical behavior that neuropsychologists intended to avoid in the first place by seeking guidance from the Ethics Code. A more beneficial approach is to expand one's understanding of the Ethics Code and to broaden one's approach to ethical decision making. This can be accomplished through the identification and examination of philosophical ethical principles, which can assist neuropsychologists in making informed choices for courses of action in dealing with situations that raise moral and ethical concerns.

All individuals have a preliminary reaction to ethical situations that reflects their initial perceptions of the situation, the totality of their prior learning, moral beliefs and values, and experience with moral reasoning, referred to as ordinary moral judgment (Beauchamp & Childress, 1983). One's moral judgment operates rather automatically and successfully in most day to day interactions and situations. However, one's own personal and cultural experiences shape moral judgment, such that each individual may view moral obligations differently from others. Consequently, ordinary moral judgment may be insufficient for guiding decisions and actions in a professional situation. The Ethics Code provides additional guidance by setting forth a set of values that are presumably shared by all psychologists, including neuropsychologists, in their roles as professionals and scientists (APA, 1992). This is not to say that personal values or moral beliefs are irrelevant to ethical decision making, but rather that these are supplementary to the Ethics Code's values and rules (APA, 1992).

Aspects of the Ethics Code have been criticized as being inadequate in specificity and open to interpretation (e.g., Artiola i Fortuny & Mullaney, 1998). However, the purpose of the Ethics Code is not to anticipate every conceivable ethical dilemma and to definitively instruct neuropsychologists about how to respond in every case. Rather, it provides expectations of psychologists for standards of conduct and allows for, and even encourages, interpretation in order to facilitate the best ethical outcome. In fact, the Preamble and general Principles of the Code are considered to be "aspirational goals to guide psychologists toward the highest ideals of psychology" (APA, 1992; p. 1598). They "should be considered by psychologists in arriving at an ethical course of action and may be considered by ethics bodies in interpreting the Ethical Standards" (APA, 1992; p. 1598). One of the strengths of the Ethics Code in facilitating decision-making about assessment, treatment, and research with culturally and linguistically diverse individuals lies in these aspirational goals and their interpretation. An even higher level of analysis that should guide ethical decision-making is derived from an understanding and appreciation of the philosophical ethical concepts underlying the Ethics Code (Beauchamp & Childress, 1994; Kitchener, 2000). These fundamental concepts can further facilitate the interpretation of the Ethical Standards of the Code in the individual case and assist the neuropsychologist in resolving complex dilemmas in their work with diverse individuals.

Ethical Principles

The 'common morality,' in its broadest sense, is a social institution with a code of learnable norms of human conduct (Beauchamp & Childress, 1994). A professional code of ethics is a statement of the common morality of the members of a given profession. The philosophical ethical principles of *respect for autonomy*, *non-maleficence*, *beneficence*, and *justice* originate in the common morality and represent the common ethical norms (Beauchamp & Childress, 1994) neuropsychologists share in carrying out their professional roles. These principles should be considered prima facie obligations, meaning they are binding unless overridden or outweighed by competing moral obligations (Kitchener, 2000). Identifying and balancing these principles is necessary in analyzing individual ethical dilemmas and in seeking the best outcome. Following is a brief description of each principle and a discussion of the relationship of the philosophical principles to the Ethics Code, in particular those standards relevant to providing services to and conducting research with individuals of diverse ethnic, cultural and linguistic backgrounds.

Respect for Autonomy

Autonomy is defined as self-determination. To recognize autonomy is to recognize the individual's right to self-governance without imposing limitations, unless an individual threatens the autonomy of others. It includes the right to develop values and make decisions, but also presumes a fundamental respect for the rights of others to make choices, even when the beliefs of others differ from one's own (Kitchener, 2000).

> APA Ethical Standard 1.09 *Respecting Others*: "In their work-related activities, psychologists respect the rights of others to hold values, attitudes, and opinions that differ from their own."
> APA Ethical Standard 1.07 *Describing the Nature and Results of Psychological Services*: "When psychologists provide assessment, evaluation, treatment, counseling, supervision, teaching, consultation, research, or other psychological services to an individual, a group, or an organization, they provide, using language that is reasonably understandable to the recipient of those services, appropriate information beforehand about the nature of such services and appropriate information later about results and conclusions."
> APA Ethical Standard 4.02 *Informed Consent to Therapy*: "(a) Psychologists obtain appropriate informed consent to therapy or related procedures, using language that is reasonably understandable to participants...."
> APA Ethical Standard 6.10 *Research Responsibilities*: "Prior to conducting research (except research involving only anonymous surveys, naturalistic observations, or similar research), psychologists enter into an agreement with participants that clarifies the nature of the research and the responsibilities of each party."

APA Ethical Standard 6.11 *Informed Consent to Research*: "(a) Psychologists use language that is reasonably understandable to research participants in obtaining their appropriate informed consent... (b) Using language that is reasonably understandable to participants, psychologists inform participants of the nature of the research..."

To respect an individual's autonomy is to respect their autonomous decision-making and to respect their rights to confidentiality, privacy, and truthfulness. Informed consent is typically addressed in the context of respect for autonomy. An individual gives informed consent if he or she is competent to act, receives a thorough disclosure, comprehends the disclosure, acts voluntarily and consents to the intervention or participation (Beauchamp & Childress, 1994).

Typically, an autonomous person is considered competent to make decisions. However, if an autonomous person does not understand the purpose of taking part in a neuropsychological evaluation, treatment, or research, and does not comprehend the planned methods, available alternatives, and the potential consequences of participating, the individual may not be competent to make a decision in that specific instance. Lack of understanding may be a linguistic issue, as in the case of an individual who does not possess sufficient comprehension of the language in which the consent process is undertaken. There may also be a constraint on understanding imposed by cultural context. An example of this is an individual who is adjusting to a new culture and lacks relevant information, such as the limits of confidentiality in some forensic situations, for deciding whether to consent to an evaluation. It is therefore necessary to undertake the consent process in a language well understood by the individual, which is typically that individual's primary language. It is further necessary to take additional steps to ensure that relevant information has been thoroughly disclosed to the individual, even though such information may seem self evident in many other cases.

By virtue of identifying with a different culture or adhering to specific cultural values and norms, an individual may display problem-solving strategies or decision-making processes that vary substantially from the neuropsychologist's expectations. Without careful analysis and efforts to understand the cultural values and decision-making considerations relevant to the patient or subject, his or her decisions might appear to reflect poor judgment. Even worse, without an understanding of the expectations for acquiring and displaying certain cognitive skills and abilities within a given culture, a neuropsychologist may inappropriately conclude that a patient is not competent. The neuropsychologist may inadvertently make decisions about the best intervention or treatment for an individual based upon the professional's own cultural perspective, experience with other patients, and beliefs about what is necessary to function adequately in the larger society within which the neuropsychologist lives and functions. Although perhaps well intentioned, it is unacceptable to act in a paternalistic fashion when the individual for whom decisions are being made is indeed autonomous and has a right to make decisions for himself or herself.

The care with which disclosure must be provided to patients and research participants from diverse backgrounds cannot be underestimated. Although assessment is a familiar component of most formal educational systems in the U.S., individuals from other cultures may not have any prior experience with testing or assessment, or the manner in which results are to be utilized. The amount of information can be overwhelming when an individual is attempting to understand both the process of assessment and the relationship of an evaluation to placement or other treatment decisions. Particularly when alterations are to be made in administration of tests or interpretation of results, the limitations of the assessment and resulting conclusions must be clearly explained to the examinee and alternatives identified as part of the consent process. A neuropsychologist who lacks knowledge of an individual's culture and background may have difficulty adequately apprising an individual of the impact of an intervention on the individual's functioning within his or her familial and other social systems. This may also be true in the identification of risks and benefits to participants in research.

Individuals who have recently immigrated and are in the process of acculturating to a new social and political environment may not realize that consent is voluntary. For example, the parents of a newly immigrated child referred for neuropsychological evaluation may not realize that they can decline the evaluation without jeopardizing the child's continued access to education or health care. Consent, when given by an individual who does not fully understand the information provided, or whose consent is not truly voluntary, cannot be regarded as properly authorized and valid.

Educating oneself regarding another individual's cultural and social perspective, values, and decision making processes and priorities, can take the form of formal academic instruction and continuing education. However, some of the most valuable resources for learning are other professionals and laypersons in the community who provide health, educational, financial, religious or other services and support to diverse populations. Taking steps to familiarize oneself with another culture by experiencing that culture firsthand is another avenue to education.

Non-maleficence and Beneficence
Non-maleficence is most clearly restated as "do no harm" and includes restraint from inflicting intentional harm as well as restraint from actions that risk harm to others (Kitchener, 2000). Beneficence includes prevention of harm, removal of harm, and promoting good, but equally important is the duty to balance possible goods against the possible harms of an action (Beauchamp & Childress, 1994). The principles of beneficence and nonmaleficence are reflected in the primary goal of the Ethics Code which is "welfare and protection of the individuals and groups with whom psychologists work" (APA, 1992; p. 1597). The principle of beneficence is generally thought to

be more demanding than the principle of nonmaleficence because it requires positive steps to help others (Beauchamp & Childress, 1983). The Preamble of the Ethics Code clearly reflects the principle of beneficence in describing the goal of psychology as the application of knowledge pragmatically to improve the condition of both the individual and society. Standards particularly relevant to working with diverse ethnic and linguistic populations are discussed below.

> APA Ethical Standard 1.04(a) *Boundaries of Competence*: "Psychologists provide services, teach, and conduct research only within the boundaries of their competence, based on their education, training, supervised experience, or appropriate professional experience."
> APA Ethical Standard 1.05 *Maintaining Expertise*: "Psychologists who engage in assessment, therapy, teaching, research, organizational consulting, or other professional activities maintain a reasonable level of awareness of current scientific and professional information in their fields of activity, and undertake ongoing efforts to maintain competence in the skills they use."
> APA Ethical Standard 1.06 *Basis for Scientific and Professional Judgments*: "Psychologists rely on scientifically and professionally derived knowledge when making scientific or professional judgments or when engaging in scholarly or professional endeavors."

Knowledge of the literature regarding individual and group differences, including ethnic, cultural and linguistic considerations, in the assessment of cognitive and neuropsychological functions is essential to maintaining expertise as a neuropsychologist and drawing sound conclusions. This is true regardless of whether or not one specializes in the assessment of ethnically or linguistically diverse populations. Some neuropsychologists may view the literature on cross cultural assessment as irrelevant to their work, particularly when dealing with an English speaking clinical or research subject. However, cultural variables that might impact assessment may be operating even when linguistic issues are not readily apparent. For example, individuals from other cultures where testing is not emphasized, may find the assessment situation highly stressful and intrusive. They may be ill prepared to participate in a neuropsychological evaluation, and this will likely impact both the process and the outcome of assessment. Neuropsychologists may be misled by what appears to be reasonably good conversational skills in an individual who speaks English as a second language and fail to provide an assessment in the language that would facilitate optimal performance. It may also be naively assumed that the same approaches and methods of assessment used with native English speakers can be used without qualification when testing individuals who speak English as a second language. A good example of this is a digit span task in which digit stimuli are individually presented to the subject. This method of digit presentation is typically unfamiliar to Spanish speakers who group numbers, such as phone numbers, when presenting them to others (e.g., three hundred fifteen, forty-six ten rather than three-one-five-four-six-one-zero). Cultural nuances, as well as linguistic idiosyncrasies, and the interaction of these variables need to be understood and addressed in the assessment (Harris et al., 2001).

> APA Ethical Standard 1.14 *Avoiding Harm*: "Psychologists take reasonable steps to avoid harming their patients or clients, research participants, students and others with whom they work, and to minimize harm where it is foreseeable and unavoidable."
>
> APA Ethical Standard 1.20 *Consultations and Referrals*: "(a) Psychologists arrange for appropriate consultations and referrals based principally on the best interests of their patients or clients, with appropriate consent, and subject to other relevant considerations, including applicable law and contractual obligations."
>
> APA Ethical Standard 1.22 *Delegation to and Supervision of Subordinates*: "(a) Psychologists delegate to their employees, supervisees, and research assistants only those responsibilities that such persons can reasonably be expected to perform competently, on the basis of their education, training, or experience, either independently or with the level of supervisions being provided. (b) Psychologists provide proper training and supervision to their employees or supervisees and take reasonable steps to see that such persons perform services responsibly, competently, and ethically. (c) If institutional policies, procedures, or practices prevent fulfillment of this obligation, psychologists attempt to modify their role or to correct the situation to the extent feasible."

When a neuropsychologist weighs the potential benefits against the potential harms of conducting an assessment with an individual whose language he or she does not speak or whose culture is not shared, the definition of harm must be carefully considered. The harms of misdiagnosing and understating or overstating a deficit are perhaps the harms most readily identified by neuropsychologists and are all relevant considerations. However, harm may also be done if an individual is not evaluated at all and perhaps misses the opportunity to participate in rehabilitation, or is referred to a psychologist who shares culture and language with the individual, but who has no expertise in neuropsychological assessment or neurobehavioral principles and makes erroneous assumptions and conclusions.

Assessing potential benefits and harms of conducting an evaluation begins with the referral question and an analysis of the needs of each individual case, the neuropsychologist's skills, and available resources. For example, a monolingual English-speaking neuropsychologist might be asked to evaluate a recently immigrated, monolingual Spanish speaker, who is charged with a criminal offense. The neuropsychologist may conclude that the risk of harms, including loss of the individual's civil rights, far outweighs the potential benefits of accepting the referral for evaluation of the individual's competency to stand trial and to participate in his own defense. This conclusion may remain even when an alternative neuropsychologist cannot be identified to whom the individual can be referred. However, the same neuropsychologist may determine that the benefits to the individual outweigh the harms when asked to evaluate an adult Spanish-speaker's cognitive and academic skills for the purpose of making recommendations for pursuit of higher education in English following a mild head injury. In the latter case, the neuropsychologist may have access to a Spanish-speaking colleague, with experience in educational assessment of non-English speakers, who would be available for consultation and close supervision to help address the referral question and to identify factors relevant to the assessment process and interpretation of results. In both of these cases, however, if another more qualified, competent neuropsychologist is available to undertake the evaluation in the examinee's preferred language, it is typically in the best interest of the examinee to refer him or her to the available neuropsychologist. For those who choose to assess the individuals referred to them, it is incumbent upon those providers to obtain consultation, additional training, and supervision to ensure that reasonable steps have been taken to avoid harming the patient.

Often, interpreters are used to facilitate a neuropsychological assessment. However, most interpreters used by neuropsychologists working with Spanish speaking patients have little or no formal training in neuropsychology (Echemendia et al., 1997). Indeed, the neuropsychologist is responsible for training the interpreter, particularly regarding the goals of assessment and the process of evaluation. The interpreter should in essence be functioning as a trained psychometrician. A psychology or special education graduate student, who speaks the language of the examinee and who has training in assessment, may be a useful and appropriate resource for test administration. While it is acceptable to utilize an interpreter to translate from one language to another during the course of a clinical or medical history interview, it is inappropriate to utilize an interpreter to translate the neuropsychologist's verbatim test instructions and test items from one language to another. Acceptable translated and adapted measures (i.e., those with demonstrated score reliability and validity) for the language and culture of the individual examinee must be identified beforehand and the interpreter/psychometrician must be familiar with the instructions and proper administration. Professional consultation can be obtained by contacting neuropsychological membership organizations, such as the National Academy of Neuropsychology, which maintain a database of neuropsychologists who conduct assessments in designated languages. Additional education and training may take the form of attendance at continuing education workshops and independent study. Suggested readings concerning cultural and linguistic considerations in cognitive and neuropsychological assessment, particularly with African American and Latino populations are provided in the Appendix.

APA Ethical Standard 1.23 *Documentation of Professional and Scientific Work:* "(a) Psychologists appropriately document their professional and scientific work in order to facilitate provision of services later by them or by other professionals, to ensure accountability, and to meet other requirements of institutions or the law."

This standard holds particular importance for the assessment of culturally and/or linguistically diverse individuals. The precise manner in which the assessment was conducted, including whether the measures used were published or were translated/adapted by the neuropsychologist or designee, and any alterations in test administration should be documented. In order to provide sufficient detail about the assessment, it is essential to specify the language in which tests were administered, whether an interpreter was used, and the language(s) in which the examinee responded and was instructed to respond. Further, the precise source of norms or other basis for interpreting results, including clinical judgment, should be documented. Cases in which individuals, in particular children, will likely undergo repeat evaluations deserve special attention in order to reduce error variance that has little to do with changes in the individual's cognitive status. While it may be necessary to make adjustments in the administration and interpretation of tests when working with diverse individuals or groups, the legitimacy and impact of these adjustments must be fully evaluated beforehand and documented (see also Ethical Standard 2.04c).

APA Ethical Standard 2.01 *Evaluation, Diagnosis, and Interventions in Professional Context:* "(b) Psychologists' assessments, recommendations, reports, and psychological diagnostic or evaluative statements are based on information and techniques (including personal interviews of the individual when appropriate) sufficient to provide appropriate substantiation for their findings."

APA Ethical Standard 2.02 *Competence and Appropriate Use of Assessments and Interventions:* "(a) Psychologists who develop, administer, score, interpret, or use psychological assessment techniques, interviews, tests, or instruments do so in a manner and for purposes that are appropriate in light of the research on or evidence of the usefulness and proper application of the techniques.

(b) Psychologists refrain from misuse of assessment techniques, interventions, results, and interpretations and take reasonable steps to prevent others from misusing the information these techniques provide...."

APA Ethical Standard 2.04 *Use of Assessment in General and With Special Populations:* "(a) Psychologists who perform interventions or administer, score, interpret, or use assessment techniques are familiar with the reliability, validation, and related standardization or outcome studies of, and proper applications and uses of, the techniques they use. (b) Psychologists recognize limits to the certainty with which diagnoses, judgments, or predictions can be made about individuals. (c) Psychologists attempt to identify situations in which particular interventions or assessment techniques or norms may not be applicable or may require adjustment in administration or interpretation because of factors such as individuals' gender, age, race, ethnicity, national origin, religion, sexual orientation, disability, language, or socioeconomic status."

APA Ethical Standard 2.05 *Interpreting Assessment Results:* "When interpreting assessment results, including automated interpretations, psychologists take into account the various test factors and characteristics of the person being assessed that might affect psychologists' judgments or reduce the accuracy of their interpretations. They indicate any significant reservations they have about the accuracy or limitations of their interpretations."

These standards address the misuse of techniques, the interpretation of results, and the steps necessary to prevent others from misusing the information these techniques yield. If a test has not been demonstrated to measure the same construct in a different population than that within which the test was developed and normed, then it may very well be invalid for use with the new population. The reliability of a test may be compromised when sources of 'error' related to language and culture are introduced. A direct translation of a stimulus item may change the difficulty level of the item, change its intent, or make it irrelevant. For example, directly translating into another language an item intended to screen for central dysarthria makes little sense. To take another example, administering tests of oral verbal fluency in another language without considering the frequency of occurrence of words beginning with specific letters or the effects of spoken word length on word generation will compromise accurate interpretation of results (Harris et al., 2001, subm. Jacobs et al., 1997; Kempler et al., 1998).

Other standards adopted by professional psychological organizations, including APA, are not part of the Ethics Code but can be considered in defining competent practice. Two documents that are of particular relevance to this discussion are the Guidelines for Providers of Services to Ethnic, Linguistic, and Culturally Diverse Populations (APA, 1991) and the International Standards and Guidelines for Adapting Educational and Psychological Tests (Hambleton, 1994; Van de Vijver & Hambleton, 1996).

The International Test Commission has set forth guidelines (Van de Vijver & Hambleton, 1996) for translating and adapting tests, which are summarized as follows: 1) the test translation methods must minimize or avoid construct, method, and item bias; 2) a thorough knowledge and understanding of the language and culture into which a test will be translated must guide the translation process; 3) the materials, methods, and techniques of administration must be familiar to the target cultural group; and 4) the ecological validity of the test must be statistically documented to assure accurate score interpretation. Test translation is also addressed in the *Standards for educational and psychological testing* (American Educational Research Association, American Psychological Association, & National Council on Measurement in Education, 1999). One particular standard, Standard 9.7, states: "When a test is translated from one language to another, the methods used in establishing the adequacy of the translation should be described, and empirical and logical evidence should be provided for score reliability and the validity of the translated test's score inferences for the users intended in the linguistic groups to be tested" (p. 99).

Factors unique to an individual such as status as a new immigrant or health and nutrition related factors must all be identified and understood so that results are interpreted in their proper context. For example, newly immigrated individuals learning to speak English as a second language may show initial steep learning curves regarding both language acquisition and acculturation that may have a bearing on interpretation of test results, particularly in the case of repeat testing several months later. This is an important consideration, for example, in the evaluation of professional athletes whose postconcussional cognitive performance is compared with baseline neuropsychological data to determine the extent of any cognitive injury and readiness to safely return to professional play. Assessment of verbal and language related functions may be particularly challenging under such circumstances and may require novel approaches, such as use of nonsense verbal stimuli to assess memory functions and repeat 'baseline' assessment during early second language acquisition.

Justice
Although each of the foregoing ethical principles is of critical importance in analyzing the dilemmas and challenges of neuropsychological assessment, treatment, and research with ethnically and linguistically diverse individuals, justice is the principle with which neuropsychologists may struggle most. There are those who find the task of providing neuropsychological services to individuals from cultures or linguistic backgrounds different than their own so daunting that without hesitation they decline to assess or treat these individuals. Paradoxically, it may be the very intention of neuropsychologists to avoid unethical behavior in working with diverse patients and subjects that ultimately may be unjust and unethical.

Justice, broadly defined, is fairness. Common to all theories of justice is a minimal principle first set forth by Aristotle which holds that equals are to be treated equally and unequals unequally (Beauchamp & Childress, 1983). The principle of formal justice holds that "no person should be treated unequally, despite all differences with other persons, until it has been shown that there is a difference between them relevant to the treatment at stake" (Beauchamp & Childress, 1983, p. 187). The principle of justice is clearly reflected in the following standards.

> APA Ethical Standard 1.08 *Human Differences*: "Where differences of age, gender, race, ethnicity, national origin, religion, sexual orientation, disability, language, or socioeconomic status significantly affect psychologists' work concerning particular individuals or groups, psychologists obtain the training, experience, consultation, or supervision necessary to ensure the competence of their services, or they make appropriate referrals."
>
> APA Ethical Standard 1.10 *Nondiscrimination*: "In their work-related activities, psychologists do not engage in unfair discrimination based on age, gender, race, ethnicity, national origin, religion, sexual orientation, disability, socioeconomic status, or any basis proscribed by law."

Material principles are principles that identify the relevant properties individuals must possess to qualify for a particular distribution of goods or services and include, for example, justice based upon need, effort, or merit (Beauchamp & Childress, 1994). When distinctions are made between classes of persons who are actually similar in relevant respects, the decision to treat them differently may be unjust. Ethnicity is an irrelevant property and it would be considered discriminatory to use ethnicity to distribute services because ethnic differences between individuals are introduced by chance and it is a property for which individuals are not responsible (Beauchamp & Childress, 1994). Other examples of irrelevant properties include IQ, disease, and native language.

Both a libertarian theory of justice, emphasizing fair or equal access to care, and an egalitarian theory, emphasizing equal distribution of health care, would support the argument that ethnicity, culture, and/or language should not exclude an individual from accessing or obtaining a neuropsychological evaluation or participating in research. If an alternative provider, with the appropriate linguistic skills, cultural knowledge, and neuropsychological expertise is not identifiable to whom a referral can be made, the principal of justice could support the argument that the neuropsychologist should acquire the training, consultation, and/or supervision to provide services to diverse individuals. This assumes, of course, that the principles of beneficence and nonmaleficence have also been considered. Taking the argument a step further, a former chairperson of the APA Ethics Committee, Karen Kitchener, is of the opinion that psychologists ought to have a commitment to fairness that goes beyond what is expected of the ordinary person. She believes that psychologists should work to ensure that individuals have access to a decent minimum of services and argues that if one's social environment has resulted in a situation wherein that person does not receive a fair share of life's benefits, then the social system is an unjust one. Further, she maintains that individuals who are committed to contributing to the welfare of others (psychologists) have a social responsibility to change that unjust system (Kitchener, 2000).

Nothing in these theories of justice would preclude a neuropsychologist from providing services using methods different from those ordinarily used, to take into account factors such as an individual's unique culture or language. Relevant methods may include restructuring one's approach to assessment to include more direct observation, collateral interviews, and less reliance upon standardized methods of assessment. On the other hand, most conceptions of justice would not provide a justification for denying services to culturally or linguistically different individuals.

Civil Rights law and institutional regulations also are intended to ensure access by ethnically and linguistically diverse individuals to services and treatment. Mandates and guidelines, such as those contained in the National Standards for Culturally and Linguistically Appropriate Services (CLAS) in Health Care, published by the U.S. Department of Health and Human Services Office of Minority Health (2000) are primarily directed at health care organizations but are also intended for use by professional organizations, quality review and peer review organizations. They may be considered in determining whether services have been offered and provided in a nondiscriminatory or just manner. The standards are intended to ensure that all people entering the health care system receive "equitable and effective treatment in a culturally and linguistically appropriate manner" (p. 80865). The CLAS Standards obligate health care entities receiving Federal assistance to ensure language assistance services, including access to bilingual staff and interpretative services at all points of contact. Further, health care organizations must assure the competence of language assistance by interpreters and bilingual staff. The CLAS standards stipulate that minor children should never be used as interpreters for their parents when the parent(s) are identified as the patient.

Neuropsychologists who practice in areas or settings where a significant proportion of the population does not share the provider's language or culture may perceive few options for addressing the needs of these individuals. Educating oneself in order to gain skills and competence to provide services to diverse individuals is a critical component in addressing inadequacies in access to care and services. Taking an active role in educating others, for example those in health care, education, and legal arenas, is also necessary in order to address the existing disparities.

Conclusion

There is no reason to expect that the ethical dilemmas in neuropsychological practice and research with diverse individuals will be any less complex than those faced in day to day living within a diverse society. Conflicts will arise that require depth of moral reasoning and ethical analysis, and careful weighing of competing needs and rights. A position has been presented here based upon work by Beauchamp and Childress (1994) and Kitchener (1984; 2000) that challenges neuropsychologists to think more broadly about the ethical considerations in providing or refusing to provide services to diverse individuals. The Ethics Code itself will not definitively instruct neuropsychologists on the course of action or inaction to take with ethnically, culturally, or linguistically diverse individuals. Neuropsychologists should not rely upon a single rule or standard in decision making any more than they should hasten to apply a single rule, observation, or test score in clinical decision making and research.

The value of the Ethics Code lies in its lack of specificity and its openness to interpretation. Each situation must be considered carefully, by consulting the Ethics Code and other relevant professional standards, but also balancing the foundational ethical principles as each potential option is considered (Kitchener, 2000). The general Principles of the Ethics Code reflect the four foundational ethical principles and derived rules, and make it clear that the psychologist is responsible to "weigh the welfare and rights of their patients or clients..." (APA, 1992; p. 1600). In other words, these Principles may come into conflict with one another, as may the foundational principles upon which they are based. Each situation must be evaluated separately and each option considered independently and thoroughly.

The assumption that the needs of ethnically and linguistically diverse individuals will automatically be met by referring these individuals to neuropsychologists who speak their same languages and share their cultural backgrounds is unrealistic. Practically speaking, there simply are not enough providers to match the multitude of cultures and languages. An ethical outcome does not automatically follow from declining to accept these cases or by referring to psychologists who share language and culture with the individuals they are asked to assess and treat.

The tools for meeting the ethical challenges of cross cultural assessment lie in achievement of competence and expertise (American Psychological Association, 1992; Canadian Psychological Association, 1991), by acculturation of providers to the individual cultures of those they serve, and expansion of the empirical knowledge base regarding cross cultural and cross linguistic issues in assessment (Harris et al., subm.). A broad view of the Ethics Code, and an understanding of the philosophical ethical principles that underlie the Ethics Code and represent the common morality of psychologists, are the surest guides for resolving the ethical dilemmas that arise in neuropsychological practice and research with diverse individuals.

References

American Education Research Association, American Psychological Association, & National Council on Measurement in Education (1999). *The standards for educational and psychological testing.* Washington, DC: American Psychological Association.

American Psychological Association (1991). *Guidelines for providers of services to ethnic, linguistic, and culturally diverse populations.* Washington, DC: American Psychological Association.

American Psychological Association (1992). Ethical principles of psychologists and code of conduct. *American Psychologist, 47,* 1597-1611.

Artiola i Fortuny, L., & Mullaney, H.A. (1998). Assessing patients whose language you do not know: Can the absurd be ethical? *The Clinical Neuropsychologist, 12,* 113-126.

Beauchamp, T.L., & Childress, J.F. (1983). *Principles of biomedical ethics,* 2nd ed. New York, NY: Oxford University Press.

Beauchamp, T.L., & Childress, J.F. (1994). *Principles of biomedical ethics,* 4th ed. New York, NY: Oxford University Press.

Canadian Psychological Association (1991). *Canadian code of ethics for psychologists.* Ottawa, Ontario: Canadian Psychological Association.

Echemendía, R., Harris, J.G., Congett, S.M., Diaz, L.M., & Puente, A.E. (1997). Neuropsychological training and practices with Hispanics: A national survey. *The Clinical Neuropsychologist, 11(3),* 229-243.

Hambleton, R.K. (1994). Guidelines for adapting educational and psychological tests: A progress report. *European Journal of Psychological Assessment, 10,* 229-244.

Harris, J.G., Echemendía, R., Ardila, A., & Rosselli, M. (2001). Cross-cultural cognitive and neuropsychological assessment. In J.J.W. Andrews, Saklofske, D., & Janzen, H. (Eds.), *Handbook of psychoeducational assessment. Ability, achievement, and behavioral assessment* (pp. 391–414). San Diego, CA: Academic Press.

Harris, J.G., Echemendía, R., Ardila, A., & Rosselli, M. (subm.). *Cognitive and neuropsychological assessment in Hispanic populations: A Review.*

Jacobs, D.M., Sano, M., Albert, S., Schofield, P., Dooneief, G., & Stern, Y. (1997). Cross-cultural neuropsychological assessment: A comparison of randomly selected, demographically matched cohorts of English- and Spanish-speaking older adults. *Journal of Clinical and Experimental Neuropsychology, 19,* 331-339.

Kempler, D., Teng, E.L., Dick, M., Taussig, I.M., & Davis, D.S. (1998). The effects of age, education, and ethnicity on verbal fluency. *Journal of the International Neuropsychological Society, 4,* 531-538.

Kitchener, K.S.(1984). Intuition, critical evaluation and ethical principles: The foundation for ethical decisions in counseling psychology. *The Counseling Psychologist, 12,* 43-55.

Kitchener, K.S. (2000). *Foundations of ethical practice, research, and teaching in psychology.* Mahwah, New Jersey: Lawrence Erlbaum Associates.

United States Department of Health and Human Services Office of Minority Health (2000). Assuring cultural competence in health care: Recommendations for national standards and an outcomes-focused research agenda. *Federal Register, 65,* 80865-80879.

Van de Vijver, F., & Hambleton, R.K. (1996). Translating tests: Some practical guidelines. *European Psychologist, 1,* 89-99.

Appendix A — Suggested Readings

Acevedo, A., Loewenstein, D.A., Barker, W.W., Harwood, D.G, Luis, C., Bravo, M., Hurwitz, D.A., Aguero, H., Greenfield, L., & Duara, R. (2000). Category fluency test: Normative data for English- and Spanish-speaking elderly. *Journal of the International Neuropsychological Society, 6,* 760-769.

American Education Research Association, American Psychological Association, & National Council on Measurement in Education (1999). *The standards for educational and psychological testing.* Washington, DC: American Educational Research Association.

American Psychological Association (1991). *Guidelines for providers of services to ethnic, linguistic, and culturally diverse populations.* Washington, DC: American Psychological Association.

Ardila, A., & Rosselli, M. (1989). Neuropsychological characteristics of normal aging. *Developmental Neuropsychology, 5,* 307-320.

Ardila, A., & Rosselli, M. (1994). Development of language, memory and visuospatial abilities in 5- to 12-year-old children using a neuropsychological battery. *Developmental Neuropsychology, 10,* 97-116.

Ardila, A., Rosselli, M., & Puente, A. (1994). *Neuropsychological evaluation of the Spanish speaker.* New York: Plenum Press.

Ardila, A., Rosselli, M., & Rosas, P. (1989). Neuropsychological assessment in illiterates: Visuospatial and memory abilities. *Brain and Cognition, 11,* 147-166.

Arnold, B.R., Cuellar, I., & Guzman, N. (1998). Statistical and clinical evaluation of the Mattis Dementia Rating Scale — Spanish adaptation: An initial investigation. *Journal of Gerontology: Psychological Sciences, 53,* 364-369.

Artiola i Fortuny, L., Heaton, R.K., & Hermosillo, D. (1998). Neuropsychological comparisons of Spanish-speaking participants from the U.S.–Mexico border region versus Spain. *Journal of the International Neuropsychological Society, 4,* 363-379.

Echemendía, R.J., Harris, J.G., Congett, S.M., Diaz, L.M., & Puente, A.E. (1997). Neuropsychological training and practices with Hispanics: A national survey. *The Clinical Neuropsychologist, 11,* 229-243.

Evans, J.D., Miller, S.W., Byrd, D.A., & Heaton, R.K. (2000). Cross-cultural applications of the Halstead-Reitan Batteries. In E. Fletcher-Janzen, T.L. Strickland, & C. R. Reynolds (Eds.), *Handbook of cross-cultural neuropsychology: Critical issues in neuropsychology* (pp. 287–303). New York, NY: Kluwer Academic/Plenum.

Fillenbaum, G.G., Huber, M., & Taussig, I.M. (1997). Performance of elderly White and African American community residents on the abbreviated CERAD Boston Naming Test. *Journal of Clinical & Experimental Neuropsychology, 19,* 204-210.

Gladsjo, J.A., Schuman, C.C., Evans, J.D., Peavy, G.M., Miller, S.W., & Heaton, R.K. (1999). Norms for letter and category fluency: Demographic corrections for age, education, and ethnicity. *Assessment, 6,* 147-178.

Harris, J.G., & Cullum, C.M. (subm.). Symbol vs. digit substitution task performance in culturally and linguistically diverse populations.

Harris, J.G., Cullum, C.M., & Puente, A. (1995). Effects of bilingualism on verbal learning and memory in Hispanic adults. *Journal of the International Neuropsychological Society, 1,* 10-16.

Harris, J.G., Echemendía, R.J., Ardila, A., & Rosselli, M. (subm.). Cognitive and neuropsychological assessment in Latino populations: A review

Harris, J.G., Echemendía, R.J., Ardila, A., & Rosselli, M. (2001). Cross-cultural cognitive and neuropsychological assessment. In J.J.W. Andrews, Saklofske,

D. & Janzen, H. (Eds.), *Handbook of psychoeducational assessmens. Ability, achievement, and behavior in children* (pp. 391–414). San Diego, CA: Academic Press.

Harris, J.G., Rojas, D., & Cory, J. (in press). Bilingualism. In B.P. Uzzell, M. Ponton, & A. Ardila (Eds.), *International handbook of cross cultural neuropsychology*. Mahwah, New Jersey: Lawrence Erlbaum Associates.

Helms, J. E. (1992). Why is there no study of cultural equivalence in standardized cognitive ability testing? *American Psychologist, 47,* 1083-1101.

Helms, J. E. (1997). The triple quandary of race, culture, and social class in standardized cognitive ability testing. In D. P. Flanagan, J. L. Genshaft, & P. L. Harrison (Eds.), *Contemporary intellectual assessment: Theories, tests, and issues* (pp. 517–532). New York: Guilford Press.

Jacobs, D.M., Sano, M., Albert, S., Schofield, P., Dooneief, G., & Stern, Y. (1997). Cross-cultural neuropsychological assessment: A comparison of randomly selected, demographically matched cohorts of English-and Spanish-speaking older adults. *Journal of Clinical and Experimental Neuropsychology, 19,* 331-339.

Kempler, D., Teng, E.L., Dick, M., Taussig, I.M., & Davis, D.S. (1998). The effects of age, education, and ethnicity on verbal fluency. *Journal of the International Neuropsychological Society, 4,* 531-538.

Loewenstein, D.A., Ardila, A., Rosselli, M., Hayden, S., Duara, R., Berkowitz, N., Linn-Fuentes, P., Mintzer, J., Norville, M., & Eisdorfer, C. (1992). A comparative analysis of functional status among Spanish- and English-speaking patients with dementia. *Journal of Gerontology, 47,* 389-394.

Loewenstein, D.A., Arguelles, T., Barker, W.W., & Duara, R. (1993). A comparative analysis of neuropsychological test performance of Spanish-speaking and English-speaking patients with Alzheimer's disease. *Journal of Gerontology: Psychological Sciences, 48,* 142-149.

Loewenstein, D.A., Rubert, M.P., Arguelles, T., & Duara, R. (1995). Neuropsychological test performance and prediction of functional capacities among Spanish-speaking and English-speaking patients with dementia. *Archives of Clinical Neuropsychology, 16,* 75-88.

Lopez, S., & Taussig, I.M. (1991). Cognitive-intellectual functioning of Spanish-speaking impaired and non-impaired elderly: Implications for culturally sensitive assessment. *Psychological Assessment, 3,* 448-454.

Maj, M., D'Elia, L., Satz, P., Janssen, R., Zaudig, M., Uchiyama, C., Starace, F., Galderisi, S., & Chervinsky, A. (1993). Evaluation of two new neuropsychological tests designed to minimize cultural bias in the assessment of HIV-1 seropositive persons: A WHO study. *Archives of Clinical Neuropsychology, 8,* 123-135.

Manly, J.J., & Jacobs, D. (in press). Future directions in neuropsychological assessment with African Americans. In Ferrarro, R. (Ed.*), Minority and cross-cultural aspects of neuropsychological assessment.* Lisse, The Netherlands: Swets & Zeitlinger.

Manly, J.J., Jacobs, D., & Mayeux, R. (1999). Alzheimer's Disease among different ethnic and racial groups. In R.D. Terry, R. Katzman, K.L. Bick, & S.S. Sisodia (Eds.), *Alzheimer's Disease,* (2nd ed., pp. 117–132). Philadelphia, PA: Lippincott Williams & Wilkins.

Manly, J. J., Miller, S. W., Heaton, R. K., Byrd, D., Reilly, J., Velasquez, R. J., Saccuzzo, D. P., Grant, I., & the HIV Neurobehavioral Research Center Group (1998). The effect of African-American acculturation on neuropsychological test performance in normal and HIV positive individuals. *Journal of the International Neuropsychological Society, 4,* 291-302.

Manly, J. J., Jacobs, D. M., Sano, M., Bell, K., Merchant, C. A., Small, S. A., & Stern, Y. (1998). Cognitive test performance among nondemented elderly African Americans and Whites. *Neurology, 50,* 1238-1245.

Manly, J. J., Jacobs, D.M., Sano, M., Bell, K., Merchant, C.A., Small, S.A., & Stern, Y. (1999). Effect of literacy on neuropsychological test performance in nondemented, education-matched elders. *Journal of the International Neuropsychological Society, 5,* 191-202.

Manuel-Dupont, S., Ardila, A., & Rosselli, M. (1992). Neuropsychological assessment in bilinguals. In A.E. Puente & R.J. McCaffrey (Eds.), *Handbook of neuropsychological assessment: A biopsychosocial perspective* (pp. 193–210). New York: Plenum Press.

Marcopulos, B.A., Gripshover, D.L., Broshek, D.K., McLain, C.A., & Brashear, H.R. (1999). Neuropsychological assessment of psychogeriatric patients with limited education. *The Clinical Neuropsychologist, 13,* 147-156.

Marcopulos, B.A., McLain, C.A., & Giuliano, A.J. (1997). Cognitive impairment or inadequate norms: A study of healthy, rural, older adults with limited education. *The Clinical Neuropsychologist, 11,* 111-131.

Mast, B.T., MacNeill, S.E., & Lichtenberg, P.A. (2000). Clinical utility of the Normative Studies Research Project test battery among vascular dementia patients. *The Clinical Neuropsychologist, 14,* 173-180.

Melendez, F. (1994). The Spanish version of the WAIS: Some ethical considerations. *The Clinical Neuropsychologist, 8,* 388-393.

Nabors, N.A., Evans, J.D., & Strickland, T.L. (2000). Neuropsychological assessment and intervention with African Americans. In E. Fletcher-Janzen, T.L. Strickland, & C.R. Reynolds (Eds*), Handbook of cross-cultural neuropsychology: Critical issues in neuropsychology* (pp. 31–42). New York, NY: Kluwer Academic/Plenum.

Norman, M.A., Evans, J.D., Miller, S.W., & Heaton, R.K. (2000). Demographically corrected norms for the California Verbal Learning Test. *Journal of Clinical & Experimental Neuropsychology, 22,* 80-94.

Ostrosky-Solis, F., Ardila, A., & Rosselli, M. (1999). NEUROPSI: A brief neuropsychological test battery in Spanish with norms by age and educational level. *Journal of the International Neuropsychological Society, 5,* 413-433.

Ostrosky-Solis, F., Canseco, E., Quintanar, L., Navarro, E., Meneses, S., & Ardila, A. (1985). Sociocultural effects in neuropsychological assessment. *International Journal of Neuroscience, 27,* 53-66.

Ostrosky-Solis, F., Lopez-Arango, G., & Ardila, A. (2000). Sensitivity and specificity of the Mini-Mental State Examination in a Spanish-speaking population. *Applied Neuropsychology, 7,* 47-60.

Perri, B., Naplin, N.A., & Carpenter, G.A. (1995). A Spanish auditory verbal learning and memory test. *Assessment, 2,* 245-253.

Pineda, D., Rosselli, M., Ardila, A., Mejia, S., Romero, M.G., & Perez, C. (2000). The Boston Diagnostic Aphasia Examination-Spanish version: The influence of demographic variables. *Journal of the International Neuropsychological Society, 6,* 802–814.

Pontón, M., Satz, P., Herrera, L., Ortiz, F., Urrutia, C.P., Young R., D'Elia, L.F., Furst, C.J., & Nameron N. (1996). Normative data stratified by age and education for the Neuropsychological Screening Battery for Hispanics (NeSB-HIS): Initial report. *Journal of the International Neuropsychological Society, 2,* 96-104.

Rey, G. J., Feldman, E., Rivas-Vasquez, R., Levin, B.E., & Benton, A.L. (1999). Neuropsychological test development and normative data on Hispanics. *Archives of Clinical Neuropsychology, 14,* 593-601.

Ross, T.P., & Lichtenberg, P.A. (1998). Expanded normative data for the Boston Naming Test for use with urban elderly medical patients. *The Clinical Neuropsychologist, 12,* 475-481.

Rosselli, M., & Ardila, A. (1991). Effects of age, education and gender on the Rey-Osterrieth Complex Figure. *The Clinical Neuropsychologist, 5,* 370-376.

Rosselli, M., & Ardila A. (1993). Developmental norms for the Wisconsin Card Sorting Test in 5- to 12-year old children. *The Clinical Neuropsychologist, 7,* 145-154.

Rosselli, M., Ardila, A., Araujo, K., Weekes, V.A., Caracciolo, V., Pradilla, M., & Ostrosky-Solis, F. (2000). Verbal fluency and repetition skills in healthy older Spanish-English bilinguals. *Applied Neuropsychology, 7,* 17-24.

Rosselli, M., Ardila, A., Florez, A., & Castro, C. (1990). Normative data on the Boston Diagnostic Aphasia Examination in a Spanish-speaking population. *Journal of Clinical and Experimental Neuropsychology, 12,* 313-322.

Rosselli, M., Ardila, A., & Rosas, P. (1990). Neuropsychological assessment in illiterates II: Language and praxic abilities. *Brain and Cognition, 12,* 281-296.

Stricks, L., Pittman, J., Jacobs, D.M., Sano, M., & Stern, Y. (1998). Normative data for a brief neuropsychological battery administered to English- and Spanish-speaking community-dwelling elders. *Journal of the International Neuropsychological Society, 4,* 311-318.

Taussig, I.M., Henderson, V.W., & Mack, W. (1992). Spanish translation and validation of a neuropsychological battery: Performance of Spanish- and English-speaking Alzheimer's disease patients and normal comparison subjects. *Clinical Gerontologist, 11,* 95-108.

Taussig, I.M., Mack, W.J., & Henderson, V.W. (1996). Concurrent validity of the Spanish language versions of the Mini-Mental State Examination, Mental Status Questionnaire, Information-Memory-Concentration Test, and Orientation-Memory-Concentration Test: Alzheimer's disease patients and nondemented elderly comparison subjects. *Journal of the International Neuropsychological Society, 2,* 286-292.

United States Department of Health and Human Services Office of Minority Health (2000). Assuring cultural competence in health care: Recommendations for national standards and an outcomes-focused research agenda. *Federal Register, 65,* 80865-80879.

Unverzagt, F.W., Hall, K.S., Torke, A.M., Rediger, J.D., Mercado, O.G., Osuntokun, B.O., & Hendrie, H.C. (1996). Effects of age, education and gender on CERAD neuropsychological test performance in an African American sample. *The Clinical Neuropsychologist, 10,* 180-190.

Van de Vijver, F., & Hambleton, R.K. (1996). Translating tests: Some practical guidelines. *European Psychologist, 1,* 89-99.

Whitfield, K.E., Fillenbaum, G.G., Pieper, C., Albert, M.S., Berkman, L.F., Blazer, D.G., Rowe, J.W., & Seeman, T. (2000). The effect of race and health-related factors on naming and memory: The MacArthur studies of successful aging. *Journal of Aging & Health, 12,* 69-89.

Chapter 12

ETHICAL ISSUES FOR THE USE OF VIRTUAL REALITY IN THE PSYCHOLOGICAL SCIENCES

Albert 'Skip' Rizzo, Maria T. Schultheis, and Barbara O. Rothbaum

Introduction

Virtual reality (VR) has undergone a transition in the past few years that has taken it out of the realm of expensive toy and into that of functional technology. Although media hype may have oversold VR's potential during the early stages of the technology's development, a uniquely suited match exists between the assets available with VR technology and applications in the psychological sciences. Virtual environments (VEs) have been developed that are now demonstrating effectiveness in a number of areas in clinical psychology and neuropsychology. These applications have shown promise for addressing: fear reduction with phobic clients (Rothbaum et al., 1997), stress management in cancer patients (Schneider & Workman, 1999), reduction of acute pain during wound care and physical therapy with burn patients (Hoffman et al., 2000), body image disturbances in patients with eating disorders (Riva et al., 1999), navigation and spatial training in children with motor impairments (Stanton et al., 2000), functional skills in persons with central nervous system (CNS) dysfunction (Brown & Stewart, 1996) and in the assessment (and in some cases, rehabilitation) of attention (Rizzo et al., 2000), memory (Brooks et al., 1999), spatial skills (McComas et al., 1998; Rizzo et al., 2001a) and executive cognitive functions (Pugnetti et al., 1998a) in both clinical and unimpaired populations. These efforts are no small feat in light of the technological challenges and funding hurdles that many of these researchers have faced in the development of this emerging technology. Also, the clinical and research targets chosen for these applications reflect an informed appreciation for the assets that are available with VR technology by clinicians/developers initially designing and using systems in this area. These initiatives give hope that the 21st century will be ushered in with new and useful tools to advance these areas that have long been mired in the methods of the past.

Continuing advances in VR technology in the future will also allow for broader human use in the general population for a variety of purposes including, training, education, entertainment and for possible self-help therapy. However, as with any application of a new technology, many unanswered questions exist that will require advance thoughtful consideration of the ethical issues relevant for its use. This is especially important in the psychological sciences where research and clinical application with human participants and patient populations requires rational determination of the possible risks and benefits. As well, larger pragmatic and societal issues for general VR use need to be addressed from our position as psychologists who are concerned about and have a professional-scientific interest in issues relevant to general human experience and its impact on mental health.

The present chapter will begin by describing the basics of what VR technology involves and how it may provide assets for assessment, rehabilitation, and treatment purposes in clinical psychology and neuropsychology. A brief overview will then follow that details some of the ethical issues relevant for its safe and effective clinical/research use during these early stages of VR application development with an eye towards larger societal issues that could have considerable relevancy as the technology evolves.

Virtual Reality: Definitions and Relevance

Virtual Reality can be generally defined as "...a way for humans to visualize, manipulate, and interact with computers and extremely complex data" (Aukstakalnis & Blatner, 1992). In essence, VR can be viewed as an advanced form of human–computer interface that allows the user to 'interact' with, and become 'immersed' within, a computer generated VE in a more intuitive and naturalistic fashion. This is achieved via the integration of real-time computer graphics and a variety of sensory input devices.

The believability of the virtual experience or sense of "presence" is supported by employing such specialized technology as head-mounted displays (HMDs), tracking systems, earphones, gesture-sensing gloves, interaction/navigational devices and sometimes haptic-feedback devices. The most commonly used technology is a combination of a HMD and tracking system which allows delivery of computer-generated images and sounds in any virtual scene, an experience that corresponds to what the individual would see and hear if the scene were real. Other methods incorporating 3D projection walls and rooms (known as CAVES), as well as basic flatscreen computer systems, have been used to create interactive scenarios for assessment, treatment and rehabilitative purposes.

Methods for navigation and interaction such as data gloves, joysticks, 3D mice, treadmills and some high-end 'force feedback' mechanisms that can provide tactile feedback have also been developed. However, challenges in existing interface design for navigation and operation still need to be addressed before a level of VE interaction is achieved that is truly intuitive and naturalistic. This will be of particular concern for persons with CNS impairments and as well for other clinical populations. For example, in order for persons with cognitive impairments to be in a position to benefit from a VR rehabilitation application, they must be capable of learning how to navigate and interact within the environment. Many modes of VE navigation (data gloves, joy sticks, space balls, etc.), while easily mastered by unimpaired users, could present problems for those with cognitive or sensorimotor difficulties. Even if patients are capable of using a VR system at a basic level, the extra non-automatic cognitive effort required to operate in a VE may serve as a distraction and limit the assessment and rehabilitation process. In this regard, Psotka (1995) hypothesizes that facilitation of a 'single egocenter' found in highly immersive interfaces serves to reduce 'cognitive overhead' and thereby enhances information access and learning. This is one area that needs attention in the current state of affairs for VR applications designed for clinical populations.

In spite of the technical challenges that currently exist for VR application development, systems currently in use are advancing new methodologies for psychological purposes. What makes VR application development in the psychological sciences so distinctively important and appealing is that it represents more than a simple linear extension of existing computer technology for human use. VR offers the potential to deliver systematic human testing, training, and treatment environments that allow for the precise control of complex dynamic 3D stimulus presentations, within which sophisticated behavioral recording is possible. When combining these assets within the context of functionally relevant, ecologically valid VEs, a fundamental advancement emerges in how human cognition and behavior can be studied, assessed, treated and/or rehabilitated (see Schultheis & Rizzo, 2001 for a detailed discussion of VR assets). In this regard, much like an aircraft simulator serves to test and train piloting ability, VEs can be developed to present simulations that assess and treat human cognitive and behavioral processes under a range of conditions that are not easily controllable in the real world. The rationales for VR applications in neuropsychological assessment, cognitive rehabilitation, and general clinical psychology will be briefly detailed in the next sections in order to put these assets into context prior to a discussion of the ethical issues that are relevant to consider in the use of VR with humans.

It is expected that with continuing advances in the underlying enabling technologies (i.e., engineering, computer science, human factors, etc.), more usable, useful, and accessible VR systems could be developed that uniquely target a wide range of physical, emotional, social, cognitive and psychological human issues and research questions. These developments have also resulted in more financially accessible low-cost PC-driven VR systems with greater sophistication and responsiveness. Such advances in both technology and access are allowing for more widespread application of VR technology in psychological research and clinical areas. However, with this emerging increase in access, the potential for uninformed and serious misapplication of the technology with particularly vulnerable clinical populations is looming. As the technology evolves, potent VE tools will become more readily available to professionals for research and clinical purposes, some of whom may not have the qualifications or expertise to deliver professional services in the area that the tool was designed to address. In addition, a growing number of VR scenarios will eventually become accessible to the general public via recorded media forms (e.g., DVD) and the Internet. The potential impact that this increased access will have on how research and clinical practice is conducted in psychology and the issues involved with general use by the population at large will need to be anticipated and analyzed from an ethical perspective. This chapter aims to address these topics.

Virtual Reality and Clinical Psychology

In the area of general clinical psychology, VR applications were initially developed in the early nineteen-nineties for exposure therapy targeting anxiety disorders. Since that time, an evolved body of literature has emerged and has provided evidence for numerous benefits in clinical psychological applications. In general, the phenomenon that users of VR can become immersed in VEs provides a potentially powerful tool. For example, VR may be used to immerse individuals in a VE that activates relevant fears, which is useful in the treatment of anxiety disorders. Alternatively, VR may be used to immerse individuals in a VE that distracts them from the real world, which can be useful in treating individuals undergoing painful medical procedures. There is a growing body of literature suggesting that the use of virtual reality in exposure therapy for specific phobias is effective. Case studies have documented the successful use of VR in the treatment of spider phobia (Carlin et al., 1997), claustrophobia (Botella et al., 1998), acrophobia (Rothbaum et al., 1995), and the fear of flying (Rothbaum et al., 1996; Smith et al., 1999). VR has also been used successfully with Vietnam veterans with posttraumatic stress disorder (Rothbaum et al., 1999a; Rothbaum et al., 2000).

Emotional processing theory as applied to anxiety disorders purports that fear memories include information about stimuli, responses, and meaning (Foa & Kozak, 1986; Foa et al., 1989). Therapy is aimed at facilitating emotional processing and modifying the fear structure. Any method capable of activating the fear structure and modifying it would be predicted to improve symptoms of anxiety. Thus, VR is a potential tool for the treatment of anxiety disorders; if an individual becomes immersed in a feared virtual environment, activation and modification of the fear structure is possible.

In a controlled study, virtual reality exposure therapy (VRE) was used to treat the fear of heights, exposing patients to virtual footbridges, virtual balconies, and a virtual elevator (Rothbaum et al., 1995). Patients were encouraged to spend as much time in each situation as needed for their anxiety to decrease and were allowed to progress at their own pace. The therapist saw on a computer monitor what the participant saw in the virtual environment and therefore was able to comment appropriately. Results showed that anxiety, avoidance, and distress decreased significantly from pre- to post-treatment for the VRE group but not for the wait list control group. Furthermore, 7 of the 10 VRE treatment completers exposed themselves to functionally meaningful height situations in real life during treatment even though they had not been specifically instructed to do so.

VRE was also compared to standard exposure (SE) therapy and to a wait list (WL) control in the treatment of the fear of flying (Rothbaum et al., 1999b; Rothbaum et al., 2000). The results indicated that each active treatment was superior to WL and that there were no differences between VRE and SE. Comparison of post-treatment data to six-month follow-up data for the primary outcome measures for the two treatment groups indicated no significant differences, indicating that treated participants maintained their treatment gains. By the six-month follow-up, 93% of treated participants had flown since completing treatment.

Researchers are also conducting innovative work integrating VR with both experientially based cognitive therapy for eating disorders (Riva et al., 1998, 1999) and with pain management protocols (Hoffman et al., 2000). Whereas the use of virtual reality exposure therapy for anxiety disorders and eating disorders capitalizes on immersing patients in the virtual world, VR for pain management benefits patients by distracting them from the real world. Comparison of distraction methods involving playing Nintendo or entering a virtual kitchen, in which patients could pick up appliances with a cyberhand or touch the body of a spider, revealed dramatic decreases in pain ratings, anxiety, and amount of time spent thinking about pain during burn care while in the virtual kitchen as compared to playing Nintendo. The patients also reported higher levels of immersion in VR as compared to video, and the level of immersion in VR increased across burn care sessions. These data are particularly important, as immersion is presumed to be a key feature of VR, though it has rarely been tested in a systematic manner.

VR has also been used to distract pediatric cancer patients during painful procedures and has been shown to significantly lower these patients' heart rates as compared to having the procedures without the VR (Gershon et al., 2001). These findings suggested that it is possible for individuals to become immersed in a virtual environment to the point that attitudes and behaviors in the real world may be changed as a result of experiences within a virtual world.

In summary, the use of VR for exposure therapy in the treatment of a variety of anxiety disorders, including specific phobia and PTSD, seems promising. In addition to efficacy, VR offers other advantages, including preserving confidentiality for the patient, increasing control of the exposure for the therapist, and increased convenience for both the therapist and the patient. Of course, there are disadvantages as well. Some patients may not be able to immerse themselves in VEs, and currently there is no data regarding who constitutes a good candidate for VR rather than in vivo exposure. Furthermore, as with any computer program, there are occasional programming glitches. Finally, the cost of VR has in the past been prohibitively expensive for the typical therapist in private practice. However, the price of using VR continues to drop and the ease of use of VR continues to improve with advancements in technology.

Virtual Reality and Neuropsychology

Neuropsychology is a branch of the psychological sciences where VR stands to have significant impact. While many VR applications have emerged in the areas of entertainment, education, military training, physical rehabilitation, and medicine, only recently has the considerable potential of VR for the study, assessment and rehabilitation of human cognitive and functional processes been recognized (Rizzo et al., in press; Rose, 1996; Pugnetti et al., 1995a). Indeed, in a U.S. National Institute of Health report of the National Advisory Mental Health Council (1995), the impact of virtual reality environments on cognition was specifically cited with the recommendation that: "Research is needed to understand both the positive and negative effects of such participation on children's and adults' perceptual and cognitive skills..." (p.51). One area where the potential for both "positive and negative effects" exists is in the application of VR for neuropsychological assessment, rehabilitation and research. In this regard, VR could serve to advance the study of brain–behavior relationships as well as produce innovative evaluation and intervention options that are unavailable with traditional methods.

Neuropsychological Assessment
In the broadest sense, neuropsychology is an applied science that evaluates how specific activities in the brain are expressed in observable behaviors (Lezak, 1995). Effective neuropsychological assessment (NA) is a prerequisite for both the scientific analysis and treatment of CNS-based cognitive/functional impairments as well as for research investigating normal functioning. The NA of persons with CNS disorders using psychometric evaluation tools serves a number of functions. These include the determination of a

diagnosis, the provision of normative data on the status of impaired cognitive and functional abilities, the production of information for the design of rehabilitative strategies, and the measurement of treatment efficacy.

NA also serves to create data for the scientific understanding of brain functioning through the examination of measurable sequelae that occur following brain damage or dysfunction. Our understanding of brain morphology and activity has undergone a revolution in the past three decades that is akin to the revolution seen in microtechnology. However, the increase in our knowledge of the genetics, chemistry, molecular biology, and the 'physics' of the brain is mitigated by our understanding of the behavior that is related to specific brain activity. For example, post-mortem studies of Alzheimer's Disease have identified the entorhinal cortex as the area where the pathological changes of AD are first noted (Braak et al., 1993). However, this is of little clinical value unless we can identify the cognitive and behavioral processes that are serviced by this region. Once such processes are identified, it becomes possible to diagnose more effectively and intervene at an earlier stage of this neurodegenerative process.

VE technology offers the potential to develop human performance testing environments that could supplement standard NA procedures that traditionally rely mainly on pencil and paper tests, behavioral observation and history taking. The capacity of VR technology to create dynamic, multi-sensory, three-dimensional (3D) stimulus environments, within which all behavioral responding can be recorded, offers clinical assessment options that are not available using traditional neuropsychological methods. In this regard, a growing number of laboratories are developing research programs investigating the use of VEs for these purposes, and a number of initial studies reporting encouraging results are now beginning to emerge (Rizzo et al., in press). This work has the potential to advance the scientific study of normal cognitive and behavioral processes, and to improve our capacity to measure and understand the impairments typically found in clinical populations with CNS dysfunction.

VE applications are now being developed and tested which focus on component cognitive processes, including attention, executive functions, memory, and spatial abilities. Functional VE assessment scenarios have also been designed to test instrumental activities of daily living such as street-crossing, automobile driving, meal preparation, supermarket shopping, use of public transportation, and wheelchair navigation. These ongoing efforts could conceivably produce new methodologies that support earlier diagnosis by improving standards for psychometric reliability and validity and that drive test development that could produce better detection, diagnosis, and mapping of the assets and limitations that occur with different forms of CNS dysfunction.

The potential for VR's impact for neuropsychological assessment was indirectly suggested early on by VR pioneer Myron Kruegar (1993) in a visionary article published in the MIT journal *Presence* ("The Experience Society"). In a prophetic statement, in the context of a discussion of VR's overall societal impact, Kruegar proclaimed that, "...Virtual Reality arrives at a moment when computer technology in general is moving from automating the paradigms of the past, to creating new ones for the future" (p. 163). In this comment Kruegar encapsulated what had also been so limited in neuropsychology's approach to using computer and information technology at that time and opened a conceptual door to VR's potential to advance the research and practice across many areas in the psychological sciences. Indeed, neuropsychology's use of technology up to that time could be characterized as mainly translating existing traditional paper and pencil tools directly into computer delivered formats.

In its defense, neuropsychology has been increasingly integrating advanced neural imaging technology tools (i.e., fMRI, SPECT, QUEEG, CT, etc.) in its quest for a better accounting of the structure and process underlying brain–behavior relationships. However, while these advances in *response* measurement have led to new findings and conceptualizations, the *stimulus* delivery end of the equation has been somewhat limited. Stimulus presentation in traditional neuropsychological applications can be characterized as mainly coming in two forms: (1) *Analog* tasks involving standardized delivery of sound, text, symbols and still/moving image stimuli, responses to which are readily quantifiable but limited in ecological validity, and (2) *Naturalistic* tasks in 'real-world' scenarios (usually requiring behavioral rating judgments) that are difficult or impractical to administer while still maintaining a systematic level of experimental control. Again, VR stands poised to fundamentally advance this area with innovative applications that leverage the immersive, involving and interactive assets available in VEs to deliver quantifiable analog-like stimulus protocols within the context of functionally relevant (and controllable) environments. Until now these features have not been pragmatically available with existing methods in neuropsychology; thus, VR now seems to have plenty to offer in this vital and challenging area of the psychological sciences.

As well, a challenge to the conceptual growth of the field of psychometric testing methods was leveled in a 1997 *American Psychologist* article by intelligence theorist Robert Sternberg in which he compared currently used intelligence and ability tests to black and white TV, rotary-dial phones, and the UNIVAC computer. His argument started by observing that the first edition of the most widely used intelligence test, the *Wechsler Adult Intelligence Scale* appeared in 1939, well before the UNIVAC. However, while computer and other information technology and telecommunication tools (i.e., TV, telephones, and sound recording) have undergone a revolution since then, with the exception of essentially cosmetic changes, tests of cognitive ability have remained essentially unchanged.

Sternberg posited that 'dynamic' interactive testing would be needed to provide a new option that could supplement traditional 'static' tests. The 'dynamic' assessment approach requires the provision of guided performance feedback as a component in tests that measure learning. This method appears well suited to the assets available with VR technology. In fact, VEs might be the most efficient vehicle for conducting dynamic testing in an 'ecologically valid' manner while still maintaining an acceptable level of experimental control. Indeed, across most NA strategies, VEs may be especially suited to improve *ecological* validity, or the degree of relevance or similarity that a test has relative to the 'real' world. This asset would allow for human cognitive/functional performance to be tested in simulated 'real-world' VE scenarios. In this way, the complexity of stimulus challenges found in naturalistic settings could be delivered while still maintaining the experimental control required for rigorous scientific analysis. Such results might have greater clinical relevance and could have direct implications for the development of more effective functional rehabilitation approaches. However, it is also important to recognize that in all cases it may not be desirable for VEs to fully 'mimic' reality.

Another strength of VEs for assessment purposes may include the capacity to present scenarios that include features not available in the 'real world'. This would be the case when 'cueing' stimuli are presented to determine what level of 'augmentative' information can be used by patients to provide insight for the development of compensatory strategies aimed at improving day-to-day functional behavior.

It is possible that the use of VE technology could revolutionize our approach to NA. However, the current status of VE technology applied to clinical populations, while provocative, is still limited by the small (but growing) number of controlled studies in this area. This is to be expected, considering the technology's relatively recent development, its high initial development costs, and the lack of familiarity with VE technology by established researchers employing the traditional tools and tactics of their fields. In spite of this, a nascent body of work has emerged which can provide knowledge for guiding future research efforts.

Finally, the possibility of linking VE assessment with advanced brain imaging and psychophysiological techniques (Pugnetti et al., 1996; Aguirre & D'Esposito, 1997) may allow neuropsychology to reach its stated purpose, that of determining unequivocal brain–behavior relationships. While pragmatic concerns need to be addressed in order for this technology to advance the science required to reach this lofty goal, the benefits that could be accrued appear to justify the effort.

VR and Cognitive Rehabilitation

Cognitive Rehabilitation (CR) can be defined as the applications of methods, following injury to the brain, which aim to restore cognitive processes or arrest the resulting decline (Parente & Herrmann, 1996). Sohlberg and Mateer (1989) suggest that cognitive rehabilitation is "...the therapeutic process of increasing or improving an individuals capacity to process and use incoming information so as to allow increased functioning in everyday life"

(p. 3). Thus, CR targets both specific component cognitive processes and fully integrated functional behaviors or Instrumental Activities of Daily Living (IADLs). Between the complexity of the subject matter and the challenges incumbent with conducting outcome research with such a hetereogenous population, considerable debate exists as to the relative effectiveness of various CR approaches (Wilson, 1997). Rather than debating the merits of any specific CR approach and for the purposes of describing the underlying rationale for VR in this chapter, we are assuming that CR subsumes strategies and processes that would be of relevance to a larger 'holistic' conceptualization of neuropsychological rehabilitation that also includes focus on vocational, self-awareness and social interaction concerns (Prigatano, 1997).

CR approaches can differ based on a variety of conceptual criteria (Kirsch et al., 1992). For the purposes of describing the application of VE technology to CR, these conceptual dimensions can be 'collapsed' into two general domains: *Restorative* approaches which focus on the systematic retraining of component cognitive processes (i.e., attention, memory, etc.) and *Functional* approaches which emphasize the stepwise training of observable behaviors, skills, and IADLs. In this regard, the restorative approach places as the primary objective the attempt to retrain individuals on how to *think*, whereas the primary emphasis of the functional approach is to teach individuals how to *do*.

Specific weaknesses have been identified in both of these approaches. One often cited criticism of restorative methods is the reliance on test materials or tasks that are essentially artificial and have little relevance to real-world functional cognitive challenges. This criticism holds that 'memorizing' increasingly difficult lists of words or activities within a therapy or school environment does not support the *transfer* or *generalization* of memory ability to the person's real-world situation (Chase & Ericsson, 1981; O'Connor & Cermack, 1987). The fundamental criticism of functional methods is that the learning of standard stereotyped behaviors to accomplish IADLs assumes that the person lives in a static world where life demands do not change, and that the person's underlying cognitive processes are not specifically addressed. This is believed to limit the flexible and creative problem-solving required to adjust to and think through changing circumstances in the real world (Kirsch et al., 1992).

The application of VE technology for the rehabilitation of cognitive/ functional deficits could serve to limit the major weaknesses of both the restorative and functional approaches, and actually produce a systematic treatment method that would integrate the best features from both methods. In essence, it may be possible for a VE application to provide systematic restorative training within the context of functionally relevant, ecologically valid, simulated environments that optimize the degree of transfer of training or generalization of learning to the person's real world environment. VEs could also serve to provide a more controlled and systematic means for *separately* administering restorative or functional techniques when this direction is deemed appropriate. An analysis of the suitability of VE technology in meeting the minimum criteria for both restorative and functional approaches can be found in a previous paper (Rizzo, 1994).

It should also be noted that underlying the goals of both of these conveniently termed treatment directions (thinking vs. doing) is the concept of *neural plasticity*. Neural plasticity refers to the capacity of the brain to reorganize or repair itself following injury through various mechanisms (i.e., axonal sprouting, glial cell activation, denervation supersensitivity, and metabolic changes) in response to environmental stimulation. Recognition of neural plasticity in response to both environmental enrichment and impoverishment has its roots in the animal literature (Renner & Rosenzweig, 1987) and detailed reviews of this increasingly favored view of the brain can be found elsewhere (Rose & Johnson, 1992). Consequently, it can be appreciated that the stimulation or 'enrichment' provided by both restorative and functional approaches may each have some effect on the physical brain structure, and hence, training with both methods would be assumed to affect brain plasticity. If this view is accepted, stimulating virtual training environments would seem well suited to support this process and new approaches to CR would be warranted.

Indeed, researchers and clinicians in neuropsychology appear to be 'wanting' for these advances. For example, in a recent National Institutes of Health (NIH) Consensus paper entitled *"Rehabilitation of Persons with Traumatic Brain Injury (TBI)"* two recommendations were made which suggest research directions that VE technology appears well poised to address. The report recommended that "Innovative study methodologies that enhance the ability to assess the effectiveness of complex interventions for persons with TBI should be developed and evaluated" and that "Innovative rehabilitation interventions for TBI should be developed and studied..." (National Institute of Health [NIH], 1998). As well, direct interest in VR for general rehabilitation purposes has also been recognized by the National Institute on Disability and Rehabilitation Research (NIDRR) which recently highlighted in their Long Range Research Plan "...The benefits of combining virtual reality with rehabilitation interventions are potentially extensive" and specifically called for research "....to determine the efficacy of virtual reality techniques in both rehabilitation medicine and in applications that directly affect the lives of persons with disabilities" (http://gcs.ed.gov/fedreg/announcement.html). These observations suggest that the discipline of cognitive rehabilitation is fertile ground for developing the innovative applications that are possible with VE technology.

Ethical Issues for the Use of VR

Thus far we have detailed some of the arguments and research findings in support of the use of VR in the psychological sciences. The feasibility of designing, developing and implementing these tools has radically advanced in the last five years and it is expected that this evolution will continue into the foreseeable future. Along the way, more sophisticated VEs that are as accessible as common word processing programs and computer/video games will appear on the clinical and societal landscape. As psychologists directly involved in the application of this technology and as members of society at large with a professional and moral–ethical responsibility for the promotion and maintenance of mental health, we are accountable to consider and address incumbent ethical concerns that surround this emerging technology. As in any area of ethical debate, clear-cut answers that cover all dilemmas are rarely found. Therefore responses to the following ten questions briefly address some of the looming ethical challenges concerning side effects, exclusionary criteria, professional practice issues and concerns regarding general societal impact for the use of this technology as it continues to evolve in the future.

1. What is the potential for VE-related side effects (Cybersickness/ Aftereffects)?
In order for VR to become a safe and useful tool for human applications, the potential for adverse side effects needs to be considered and addressed. This is a significant concern as the occurrence of side effects could limit the applicability of VEs for certain clinical populations. Two general categories of VE-related side effects have been reported: cybersickness and aftereffects.

Cybersickness is a form of motion sickness with symptoms reported to include nausea, vomiting, eyestrain, disorientation, ataxia, and vertigo (Kennedy et al., 1994). Cybersickness is believed to be related to sensory cue incongruity. This is thought to occur when there is a conflict between perceptions in different sense modalities (auditory, visual, vestibular, proprioceptive) or when sensory cue information in the VE is incongruent with what is felt by the body or with what is expected based on the user's history of 'real world' sensorimotor experience (Reason, 1970). However, the simple explanation of 'sensory cue incongruity' influencing cybersickness in VEs requires further study in view of the observation that highly 'congruent' VEs sometimes produce these ill-effects and, conversely, incongruent scenarios may not produce them (Nat Durlach, personal communication, 1999).

Aftereffects may include such symptoms as disturbed locomotion, changes in postural control, perceptual-motor disturbances, past pointing, flashbacks, drowsiness, fatigue, and generally lowered arousal (Rolland et al., 1995; DiZio & Lackner, 1992; Kennedy & Stanney, 1996). The appearance of aftereffects may be due to the user adapting to the sensorimotor requirements of the VE, which in most cases is an imperfect replica of the non-VE world. Upon leaving the VE there is a lag in the readaptation to the demands of the non-VE, and the occurrence of aftereffects may reflect these shifts in sensorimotor response recalibration. The reported occurrence of side effects in virtual environments in unimpaired populations varies across studies, depending upon such factors as the type of VE program used, technical drivers (i.e., vection, response lag, field of view, etc.), the length of exposure time, the person's prior experience using VEs, active vs. passive movement, gender, and the method of measurement used to assess occurrence (Hettinger, 1992; Kolasinski, 1995; Regan & Price, 1994). It has been suggested that side effects can be reduced via gradual repeated exposures to VEs and by the provision of more optimal levels of user initiated control over movement in the virtual environment (Stanney & Kennedy, 1997). These issues should be investigated further in order to determine what effective methods exist to reduce side effects that could limit the feasibility of VEs for applications with clinical populations.

A recent review of this area (Stanney et al., 1998) targets four primary issues in the study of VE-related side effects that may be of particular value for guiding feasibility assessments with different clinical populations. These include: "(1) How can prolonged exposure to VE systems be obtained? (2) How can aftereffects be characterized? (3) How should they be measured and managed? (4) What is their relationship to task performance?" (p. 6). These questions are particularly relevant to developers of clinical VEs, as these systems are primarily designed to be used by persons with some sort of defined diagnosis or impairment. It is possible that these users may have increased vulnerability and a higher susceptibility to VE-related side effects, and ethical clinical vigilance to these issues is essential. Particular concern may be necessary for neurologically impaired populations, some of which display residual equilibrium, balance, perceptual, and orientation difficulties. It has also been suggested that subjects with unstable binocular vision (which sometimes can occur following strokes, TBI, and other CNS conditions) may be more susceptible to post-exposure visual aftereffects (Wann & Mon-Williams, 1996). Unfortunately, statistics on the occurrence of side effects with clinical populations have been inconsistently reported in the published literature to date. This is an aspect of data reporting on VEs that should be changed. Some type of assessment and reporting of VE-related side effects, whether using "in-house" designed ratings scales or standardized subjective and objective measures (Kennedy et al., 1993), should be standard procedure for presenting results on systems in this area.

Thus far, anecdotal reports of flatscreen scenarios used with clinical populations have not indicated problems with these less immersive systems. However, it does not appear that much systematic assessment has occurred and, in some cases, the verbal reports of the patients may have been compromised. Also, most clinical applications appear to use short periods of exposure (10–20 minutes) and this may have served to mitigate the occurrence of side effects based on the scant reporting in this literature. In one of the first studies to present systematic data for a HMD system used with populations having CNS dysfunction, 11 neurological patients were compared with 41 non-neurologically impaired subjects regarding self-reported occurrence of side effects (Pugnetti et al., 1995b). Subjects were tested in a VE specifically designed to target executive functioning with CNS populations. The results suggest a reduced occurrence of VE-related side effects relative to other studies using the same assessment questionnaire, the Simulator Sickness Questionnaire (Kennedy et al., 1993), with an overall rate of 17% for the total sample. The authors concluded that the neurologically impaired subjects appeared to be at no greater risk for developing cybersickness than the non-neurologically compromised group.

In a more recent study, Pugnetti et al. (1998b) reported side effect results comparing 36 patients having mixed neurological diagnoses, with 32 normal controls for a 30-minute VE exposure using the system described above. Using a variety of self-report questionnaires, assessments were conducted prior, during, and following VE usage and no differences were found between the groups on any of the side effect measures. It is important to note, though, that the patient group was recruited from those with stable neurological conditions (good bilateral visual acuity, no epilepsy, preserved dominant handedness, and no psychiatric, vestibular, or severe cognitive disorders), and this screening procedure may have contributed to the low level of side effect occurrence. The screening of patient groups, as was prudently done by these authors, may be the safest course of action until more specific and 'cautiously' acquired data becomes available from more impaired populations, particularly regarding the objective assessment of perceptual aftereffects.

While these initial findings are encouraging, further work is necessary to specifically assess how the occurrence of side effects is influenced by factors such as the type and severity of neurological trauma, specific cognitive impairments, psychological/emotional factors, length of time within the VE, previous VE exposure and characteristics of the specific VE program. This is an essential step in determining the conditions where VEs would be of practical value with clinical groups. A useful tool for monitoring VE-related side effects is the Simulator Sickness Questionnaire (SSQ) (Kennedy et al., 1993). While more involved 'objective' measures may exist, particularly for the measurement of aftereffects, SSQ data is relatively simple to collect and may serve as a low-cost method to begin to specify and document the basic occurrence of VE side effects in clinical populations. Until we have better data on these issues, extra caution may be needed with some applications. For example, since we couldn't be confident regarding the absence of potential perceptual aftereffects occurring in a recent study with an elderly group (+65years old) testing visuospatial abilities, we had funding built into our grant to provide transportation to *and* from the test site, thereby minimizing any possible risk for altered driving behavior resulting from the VR exposure. Concerns, such as these, must be addressed in order to assure a positive course for developing VE applications for all persons and particularly with clinical groups.

2. *What special considerations are needed for VR applications among individuals with altered awareness or reality-testing?*
The immersive and interactive features that add to the 'realism' of VEs are two of the most appealing benefits of using this technology for clinical appli-

cations. However, it is the multidimensional and multisensory aspects of VR that also hold the potential to be harmful for some clinical populations. In particular, specific considerations should be given when working with individuals who may have psychiatric conditions resulting in distorted reality testing or individuals with cognitive impairments who may have altered awareness. Specifically, such impairments may result in increasing an individuals vulnerability for negative behavioral responses following exposure to VEs or the development of a propensity for escaping from reality through the use of VEs.

Altered Sense of Reality. One creative VR application, proposed by some, is its use to understand different mental states, such as hallucinations, delusions and altered states (Tart, 1990). While, it can be argued that individuals with intact mental functioning are able to distinguish between virtual and real environments and efficiently detect errors or distortions, individuals whose judgement is already impaired may be at a high risk for further distortion of their reality testing. For example, difficulties in detecting experiences between real and virtual environments could lead to misinterpretation of sequence of events, and/or the development of paranoid delusions.

In addition, because VR protocols are more dynamic than traditional psychological or psychiatric approaches, the level of stress induced, as well as the lure of an alternate environment, would be hard to predict for individuals who are faced with the daily struggle of coping with visual or auditory hallucinations. As such, these individuals may be at higher risk for negative behavioral and psychophysiological responses. Finally, it should be considered that as this technology becomes more accessible, it is possible that individuals may seek to enter virtual environments in order to increase their own understanding of their psychological processes (Whalley, 1995). Such independent exploration, which lacks the therapeutic support and guidance, could prove to be detrimental to individuals with altered levels of reality-testing.

Limited Self-Awareness. Increasing awareness of deficits is a common goal in the rehabilitation of cognitively impaired populations. Prior studies incorporating awareness-building have demonstrated the benefits of increasing an individuals awareness of deficits for improving functional outcome. The added level of 'realism' that can be delivered with VR may allow for a higher level of awareness training. Therefore, ethical considerations for the overall consequences of increased awareness require attention.

For example, while traditional neuropsychological testing can elicit feelings of frustration, anxiety or concerns about performance, typically this response is task-specific and often is not generalized to daily activities by the patient. Subsequently, patients rely on feedback from clinicians to help them understand how their impairments will relate to their day-to-day functioning. The use of VEs offers a medium for patients to directly experience their impairments in 'real-world' situations. As a result, a new level of response to this awareness of deficit can be anticipated. For example, in assessment of driving capacity in cognitively compromised populations, traditional measures (e.g., paper and pencil tests, computer tests), often are not easily associated with actual driving behaviors by the patients. In contrast, with VR's realism, patients can more easily associate their poor performance on a VR driving simulator with 'real-world' driving. The impact of this awareness may be beneficial for some but potentially harmful for others. For example, poor performance may elicit increased anxiety and/or concerns regarding driving capacity, which may result in a choice to discontinue driving. Depending on the circumstances, this could significantly alter an individual's lifestyle, such as altered vocational situations, reliance on external support for transportation, added demands on family members, and possible negative emotional reactions (i.e., depression, isolation) to the loss of independence. As such, the evaluation of these types of potential responses to VR should be conducted both before *and* after VR exposure, as part of standard protocol.

In addition to increased awareness, individuals with physical and/or cognitive disabilities may also be more vulnerable to 'escapism' via exposure to VEs. For example, the application of VR for simulated walking by individuals with spinal cord injury has been proposed (Riva, 2000). While therapeutic benefits may be the fundamental intention, one can predict that the VE could be more enticing and positive than the real world. The question then arises, will the patient, with time, choose to escape from the confines of a wheelchair and the reality of the real world and choose to spend more and more time in the virtual world? As well, if it is argued that behavior is influenced by experience, it could be anticipated that individuals with such disabilities may demonstrate changes in their behavior in response to the VR exposure. That is, continued exposure to life without disability in the VR may result in individuals experiencing increased difficulties in accepting their disabilities in the 'real world'.

Loss of Choice. Finally, with both altered reality testing and impaired awareness the question of choice must be addressed. This can be considered both from a clinical and legal point of view. First, from a clinical perspective, the choice of the virtual experience to be administered to patients is often dependent upon several factors: the computer, the skill of the designer, and preferences of the supervising clinician. Subsequently, for the patient there is a restriction of choice that can unfortunately allow for opportunities of abuse. In addition, it should be considered that because VEs are limited to the designer's interpretation, the meaning of these experiences imposed by the patient may not agree with those imposed by the designer. The result may be negative experiences and subsequent maladaptive behaviors.

Since so many factors can limit, control, and /or determine a VE experience, issues of accountability, responsibility and liability predominate. From a legal perspective, an additional level of consideration is required for these vulnerable populations.

3 Using VR out of your area of expertise: Who is qualified to treat with VR?
Principle A of the *Ethical principles of psychologists and code of conduct* (American Psychological Association, 1992) regards competence. It reads:

> *"Psychologists strive to maintain high standards of competence in their work. They recognize the boundaries of their particular competencies and the limitations of their expertise. They provide only those services and use only those techniques for which they are qualified by education, training, or experience. Psychologists are cognizant of the fact that the competencies required in serving, teaching, and/or studying groups of people vary with the distinctive characteristics of those groups. In those areas in which recognized professional standards do not yet exist, psychologists exercise careful judgment and take appropriate precautions to protect the welfare of those with whom they work. They maintain knowledge of relevant scientific and professional information related to the services they render, and they recognize the need for ongoing education. Psychologists make appropriate use of scientific, professional, technical, and administrative resources."*

Ethical Standard 1.04 further expounds on the Boundaries of Competence:

> *(a) Psychologists provide services, teach, and conduct research only within the boundaries of their competence, based on their education, training, supervised experience, or appropriate professional experience.*
> *(b) Psychologists provide services, teach, or conduct research in new areas or involving new techniques only after first undertaking appropriate study, training, supervision, and/or consultation from persons who are competent in those areas or techniques.*
> *(c) In those emerging areas in which generally recognized standards for preparatory training do not yet exist, psychologists nevertheless take reasonable steps to ensure the competence of their work and to protect patients, clients, students, research participants, and others from harm.*

It is clear from the spirit of these ethical principles and standards that a professional should practice only within the realm of his or her expertise. This has come up repeatedly in the area of virtual reality exposure therapy. In the first published manual for providing virtual reality exposure therapy for anxiety disorders, this caution was included:

> *"The Virtually Better^{TM} virtual reality exposure therapy system is intended to be used as a tool by experienced clinicians who are also experienced in delivering exposure therapy. This is intended as a com-*

ponent of a comprehensive treatment program. If you are unsure, please seek supervision from an experienced clinician. Virtually Better^TM should be considered essentially equivalent to in vivo exposure. Although research has not addressed this equivalence, if you would not be qualified to take a patient out for in vivo exposure, you should not attempt Virtually Better^TM exposure, either" (Rothbaum et al., 1999b).

Virtual reality should be approached as a tool to be used by clinicians experienced with the types of patient problems and treatment they are treating. It is not meant to be a convenient way of attracting new patients or of administering a new type of therapy that they are not qualified to provide. As an example, as described above, there is mounting evidence of the efficacy of VR exposure therapy. As mentioned in the caveat quoted from the treatment manual above, therapists should only attempt to use VR for exposure therapy if they are qualified to provide exposure therapy. Likewise, clinicians should only use the VR applications for ADHD or neuropsychological testing if these are areas of expertise. As the use of therapeutic VR expands, it will be incumbent upon clinical training programs to train future professionals in its competent and ethical use.

4. Will therapists use VR at the expense of the normal therapist–client relationship?

Much has been written about the therapeutic relationship between a patient and therapist, and it is an important variable in treatment. A discussion of the intricacies of the therapeutic relationship is beyond the scope of this chapter, but the impact of introducing technology such as VR should be examined. As in any social interaction, non-verbal communication is of paramount importance in the therapist–patient dyad. Much of this non-verbal communication comes from facial expressions, body postures, hand gestures, and intonations. If patients are wearing head-mounted displays, they cannot see the therapist and therefore lose all of the non-verbal communication absorbed visually. If it is a loud virtual environment, such as the virtual Vietnam or even the virtual airplane, the therapist may be talking to the patient through a microphone connected to the earphones. Although they can still carry on a conversation, some of the natural inflections are stilted and the therapist is speaking over the background noise of the virtual environment. The use of such technology definitely impacts on the therapeutic relationship. It may allow avoidant patients to 'hide' behind the technology. Very avoidant patients may focus on the details of the technology (e.g., "Is this stereoscopic?"; "What's the field of view in this?") to avoid processing the feared stimuli. The astute therapist should deal with this avoidance rather than engage in a technical discussion. The use of such technology may also allow therapists who might be less than comfortable with interpersonal issues to hide behind the technology or to become comfortable with a routine use of VR instead of assessing the needs of the patient on an ongoing basis.

This is not to say that the use of VR must by definition lead to the loss of the normal therapist-patient relationship. Presumably, VR was not introduced immediately upon the first visit, so there were likely several sessions of standard information gathering and skills training before the patient was ready for VR exposure. Within one session, there is still conventional conversation at the beginning of the session and at the end of the session. In fact, VR could possibly add to the therapeutic relationship if the therapist is very skilled at the presentation of feared stimuli at precisely the right moment and right intensity for a therapeutic exposure and processes the session sensitively afterwards. Just as standard exposure therapy is different from 'talk therapy' and often occurs outside of the office and therefore fosters slightly different dynamics, so does the introduction of VR. Therapists should be cautioned not to hide behind the technology or let the technology dominate the session. Again, VR should be approached as a tool to be used to enhance therapy rather than as the therapy itself.

5. *Will therapists rely on VR as a substitute for good clinical skills or to mask shoddy service?*
Related to this issue is Ethical Standard 1.05 (*Maintaining Expertise*):

> "*Psychologists who engage in assessment, therapy, teaching, research, organizational consulting, or other professional activities maintain a reasonable level of awareness of current scientific and professional information in their fields of activity, and undertake ongoing efforts to maintain competence in the skills they use.*"

Also, Ethical Standard 1.14 (*Avoiding Harm*) states:

> "*Psychologists take reasonable steps to avoid harming their patients or clients, research participants, students, and others with whom they work, and to minimize harm where it is foreseeable and unavoidable.*"

And Standard 2.02 (*Competence and Appropriate Use of Assessments and Interventions*) states:

> "*(a) Psychologists who develop, administer, score, interpret, or use psychological assessment techniques, interviews, tests, or instruments do so in a manner and for purposes that are appropriate in light of the research on or evidence of the usefulness and proper application of the techniques.*
> *(b) Psychologists refrain from misuse of assessment techniques, interventions, results, and interpretations and take reasonable steps to pre-*

vent others from misusing the information these techniques provide. This includes refraining from releasing raw test results or raw data to persons, other than to patients or clients as appropriate, who are not qualified to use such information." (See also Standards 1.02, *Relationship of Ethics and Law,* and 1.04, *Boundaries of Competence.*)

As discussed above and as is made clear in the Ethics Code, therapists should use VR to enhance therapy rather than substitute for it. It would not be advised to obtain the VR hardware and software to rejuvenate a floundering practice if the problem is the competence level of the clinician. Therapists must be thoroughly trained in the assessment or therapy they are delivering and use VR for the advantages it affords, such as control over stimuli for assessment or treatment, ease of exposure, or cost-effectiveness. It would not be ethical to obtain the VR technology and use it as a substitute for clinical competence. To misquote a colleague, bad therapy with VR is still just bad therapy.

6. *Will continued VR access lead to cases of faulty self-diagnosis and self-treatment?*

Although the current therapeutic uses of VR still require a clinician to be present, future uses will probably not have this requirement. Individuals will be able to download or purchase locally VR assessment and therapeutic tools. Will this contribute to faulty self-diagnosis and inadequate self-treatment? Probably to a small degree, but also likely not more than currently exists in the self-help arena. One cannot overemphasize the importance of self-help programs. The fact of the matter is that most people 'cure' themselves of their problems without ever seeking professional assistance. Anything that aids in this process can only be seen as advantageous. It is true that many people who rely on self-help programs may not meet diagnostic criteria for their 'disorders,' but significant distress and interference can result even from subclinical syndromes and, therefore, these individuals have much to gain from any intervention. A self-help intervention for the fear of public speaking, for example, will likely attract more people than would meet DSM criteria for social phobia, but that is not to say these individuals would not profit from such a program. One of the most significant problems with self-help programs in general is compliance. In this way, the attraction of the VR graphics and technology may hold an advantage of keeping people engaged long enough to profit from the program.

7. *What are the risks of overstated claims in the application of VR to medical research?*

The history of medicine serves to provide numerous examples of the over-exploitation of new technologies. As is commonly the case, the introduction of a new application is often met with an atmosphere of optimistic overexpectation and urgency for implementation. Given it's considerable potential to increase our understanding of human function and to serve as a powerful treatment tool, VR is a current technology that clinicians and researchers are implementing in medical studies. As such, consideration of the potential ethical dilemmas that could arise from this overexpection and urgency is warranted.

The medical use of electricity has served as an example of a commonly accepted procedure in the nineteenth century, during which time clinicians who had minimal to no experience in the physics of electricity applied this technique to patients (Whalley, 1995). Similarly, with today's growing interest in the use of VR for medical research and treatment, consideration of who implements these procedures and how they are implemented must be addressed. The foundation of completed studies can serve to demonstrate that successful and safe use of VR environments for assessment or treatment of clinical populations will require an integrated foundation of knowledge. To date, most protocols have combined the expertise of clinicians, programmers and engineers. Given the encouraging findings from initial VR studies, it is necessary to consider that numerous underlying gains which may lead scientists to 'rushing into' the application of this technology and potentially making premature and overstated claims about its benefit.

It can be argued that scientists often are at risk of being too enamoured or wedded to their ways of thinking. This is a problem that has been around prior to VR. However, the enthusiasm for the use of VR in research does raise the question of how well researchers will know this technology, it's capabilities and limitations, prior to it's application. The potential dangers of limited knowledge are twofold. First, because control of both the stimulus (input) and the desired outcome variables are at the disposal of the researcher, limited knowledge regarding the impact of VR technology on human performance could lead to inaccurate interpretations and conclusions. In addition, the probability of exposing patients to unnecessary risks would be increased. The importance of understanding the underlying mechanisms of new technologies is not unique to VR and has been underscored by others (Whitbeck & Brooks, 1982; Whitbeck, 1993). Second, it is important to recognize that the introduction of new technologies often highlights capabilities and not limitations. Such a skewed perspective could result in a failure to pay attention to the scientific and clinical needs. Therefore, to ensure that the appropriateness of the application does not get overlooked, the question of how this new capacity influences the focus of research should be considered. Given the rapidly advancing changes in VR, the importance of recognizing both strengths and limitations can help researchers to better match VR's capabilities to investigative and scientific needs.

In addition to potentially premature and ill-judged clinical applications, it is important to recognize the possible secondary gains for researchers using this new technology. In a field where competition between institutions is openly acknowledged, and where funding sources are often dependent upon public funds, there is considerable pressure for researchers to achieve the highest level of expertise and to conduct studies that are at the forefront of scientific research. As such, the application of promising, innovative technologies such as VR could be considerably appealing to researchers. Claims of 'expertise' or 'specialization' could serve to further the careers of researchers and attract funding sources to institutions.

Concerns regarding medical paternalism and misuse of VR technology have been recognized by many researchers (Kallman, 1993; Whalley, 1995). Subsequently, it is timely to examine the ethical issues that may arise in the development and application of VR to clinical research and treatment. VR possesses enormous potential to improve our current scientific protocols and enhance our understanding of various medical issues; it would be a pity if such opportunity were delayed or lost as a result of unresolved ethical issues.

8. *Will certain individuals prefer to spend time in virtual environments and interact with Virtual Human Representations (Avatars) to the exclusion of interactions in the 'real' world and relationships with 'real' people?*
As the underlying enabling technologies evolve, ever more realistic and compelling VEs will be created, and many of these scenarios will be inhabited with very convincing and believable virtual human representations or 'Avatars'. Already we have seen the initial use of avatars on the Internet for news presentations (Ananova, 2001), representing participants in chatroom interaction (Damer, 1998), and for avatar-delivered email messaging that allows for the transmission of 3D photorealistic renditions of faces capable of delivering voice messages. The use of avatars has also emerged as a 'hot topic' for enhancing interaction in virtual environments and for promoting better forms of human-computer interaction (Rizzo et al., 2001b). In fact, some of the major information technology corporations are looking to create computer systems that integrate avatar 'technology' as part of a long-term view toward modeling human-computer interaction after human-human interaction. This direction aims to maximize naturalistic 'engagement' between humans and computational devices by leveraging human cognitive, perceptual and social attributes in a way that promotes interaction with technology in a social manner (Turk & Robertson, 2000). This effort to support more naturalistic engagement between these two complex 'systems' is seen quite poignantly in a statement from the IBM Almaden website on the area of 'emotional computing' in the following statement:

> "Just as a person normally expects a certain kind of engagement when interacting with another person, so should a person be able to expect similar engagement when interacting with a computational device. Such engagement requires the computer to carefully observe the user, anticipating user actions, needs, and desires. Such engagement enables users to begin to build personal relationships with computers" (IBM, 1999).

By integrating such emotional computing concepts with avatar delivery formats (e.g. users giving voice commands to a virtual avatar instead of using a keyboard or mouse), we will see much more opportunity for human interaction and 'bonding' with avatars on the Internet and in VEs in the future. It will also be possible for users to 'select' both appearance and 'personality' features for these avatars to suit specific user-determined needs, tastes and preferences. Already, advanced research is demonstrating the feasibility of developing avatars that are 'fueled' with Artificial Intelligence (AI), aimed at fostering more 'authentic' real time interaction between 'real' humans and virtual characters for training purposes. For example, Rickel and Johnson (1999) have reported success in the implementation of an AI avatar named 'Steve' who serves the role as 'instructor' for a virtual training environment targeting the operation and maintenance of equipment on a battleship. As well, similar avatar applications for testing and training tactical decision-making tasks, such as crisis response in U.S. Army peacekeeping operations, are under development (Swartout et al., in press). These applications could be said to emulate the type of interactions that occur with holographic characters that are often portrayed on the 'holodeck' in various versions of the science 'fiction' TV franchise/series 'Star Trek.'

On the positive side, more believable virtual humans inhabiting VEs would open up possibilities for scenarios that allow for assessment and intervention strategies that involve social interaction, naturalistic communication and more 'personal' guidance/instruction. Populating VEs with avatars could also serve to enhance a sense of realism that may in turn promote the experience of presence in VR. For example, VEs designed to target certain anxiety disorders might directly benefit from the presentation of virtual humans that are capable of some form of interaction, speech, and ability to recognize and emit typical non-verbal social communication via facial expressions and hand/body gesture cues. Early research in this area is investigating the use of video and computer graphics methods to render virtual humans for treatment of public speaking and social phobias (Anderson et al., 2000; Pertaub & Slater, 2001; Wiederhold et al., 2000), as well as for a variety of social psychology research applications (Blascovich et al., in press). The capacity to easily render avatars that are modeled after 'real' persons in the user's everyday life might also create new possibilities for mental health applications that could utilize more realistic 'role-playing' strategies.

However, the 'creation' of avatars at this level could also be 'challenging' to humans' general self-perceptions on a number of existential and ethical levels, and a truly visionary and involved treatment of these issues can be found in Kurzweil (1999). One of the key concerns in the future may involve the clinical and social ramifications of chronic use or 'addiction' to 'fantasy' VEs and the avatars that inhabit them, at the expense of involvement in the real world and relationships with real persons. While limitations in the state of current VR technology make it doubtful that these issues will be of immediate concern, as the technology evolves and VEs begin to rival (or exceed) the experiences that are available in a person's real world, there will undoubtedly be individuals who will develop preferences for the sensory, intellectual and personal control options that will be afforded in a synthetic virtual world.

This issue has already received considerable popular media press (and some academic attention) as it pertains to the current topic of 'Internet Addiction' (cf. Young, 1999). As new information technologies become integrated into the sociocultural landscape, questions are commonly posed as to whether people will become so involved in their activities in cyberspace that they will in turn neglect their social and functional involvement in the 'real world'. Efforts to examine the relationship between Internet use and measures of social interaction and participation in other activities have produced a few large scale studies with contradictory results (Miller & Dunn, 2000) and no shortage of heated debate. Similar concerns were raised with the previous introduction of popular media forms (TV, video games) and as well with the rapid adoption of everyday assistive technology devices (calculators, cell phones). Along the way, TV has produced its share of 'couch potatoes' and 'CNN junkies,' while the use of personal calculators never actually produced a generation of children who were unable to do simple addition. The question as to whether a frequently engaged activity becomes a pastime, a passion or a personal addiction warranting a DSM-IV designation becomes a very contentious and thorny area that oftentimes becomes rooted in relativist philosophy steeped in personal value judgments. However, these existing forms of entertainment and assistive devices are easily seen to allow for interaction and shared experiences with other people and provide a modicum of convenience for modern living.

In contrast, the concern about persons who might prefer to spend time in VE's and form relationships with the 'artificially intelligent and personable' characters that may inhabit them seems to strike a unique chord in everyday judgments about pathological interests. Out of this concern it becomes possible to quickly view these activities as a threat to psychological well-being by way of providing an unhealthy substitute for physical proximity and interaction with 'real' humans that could promote or exacerbate social withdrawal or other forms of psychological disturbance. Yet, we can observe socially-evolved Internet communities based on shared interests, as well as highly structured distributed internet gaming societies that serve as meaningful personal and social outlets for many participants without ever requiring face-to-face interaction. These issues are particularly challenging to address due to the rapid onset of the information technology revolution. Essentially, the psychological sciences are still trying to make sense of how much of the knowledge acquired over a century of empirical study in the real world can be usefully applied to predict the impact of activities in cyberspace on psychological processes. Currently, no fully satisfying or comprehensive answers exist for these questions, nor are they expected to appear in the near future.

An early test case for these issues currently exists in Japan where there is considerable controversy raging over the existence of a condition among adolescents popularly termed *"hikikomori"*, characterized by a lack of social communication skills and withdrawal. While no systematic research has examined this condition scientifically, social critics have linked its occurrence generally to the widespread use of digital media and communication devices that are currently quite popular with children in Japan. More specifically, this social commentary has increasingly focused on the popularity of "Love Simulation Games" (Kato, 1997). These interactive computer games involve the creation of thematic gaming scenarios where the 'player' meets and evolves relationships with avatar representations of members of the opposite sex, each having differentially programmed personalities. The player makes an initial judgment as to which one he or she would like to form a relationship with, and various choice points occur in the 'game' (i.e., giving presents, having 'conversations,' planning dates, doing favors, etc.) that determine various outcomes. The player interacts with the characters, and the game is won or lost based on by whether the sought-after avatar selects the player to be their 'steady' at the end of the game. The popular image of the ill effects of this sort of gaming is the perception that adolescents with fears of failing at social interactions will immerse themselves in the many 'Love-simulation' games that are available, in the absence of taking the risks that are involved in pursuing and forming relationships with 'real' peers.

It is clear that many alternative views of these 'relational' activities are possible. However, the previous discussion suggests one possible way that, even at the currently limited and unnaturalistic level of the interaction that is available with 2D computer game avatars, involvement with the virtual characters that 'populate' these thematic gaming environments occurs, which is being seriously questioned (whether correctly or incorrectly). While the focused scope of this chapter precludes in-depth coverage of this area, it is not hard to imagine the possible socioethical issues that will emerge when exotic VEs become available (beyond what is available to the user in their real world) that allow for behavior with custom-tailored avatars which is devoid of immediate real-world consequences. As psychologists, it will become increasingly necessary to consider possibilities that are both positive (i.e., social skills training, entertainment in imaginative growth-fostering VEs, etc.) and negative (i.e., increases in social isolation, playing out of 'pathological' exploitive impulses), with an appreciation of both the personal choice and real world mental health issues in the balance.

9. *What are the potential human and societal consequences that could occur with the creation of VEs that involve violent or dehumanizing content and how are they to be anticipated and investigated?*

As with most tools that result from human scientific and technological achievement, the use of VR can be seen as a 'double-edged sword'. Indeed, many of the attributes that make VR such a promising tool for targeting useful goals and purposes could also serve to produce scenarios with the potential for negative consequences. Similar to the topics presented in the last section, the question here concerns the possibility that VR use could have a negative impact on real world attitudes and behavior. One of VR's assumed assets is its capacity to deliver high fidelity training or rehabilitation environments that are designed to promote transfer of VR-acquired learning or behavior to the real world. Ordinarily this asset is expected to support 'positive' outcomes and to promote human welfare, but it is not hard to imagine the development of scenarios that could serve less 'noble' purposes. One highly visible concern is in the creation of VEs that involve violent content or allow for engagement in other forms of 'dehumanizing' behavior, as has already occurred with less immersive computer games (e.g., 'first-person' shooting scenarios). In this regard, there exists a long history of research and contentious debate concerning the effects of *exposure* to violent content in other popular media forms (i.e., television, film, gaming, etc.), particularly with children. An extensive and diverse literature has evolved in this area over the last 40 years, initially gaining visibility with the early work of Bandura and colleagues on the effects of 'modeling' on the expression of aggressive behavior (Bandura & Walters, 1959; Bandura et al., 1961). More recently, in the wake of a rash of school shootings in the U.S., this issue has been thrust into the glare of the popular media spotlight. These recent events have reinvigorated the debate concerning what role exposure to media violence may play in the occurrence of such tragic incidents (Calvert, 2001).

The purpose of this section is not to weigh in on the issue of whether certain media content directly influences or causes violent, anti-social or otherwise unhealthy or 'undesirable' behavior. Rather, we will briefly address the issues specific to VR use, particularly in view of its immersive and interactive features, that are relevant to envision a research agenda to rationally examine VR's potential impact on negative or socially undesirable behavior. These topics will increase in relevance (and visibility) as VR technology advances and becomes more accessible, especially with the arrival of next-generation gaming platforms that will soon be capable of delivering compelling VEs (Macedonia, 2000). As this gaming infrastructure becomes integrated into the 'digital homestead,' it is naïve to believe that game developers will ignore the future commercial potential for creating VEs that immerse players in violent or antisocial digital content. Already computer gaming has approached the 'Hollywood' film industry in total entertainment market share, and much of this may be due to the seemingly universal popularity of games that present highly realistic depictions of graphic violence.

If history is any predictor of future design, marketing, and consumer trends in the computer gaming industry, VR gaming scenarios will likely 'advance' along a path similar to that which produced the 'Pong' to 'Space Invaders' to 'Duke Nukem' evolution. While emotion-driven and value-laden viewpoints often serve to promote wide social awareness of the problems that could occur with the popular adoption of any emerging technology, reasonable answers to these questions will require rigorous scientific investigation.

A thoughtful and rationally planned scientific agenda to guide research examining VR's potential negative impact is needed in order to integrate perspectives from many areas of the psychological sciences (i.e., social psychology, neuropsychology, communications theory, forensics, etc.).

A reasonable starting point for this agenda may be found in the examination of VR's specific characteristics in comparison to already existing forms of popular media. Unlike television or cinema, which essentially involve passive exposure or consumption of content, VR allows for more naturalistic interaction *within* the content. The difference between the passive viewing experience that is afforded by TV or cinema and the immersive/interactive features of a VE can be intuitively grasped by considering the difference between observing activity in an aquarium through a window vs. actually swimming within it. Such a capacity for immersive interaction may foster a sense of presence within a simulated VE that promotes an active behavioral learning experience that is supported by potent *procedural* learning mechanisms.

From a neuropsychological perspective, procedural or skill learning/ memory (Cohen & Squire, 1980; Charness et al., 1988) involves the capacity to learn rule-based or automatic procedures including motor skills, certain kinds of rule-based puzzles, and sequences for running or operating things (Sohlberg & Mateer, 1989). This type of 'hands-on' experiential learning is based in very old neural circuitry that is initially responsible for basic acquisition of skills that are necessary for survival in young organisms, yet its functional value continues throughout the lifespan. In fact, the survival relevance of procedural learning can be inferred when viewed in contrast to *declarative,* or fact-based memory, which is usually more impaired in persons with CNS dysfunction and less amenable to rehabilitative improvement (Sohlberg & Mateer, 1989). As well, procedural learning may occur without any recollection of the actual training. This is commonly referred to as *implicit* memory (Graf & Schacter, 1985), and its presence is indicative of a relatively 'sturdy' ability to process and retain new material without the person's conscious awareness of when or where the learning occurred. These learning concepts are of particular relevance when considering the potential impact of immersive interactive VE scenarios that, for better or worse, may produce 'reflexive' behavioral responding operating beneath a person's awareness level. As such, some important initial research questions for psychologists concerned with these issues would include the following:

(1) Will procedural skill acquisition for violent or undesirable behaviors acquired in a VE produce a higher likelihood that these behaviors will be manifested in real world behavior?

(2) Human judgment processes may function to generally inhibit impulsive aggressive behavior under normal conditions. However, in high arousal situations, would implicit encoding of violent behavior patterns that are well practiced and overlearned in VEs serve to increase the likelihood of aggressive reaction/reflex responding by placing these behavioral pro-

pensities in a higher 'position' in a person's response hierarchy? Would this learning promote a higher likelihood of aggression in certain stressful or highly charged emotional contexts (e.g., reflexively delivering a kung-fu kick to someone when in disagreement, instead of responding with a persuasive verbal argument)?

(3) Are there populations where such 'reflexive' responding (number 2 above) would be more likely to occur, such as with children or individuals having certain neuropsychological or psychiatric diagnoses (i.e., dysexecutive syndrome, antisocial personality disorder, etc.)?

(4) Would highly proceduralized interactive 'exposure' to graphically rich violence or other dehumanizing activities serve to diminish or habituate a person's sensitivity to horrific events in the real world or would this activity serve to support an empathy-building function by way of exposing the user to a less "sanitized" depiction and *experience* of consequences than is typically seen with the passive observation of TV or cinema.

(5) Would a 'super-cathartic' effect occur due to proceduralized simulated engagement in such violent activities that would serve to 'run off' aggressive or maladaptive impulses and lead to an actual decrease in subsequent negative real world behavioral manifestations?

Clearly, it will be incumbent on the psychological sciences to begin to address these questions as advances in VR technology allow for more realistic and compelling scenarios to become widely accessible to the general public. The development of a research agenda to address these ethical concerns at the societal level as well as for individual human use falls squarely on the scientific and professional skills of psychologists. These issues are complex and diverse, and require a perspective that integrates the diverse specialized knowledge found across the many areas of psychology. While many benefits may be derived from the thoughtful use of VR, we cannot expect these to come without certain risks. It is to be expected that *unintended* risks will always exist in the mainstream distribution of products derived from any noteworthy human achievement. However, it is the *unanticipated* risks that reveal a lack of ethical responsibility and have the most potential to do harm. In this regard it has been the purpose of this section to reduce this potential by anticipating these risks and focusing awareness on the other edge of the VR 'sword.'

10. Will 'Universal Access' prevail or will a 'Digital Divide' emerge regarding the availability of these forms of VR assessment and treatment?

As is apparent from the previous discussion, we are experiencing the emergence of an information society, increasingly based on the production and exchange of information. As this vision unfolds, those who are able to thoughtfully design, develop and apply information technology and telecommunications (IT&T) will be in a position to drive fundamental advances for promoting human welfare. However, in order to maximize the potential benefits of this paradigm shift for those with special needs, it is necessary to focus efforts on the development and application of more usable and accessible IT&T. This direction fits well with the 'Information Society for All' concepts that have recently been addressed in the human-computer interaction literature (HCI) (Stephanidis et al., 1998). Efforts in this area support the development of IT&T that accommodates the broadest range of human abilities, skills, requirements and preferences. The potential results of such efforts could substantially redefine the assessment and rehabilitative strategies that are used in the area of disabilities, particularly with clinical populations having (CNS) dysfunction. However, in all areas where humans have access to resources, there are the 'haves' and the 'have-nots.' Information technology resources are no different, and the potential for inequity in this area has been recognized as a challenge to be considered (U.S. Department of Commerce, 2000a). This issue is clearly addressed in a series of U.S. government and international reports and is nicely summed up in the following:

> "In just about every country, a certain percentage of people has the best information technology that society has to offer. These people have the most powerful computers, the best telephone service and fastest Internet service, as well as a wealth of content and training relevant to their lives. There is another group of people. They are the people who for one reason or another don't have access to the newest or best computers, the most reliable telephone service or the fastest or most convenient Internet services. The difference between these two groups of people is what we call the Digital Divide" (U.S. Department of Commerce, 2000b).

Up to now, discussion of the Digital Divide has mainly centered on the Internet and computer system access. However, it is not difficult to imagine how this issue will take on added relevancy if VR tools are proven to be more effective than traditional approaches, yet are only selectively available to certain socioeconomic classes. The potential exists for the public to perceive VR as a more technically complex and 'sexy' approach, and this perception could serve to push its application into the realm of a more costly alternative to standard assessment and treatment approaches. In essence, will a digital divide occur in the access to sophisticated VR scenarios for assessment/diagnosis, education, therapy and personal growth promoting applications? Will we see access to these forms of technology-supported services limited to delivery by private practitioners as a more exclusive and costly 'specialty' approach? Will community-based mental health clinics or educational institutions serving lower socioeconomic communities (that often are lucky to have any access to computers for even administrative needs) fall into the future as VR 'have-nots'? Although some may support the notion that market forces will drive availability to all in need as the demand becomes more substantial, this has not been the case in the managed care era of medical treatment.

While the purpose of this chapter is not to promote a political agenda, it is our view that ethical concerns regarding fair access to services will need to be addressed, particularly if VR applications are found to be more efficacious than less expensive standard methods. Perhaps with continuing reductions in computing costs, this point will become moot as the technology 'trickles down' to all sectors of society. However, advanced consideration and monitoring of digital divide indicators by psychologists (as well as other health care and educational professionals) is recommended. This could serve to promote the ethical ideals embodied in Universal Access principles to enhance availability of clinical and educational services by supporting access to emerging information technologies.

Conclusion

VR appears to hold considerable promise for practitioners and researchers in neuropsychology and throughout the psychological sciences. With careful consideration of the ethical issues discussed in this chapter, the potential for improved understanding and treatment of our patients appears great.

References

Aguirre, G.K., & D'Esposito, M. (1997). Environmental knowledge is subserved by separable dorsal/ventral neural areas. *Journal of Neuroscience, 17,* 2512-2518.

American Psychological Association (1992). Ethical principles of psychologists and code of conduct. *American Psychologist, 47,* 1597-1611. Ananova (2001). *ANANOVA.* Available at: http://www.ananova.com/home.htm?79477.

Anderson, P., Rothbaum, B.O., & Hodges, L.F. (2000). Social phobia: Virtual reality exposure therapy for fear of public speaking. Paper presented at the Annual Meeting of the American Psychological Association, Washington, DC.

Aukstakalnis, S., & Blatner, D. (1992). *Silicon mirage: The art and science of virtual reality.* Berkeley, CA: Peachpit Press.

Bandura, A., Ross, D., & Ross, S.A. (1961). Transmission of aggression through imitation of aggressive models. *Journal of Abnormal and Social Psychology, 63,* 575-582.

Bandura, A., & Walters, R.H. (1959). *Adolescent aggression.* New York: Ronald.

Blascovich, J., Loomis, J., Beall, A.C., Swinth, K.R., Hoyt, C.L., & Bailenson, J.N. (in press). Immersive virtual environment technology as a methodological tool for social psychology. *Psychological Inquiry.*

Botella, C., Banos, R.M., Perpina, C., Villa, H., Alcaniz, M., & Rey, A. (1998). Virtual reality treatment of claustrophobia: A case report. *Behaviour Research and Therapy, 36,* 239-246.

Braak, H., Braak, E., & Bohl, J. (1993). Staging of Alzheimer-related cortical destruction. *European Neurology, 33,* 403-408.

Brooks, B.M., McNeil, J.E., Rose, F.D., Greenwood, R.J., Attree, E.A., & Leadbetter, A.G. (1999). Route learning in a case of amnesia: A preliminary investigation into the efficacy of training in a virtual environment. *Neuropsychological Rehabilitation, 9,* 63-76.

Brown, D.J., & Stewart, D.S. (1996). An emergent methodology for the design, development and implementation of virtual learning environments. In P. Sharkey (Ed.), *Proceedings of the first European conference on disability, virtual reality and associated technology* (pp. 75-84). Reading, UK: The University of Reading.

Carlin, A. S., Hoffman, H. G., & Weghorst, S. (1997). Virtual reality and tactile augmentation in the treatment of spider phobia: A case report. *Behavior Research and Therapy, 35,* 153-158.

Calvert, S.L. (in press). The social impact of virtual reality. In K. Stanney (Ed.), *The handbook of virtual environments.* New York: Erlbaum.

Charness, N., Milberg, W., & Alexander, M. P. (1988). Teaching an amnesic a complex cognitive skill. *Brain Cognition, 8,* 253-272.

Chase, W.G., & Ericsson, K.A. (1981). Skilled memory. In J. R. Anderson (Ed.), *Cognitive skills and their acquisition.* Hillsdale, NJ: Erlbaum.

Cohen, N.J., & Squire, L.R. (1980). Preserved learning and retention of pattern-analyzing skill in amnesia: Dissociation of "knowing how" and "knowing that." *Science, 210,* 207-209.

Damer, B. (1998). *Avatars!* Berkeley, CA: Peachpit Press.

DiZio, P., & Lackner, J.R. (1992). Spatial orientation, adaptation, and motion sickness in real and virtual environments. *Presence: Teleoperators and Virtual Environments,1,* 323.

Foa, E.B., & Kozak, M.J. (1986). Emotional processing of fear: Exposure to corrective information. *Psychological Bulletin, 99,* 20-35.

Foa, E.B., Steketee, G., & Rothbaum, B. (1989). Behavioral/cognitive conceptualizations of post-traumatic stress disorder. *Behavior Therapy, 20,* 155-176.

Gershon, J., Zimand, E., Pickering, M., Lemos, R., Hodges, L., & Rothbaum, B.O. (2001). *Virtual reality as a distractor during an invasive medical procedure for pediatric cancer patients.* Paper presented at the 35th Annual Convention of the Association for the Advancement of Behavior Therapy, Philadelphia, PA. November 15–18, 2001.

Graf, P., & Schacter, D.L. (1985). Implicit and explicit memory for new associations in normal and amnesic patients. *Journal of Experimental Psychology: Learning, Memory, and Cognition, 11,* 501-518.

Hettinger, L.J. (1992). Visually induced motion sickness in virtual environments. *Presence: Teleoperators and Virtual Environments, 1,* 306-307.

Hoffman, H.G., Doctor, J.N., Patterson, D.R., Carrougher, G.J., & Furness, T.A. (2000). Virtual reality as an adjunctive pain control during burn wound care in adolescent patients. *Pain, 85,* 305-309.

Horowitz, M.J., Wilner, N., & Alvarez, W. (1979). Impact of Events Scale: A measure of subjective distress. *Psychosomatic Medicine, 41,* 207-218.

IBM (1999). *Almaden Computer Science Research.* Available at: *http://www. almaden.ibm.com/cs/blueeyes/suitor.html*

Kallman, E.A. (1993). Ethical evaluation: A necessary element in virtual environment research. *Presence, 2,* 143-146.

Kato, S. (1997). Girl Simulation games and its 10 year history. *Game Critique, 14,* 138-140.

Kennedy, R.S., Berbaum, K.S., & Drexler, J. (1994). *Methodological and measurement issues for identification of engineering features contributing to virtual reality sickness.* Paper presented at: Image 7 Conference. Tucson, AZ.

Kennedy, R.S., Lane, N.E., Berbaum, K.S., & Lilienthal, M.G. (1993). Simulator sickness questionnaire: An enhanced method for quantifying simulator sickness. *International Journal of Aviation Psychology, 3,* 203-220.

Kennedy, R.S., & Stanney, K.M. (1996). Postural instability induced by virtual reality exposure: Development of certification protocol. *International Journal of Human-Computer Interaction, 8,* 2547.

Kirsch, N.L., Levine, S. P., Lajiness-O'Neill, R., & Schnyder, M. (1992). Computer-assisted interactive task guidance: Facilitating the performance of a simulated vocational task. *Journal of Head Trauma Rehabilitation, 7*(3), 13-25.

Kolasinski, G. (1995). *Simulator sickness in virtual environments* (Tech Report 1027). Orlando: United States Army Research Institute for the Behavioral and Social Sciences.

Kurzweil, R. (1999). *The age of spiritual machines*. New York: Penguin Putnam Inc.

Krueger, M.W. (1993). The experience society. *Presence: Teleoperators and Virtual Environments, 2,* 162-168.

Lezak, M.D. (1995). *Neuropsychological assessment*. New York: Oxford University Press.

Macedonia, M. (2000). The empire strikes back...with the X-Box. *Computer Society Magazine*, June,104-106.

McComas, J. Pivik, J., & Laflamme, M. (1998). Children's transfer of spatial learning from virtual reality to real environments. *CyberPsychology and Behavior, 1,* 2.

Miller, G., & Dunn, A. (2000). Internet's toll on social life? *Los Angeles Times*, October 26, 2000: 1.

National Institutes of Health (1995). *Basic behavioral science research for mental health: A national investment*. A report of the U.S. National Advisory Mental health Council (NIH Publication No. 95-3682). Rockville, MD: Author.

National Institutes of Health (1998). *Rehabilitation of persons with traumatic brain injury. Consensus Statement*. October 26 - 28, 16(1). Available at: *http:// consensus nih.gov*.

O'Connor, M., & Cermack, L.S. (1987). Rehabilitation of organic memory disorders. In M. J. Meier, A. L. Benton, & L. Diller (Eds.), *Neuropsychological rehabilitation*. New York: Guilford.

Parente, R., & Herrmann, D. (1996). *Retraining cognition: Techniques and applications*. Gaithersburg, MD: Aspen Publishing Inc.

Pertaub, D.P., & Slater, M. (2001). *An experiment on fear of public speaking in virtual reality*. Paper presented at the 9th Annual Medicine Meets Virtual Reality Conference, Newport Beach, CA.

Prigatano, G.P. (1997). Learning from our successes and failures: Reflections and comments on "Cognitive Rehabilitation: How it is and how it might be." *Journal of the International Neuropsychological Society, 3,* 497-499.

Psotka, J. (1995). Immersive training systems: Virtual reality and education and training. *Instructional Science, 23,* 405-431.

Pugnetti, L., Mendozzi, L., Motta, A., Cattaneo, A., Barbieri, E., & Brancotti, A. (1995a). Evaluation and retraining of adults' cognitive impairments: Which role for virtual reality technology? *Computers in Biology and Medicine, 25,* 213-227.

Pugnetti, L., Mendozzi, L., Motta, A., Cattaneo, A., Barbieri, E., Brancotti, A., & Cazzullo, C.L. (1995b). *Immersive VR for the retraining of acquired cognitive defects*. Paper presented at the Medicine Meets Virtual Reality 3 Conference. San Diego, CA.

Pugnetti, L., Mendozzi, L., Barberi, E., Rose F.D., & Attree, E.A. (1996). Nervous system correlates of virtual reality experience. In P. Sharkey (Ed.), *Proceedings of the first European conference on disability, virtual reality and associated technology* (pp. 239 - 246). Reading, UK: The University of Reading.

Pugnetti, L., Mendozzi, L., Attree, E.A., Barbieri, E., Brooks, B.M., Cazzullo, C.L., Motta, A., & Rose. F.D. (1998a). Probing memory and executive functions with virtual reality: Past and present studies. *CyberPsychology and Behavior, 1, 2.*

Pugnetti, L., Mendozzi, L., Barbieri, E., & Motta, A., Alpini, D., Attree, E.A., Brooks, B.M., & Rose, F.D. (1998b). Developments of a collaborative research on VR applications for mental health. In P. Sharkey, F.D. Rose, & J. Lindstrom (Eds.), *Proceedings of the 2nd European conference on disability, virtual reality and associated techniques* (pp. 77-84). Reading, UK: University of Reading.

Reason, J.T. (1970). Motion sickness: A special case of sensory rearrangement. *Advancement in Science, 26,* 386-393.

Regan, E., & Price, K.R. (1994). The frequency of occurrence and severity of side-effects of immersion virtual reality. *Aviation, Space, and Environmental Medicine, 65,* 527-530.

Renner, M.J., & Rosenzweig, M.R. (1987). *Enriched and impoverished environments: Effects on brain and behaviour.* New York: Springer-Verlag.

Rickel, J., & Johnson, W.L. (1999). Animated agents for procedural training in virtual reality: Perception, cognition, and motor control. *Applied Artificial Intelligence, 13,* 343-382.

Riva, G. (2000). Virtual reality in rehabilitation of spinal cord injuries: A case report. *Rehabilitation Psychology, 45,* 81-88.

Riva, G., Bacchetta, M. Baruffi, M., Rinaldi, S., & Molinari, E. (1998). Experiential cognitive therapy: A VR based approach for the assessment and treatment of eating disorders. In G. Riva, B. Wiederhold, & E. Molinari (Eds.), *Virtual environments in clinical psychology and neuroscience: Methods and techniques in advanced patient-therapist interaction* (pp. 120-135). Amsterdam: IOS Press.

Riva, G., Bacchetta, M. Baruffi, M., Rinaldi, S., & Molinari, E. (1999). Virtual reality based experiential cognitive treatment of anorexia nervosa. *Journal of Behavior Therapy and Experimental Psychiatry, 30,* 221-230.

Rizzo, A.A. (1994). Virtual reality applications for the cognitive rehabilitation of persons with traumatic head injuries. In Murphy, H.J. (Ed.), *Proceedings of the 2nd international conference on virtual reality and persons with disabilities.* Northridge: CSUN.

Rizzo, A.A., Buckwalter, J.G., Bowerly, T., McGee, J., van Rooyen, A., van der Zaag, C., Neumann, U., Thiebaux, M., Kim, L., Pair, J., & Chua, C. (2001a). Virtual environments for assessing and rehabilitating cognitive/functional performance: A review of projects at the USC Integrated Media Systems Center. *Presence: Teleoperators and Virtual Environments 10,* 359–374.

Rizzo, A.A., Buckwalter, J.G., Bowerly, T., van der Zaag, C., Humphrey, L., Neumann, U., Chua, C., Kyriakakis, C., van Rooyen,, A., & Sisemore, D. (2000). The virtual classroom: A virtual reality environment for the assessment and rehabilitation of attention deficits, *CyberPsychology and Behavior, 3,* 483-501.

Rizzo, A.A., Buckwalter, J.G., & van der Zaag, C. (in press). Virtual environment applications for neuropsychological assessment and rehabilitation. In K. Stanney (Ed.), *Handbook of virtual environments.* New York: Earlbaum.

Rizzo, A.A., Neumann, U., Enciso, R., Fidaleo, D., & Noh, J.Y. (2001b). Performance driven facial animation: Basic research on human judgments of emotional state in facial avatars. *CyberPsychology and Behavior, 4,* 471–488.

Rolland, J.P., Biocca, F.A., Barlow, T., & Kancherla, A. (1995). Quantification of adaptation to virtual-eye location in see-thru head-mounted displays. *Proceedings of the IEEE virtual reality annual international symposium '95* (pp. 55-66). Los Alamitos, CA: IEEE Computer Society Press.

Rose F.D. (1996). Virtual reality in rehabilitation following traumatic brain injury. In P. Sharkey (Ed.), *Proceedings of the first European conference on disability, virtual reality and associated technology* (pp. 5-12). Reading, UK: The University of Reading.

Rose, F.D., & Johnson, D.A. (1992). *Brain injury and after.* Chichester: Wileys.

Rothbaum, B.O., Hodges, L.F., Alarcon, R., Ready, D., Shahar, F., Graap, K., Pair, J., Hebert, P., Gotz, D., Wills, B., & Baltzell, D. (1999a). Virtual reality exposure therapy for PTSD Vietnam veterans: A case study. *Journal of Traumatic Stress, 12*, 263-271.

Rothbaum, B.O., Hodges, L.F., & Kooper, R. (1997). Virtual reality exposure therapy. *Journal of Psychotherapy Practice and Research, 6*, 291-296.

Rothbaum, B.O., Hodges, L.F., Kooper, R., Opdyke, D., Williford, J., & North, M.M. (1995). Effectiveness of virtual reality graded exposure in the treatment of acrophobia. *American Journal of Psychiatry, 152*, 626-628.

Rothbaum, B.O., Hodges, L.F., & Smith, S. (1999b). Virtual reality exposure therapy abbreviated treatment manual: Fear of flying application. *Cognitive and Behavioral Practice, 6*, 234-244.

Rothbaum, B.O., Hodges, L.F., Smith, S., Lee, J.H., & Price, L. (2000). A controlled study of virtual reality exposure therapy for the fear of flying. *Journal of Consulting and Clinical Psychology, 68*, 1020-1026.

Rothbaum, B.O., Hodges, L., Watson, B.A., Kessler, G.D., & Opdyke, D. (1996). Virtual reality exposure therapy in the treatment of fear of flying: A case report. *Behaviour Research and Therapy, 34*, 477-481.

Schneider, S.M., & Workman, M.L. (1999). Effects of virtual reality on symptom distress in children receiving chemotherapy. *CyberPsychology and Behavior, 2*, 125-134.

Schultheis, M.T., & Rizzo, A.A. (2001). The application of virtual reality technology in rehabilitation. *Rehabilitation Psychology, 46*, 296–311.

Smith, S., Rothbaum, B.O., & Hodges, L.F. (1999). Treatment of fear of flying using virtual reality exposure therapy: A single case study. *The Behavior Therapist, 22*, 154-158.

Sohlberg, M.M., & Mateer, C.A. (1989). *Introduction to cognitive rehabilitation: Theory and practice.* New York: The Guilford Press.

Stanney, K.M., & Kennedy, R.S. (1997). The psychometrics of cybersickness. *Communications of the ACM 40*(8), 67-68.

Stanney, K.M., Salvendy, G., Deisigner, J., DiZio, P., Ellis, S., Ellison, E., Fogleman, G., Gallimore, J., Hettinger, L., Kennedy, R., Lackner, J., Lawson, B., Maida, J., Mead, A., Mon-Williams, M., Newman, D., Piantanida, T., Reeves, L., Riedel, O., Singer, M., Stoffregen, T., Wann, J., Welch, R., Wilson, J., & Witmer, B. (1998). Aftereffects and sense of presence in virtual environments: Formulation of a research and development agenda. Report sponsored by the Life Sciences Division at NASA Headquarters. *International Journal of Human-Computer Interaction, 10*, 135-187.

Stanton D., Wilson P., Foreman N., & Duffy H. (2000). Virtual environments as spatial training aids for children and adults with physical disabilities. In P. Sharkey, A. Cesarani, L. Pugnetti, & A. Rizzo (Eds.), *Proceedings of the 3rd international conference on disability, virtual reality, and associated technology.* Reading, UK: University of Reading.

Stephanidis, C., Salvendi, G., Akoumianakis, D., Bevan, N., Brewer, J., Emiliani, P.L., Galetsas, A., Haataja, S., Iakovidis, I., Jacko, J.A., Jenkins, P., Karshmer, A.I., Korn, P., Marcus, A., Murphy, H.J., Stary, S., Vanderheiden, G., Weber, G., & Ziegler, J. (1998). Toward an information society for all: An international research and development agenda. *International Journal of Human-Computer Interaction, 10*, 107-134.

Sternberg, R.J. (1997). Intelligence and lifelong learning: What's new and how can we use it? *American Psychologist, 52*, 1134-1139.

Swartout, W., Hill, R., Gratch, J., Johnson, W.L., Kyriakakis, C., LaBore, C., Lindheim, R., Marsella, S., Miraglia, D., Moore, B., Morie, J., Rickel, J., Thiébaux, M., Tuch, L., & Whitney R. (2001). Toward the Holodeck: Integrating graphics, sound, character and story. Paper presented at the 5th International Conference on Autonomous Agents, Montreal CN, May 28–June 1, 2001.

Turk, M., & Robertson, G. (2000). Perceptual user interfaces. *Communications of the ACM, 43(3)*, 33-34.

Tart, C. (1990). Multiple personality, altered states and virtual reality: The world simulation process approach. *Dissociation, 3*, 222-233.

US Department of Commerce (2000a). *Falling through the Net, toward digital inclusion*. National Telecommunications and Information Administration. Available at: *http://www.ntia.doc.gov/ntiahome/fttn00/contents00.html*.

US Department of Commerce (2000b). *Closing the digital divide*. Available at: *http://www.digitaldivide.gov/about.htm*.

Wann, J.P., & Mon-Williams, M. (1996). What does virtual reality NEED? Human factors issues in the design of three dimensional computer environments. *International Journal of Human-Computer Studies, 44*, 829-847.

Whalley, L.J. (1995). Ethical issues in the application of virtual reality to medicine. *Computer, Biology and Medicine, 25*, 107-114.

Whitbeck, C. (1993). Virtual environments: Ethical issues and significant confusions. *Presence, 2 (2)*, 17-52.

Whitbeck, C., & Brooks, R. (1982). Criterion for evaluating a computer aid to clinical reasoning. *Journal of Medicine and Philosophy, 9*, 51-65.

Wiederhold, B., Riva, G., Choi, Y.H., & Wiederhold, M. (2000). *Virtual reality exposure therapy in the treatment of panic disorder with agoraphobia*. Paper presented at the 34th Annual Convention of the Association for the Advancement of Behavior Therapy, New Orleans, LA.

Wilson, B.A. (1997). Cognitive rehabilitation: How it is and how it might be. *Journal of the International Neuropsychological Society, 3*, 487-496.

Young, K.S. (1999). Introduction to theme issue on Internet addiction entitled: The research and controversy surrounding Internet addiction. *CyberPsychology and Behavior, 2*, 381-383.

Appendix — Institutional Review Boards and Virtual Reality: Helpful Tips

In general, the primary responsibilities of Institutional Review Boards (IRBs) include overseeing the protection of the rights and welfare of human subjects involved in research studies and upholding federal regulations set forth by the Department of Health and Human Services and the Food and Drug Administration. To this end, specific risks, benefits and appropriate safeguards require careful consideration when new procedures or protocols are employed. Given the increasing number of VR applications within clinical research and treatment, we offer the following 'IRB Tips' for the preparation of VR protocols:

(1) *Conduct ethical analysis.* As with any research consideration, determining ethicality, should begin with a clear description of the protocol under consideration and the list of potential affected parties and stakeholders. Thorough evaluation of each step of the process, identifying both the risks and the benefits for all parties involved, can help to generate a rational foundation for choices at each level of the procedure.

(2) *Consideration of the unique risks of VR exposure.* As discussed earlier in this chapter, VR exposure has been associated with some side effects (i.e., simulator sickness, escapism) that may not be an issue in more traditional protocols.

(3) *Plan for the unexpected.* Because VR is continuing to evolve, not all of the questions regarding the consequences of VR exposure have been answered. As such, a thorough evaluation of all possible negative reactions should be conducted prior to initiation of protocol

(4) *Integrate safeguards into your protocol.* Although much remains to be learned about VR exposure, some side effects have been consistently noted, and subsequent procedures for minimizing risk to these side effects have been developed. Inclusion of the most recent screening procedures (i.e., Simulator Sickness Questionnaire) should be standard in all VR protocols.

(5) *Identify your most vulnerable groups.* As discussed earlier, some clinical populations (e.g., impaired awareness, psychiatric) may be at a higher risk for negative experiences when exposed to VR. As such, researchers should consider the need for inclusion of such populations, and when necessary identify the additional steps taken to minimize risks among these individuals.

(6) *Clearly define the need for VR.* As VR continues to evolve, new environments and applications will continue to be developed. Consideration and justification for the appropriateness of the addition of VR to protocols should be addressed in all newly proposed applications. Unnecessary exposure to risk is a justifiable limitation to any research protocol.

(7) *Explaining your protocol.* Although improving, VR and the hardware required for delivering VR environments (i.e., HMDs) still remain in the 'futuristic technology' domain for many clinical disciplines and laymen.

As such, description of the VR component of research protocols should be clear and concise with minimal jargon. In many cases, the use of diagrams for explaining hardware is often useful.

(8) *Defining your data.* Because VR affords an environment where all behavioral responses can be recorded throughout the virtual experience, variables to be measured in the VE should be clearly identified. These variables should be hypothesis driven and based on prior research or knowledge. The unique feature of recording all and any possible responses sets up an opportunity for 'fishing expeditions' which could subsequently lead to unnecessary exposure and abuse of this technology.

(9) *Identify responsibility, liability and accountability.* Given the fact that much remains to be learned regarding medical applications of VR, identification of procedures to address any significant complications should be clearly identified in the early stages of the protocol development.

Chapter 13

ADDRESSING PERCEIVED ETHICAL VIOLATIONS IN CLINICAL NEUROPSYCHOLOGY

Cecilia Deidan and Shane Bush

Introduction

The role of the neuropsychologist has evolved considerably in recent years in both the clinical and medical–legal arenas. Neuropsychologists are relied upon by neurologists, neurosurgeons, primary care physicians, pediatricians, physiatrists, psychiatrists, educators, attorneys, and others to assist in determining the presence and nature of brain dysfunction and in establishing and conducting courses of rehabilitation. The role of the clinical neuropsychologist often involves reviewing medical, academic, psychosocial, and legal history; interviewing the patient and collateral sources; observing the patient's behavior; and conducting a comprehensive neuropsychological evaluation as a means of rendering a clinical opinion or judgment. Each of these aspects of practice involves potential ethical decision-making challenges and potential areas for colleagues to neglect adherence to the APA Ethical Principles and Code of Conduct (APA, 1992).

Ethical decision-making is based upon logic and reasoning. The scientist–practitioner model of education and training (Pepinsky & Pepinsky, 1954) equips neuropsychologists with the skills needed to formulate clinical impressions and hypotheses concerning the nature, origin, and treatment of a patient's reported cognitive and/or neurobehavioral disturbances. These skills include the ability to (a) formulate hypotheses about the patient, (b) gather data, (c) formulate hypotheses about the patient's presenting symptoms or concerns, and (d) test the hypotheses or impressions in a logical, methodical, and scientific manner. However, even with these skills neuropsychologists may fail to recognize a critical factor inherent in the neuropsychological evaluative process; specifically, errors in judgment or inferential bias. These errors may result in ethical violations, and they may bias the way we view or respond to violations by others. Additionally, as Treppa (1998) points out, most psychologists do not have sufficient graduate training on how to take one's personal or professional biases into account when making decisions about ethical issues.

The purpose of this chapter is to describe a process of evaluating and addressing potential ethical violations in clinical neuropsychology. To accomplish that goal, we present common errors in the reasoning process (inferential biases) that can lead to unethical practice or to errors in one's approach to addressing the possible ethical violations of others. We then tie the reasoning process into specific recommendations and illustrative cases.

Inferential Biases

The same processes that are used in making judgments or inferences about people in day-to-day interactions are used by clinicians in their practice and may inadvertently result in ethical violations (Chapman & Chapman, 1969; Mahoney, 1977; Meehl, 1954; Routh & King, 1972; Tversky & Kahneman, 1971). The use of general rules (e.g., heuristics) can often result in biases in the inferential process (Faust, 1986; Kahneman & Tversky, 1973; Turk & Salovey, 1985). Such inferential biases include those related to: (a) the availability and representative heuristic; (b) fundamental attribution error; (c) anchoring, prior knowledge, and labeling; (d) confirmatory hypothesis testing; and (e) reconstructive memory. Negative consequences of bias in psychological and neuropsychological practice have been identified, and the consequences may include misdiagnoses, inappropriate treatments, inaccurate expert opinions, and exacerbation of a patient's problems (e.g., Darley & Gross, 1983; Sweet & Moulthrop, 1999).

The need to increase awareness of the pitfalls of inferential bias in the field of neuropsychology is as clear as it has been in the field of psychology in general (e.g., Arnoult & Anderson, 1988; Leary & Miller, 1986). However, merely *knowing* that bias exists and can be a threat to a clinician in formulating his or her judgments is not sufficient to avoid falling prey to such biases (Wiggins, 1981). Strategies have been proposed that are aimed at bias minimization, including using disconfirmatory strategies and writing out explicit arguments for and against proposed hypotheses (Arkes, 1981; Arnoult & Anderson, 1988; Dawes, 1982; Faust, 1986; Fischoff, 1982; Leary & Miller, 1986). Recently, self-examination questions have been proposed as a means of identifying bias when formulating opinions in the course of forensic neuropsychological evaluations (Sweet & Moulthrop,

1999). This type of self-examination may also be applied to ethical decision-making.

Availability and Representative Heuristics

The availability heuristic (Kahneman & Tversky, 1973) occurs when an individual attempts to determine how likely it is that a particular event or situation will occur. This heuristic involves basing judgment on how easily information comes to mind (information saliency; Morrow & Deidan, 1992). If pertinent information is available in memory, situations are perceived as being likely to occur (Nisbett & Ross, 1980), and an individual's search for less salient, less consistent information is not likely to occur (Taylor & Fiske, 1978).

The availability heuristic may bias neuropsychologists toward judging certain diagnoses as being more common that they actually are. For instance, a neuropsychologist working primarily with geriatric patients who have dementia may view dementia as more common in the elderly in general than it actually is. Such a bias may affect his or her clinical judgment, resulting in an overestimation of the presence of the diagnosis and a decreased likelihood that diagnostic conditions with better prognoses will be considered.

The representative heuristic (Kahneman & Tversky, 1973) involves categorizing information or events based on how well they meet the characteristics of various groups (i.e., goodness of fit). What are perceived as the salient features of an object are compared with the characteristics of certain groups to determine if the object fits into the category. For example, a child may determine that an unfamiliar animal is a bird because it meets the salient criteria of the bird category (e.g., wings, beak, ability to fly; Morrow & Deidan, 1992). The representative heuristic may influence the neuropsychological evaluation in a number of ways. For example, a neuropsychologist may perceive that his or her patient matches stereotypical characteristics concerning gender, race, and socioeconomic status (Brown, 1970; Sharf & Bishop, 1979). Another example of the representative bias would be the tendency for a neuropsychologist to classify patients as either 'good patients' (nonmalingers) or 'bad patients' (malingers) based on their experience with similar patients (Strupp, 1958). This type of bias may lead the neuropsychologist not to consider factors that would influence the probability of events, such as the base rates of disorders or the reliability and validity of information obtained (Kruglanski & Ajzen 1983).

Neuropsychologists use both availability and representative heuristics when formulating hypotheses and making clinical decisions (Cantor et al., 1980; Turk & Salovey, 1985). For example, diagnoses that are given more frequently by a neuropsychologist are more salient to that neuropsychologist. Therefore, future patients will have a higher probability of receiving those diagnoses than diagnoses that the neuropsychologist is less familiar with or uses less frequently (Higgins & King, 1981).

For instance, a neuropsychologist that works in an acute rehabilitation setting primarily with individuals who have sustained traumatic brain injuries will likely see restlessness and agitation exacerbated by excessive environmental stimulation. The neuropsychologist may address such behavior by reducing the amount of stimulation to which the patient is exposed, such as ensuring that the environment is quiet and free of excessive visual stimulation (Bush & Coben, 1997). Similarly, if a patient with a left hemisphere cerebrovascular accident and expressive aphasia were admitted to that neuropsychologist's unit and evidenced restlessness and agitation when interacting with others, the neuropsychologist employing the availability and representative heuristics would remove that patient to a quiet environment and reduce the light. However, the patient with aphasia may have become agitated because the staff did not understand their need to use the restroom.

Additionally, certain diagnoses will be more salient to some neuropsychologists than to others due to differences in theoretical orientations or philosophical positions (Bishop & Richards, 1984; Langer & Abelson, 1974; Mahoney 1977; Snyder 1977), which will inevitably lead to a higher rate of certain diagnoses. The proclivity toward bias during the formation of diagnoses led Grosz and Grossman (1964) to conclude that "Such judgements may be less informative about the patient they are meant to describe than about the clinician who makes them" (p. 112).

In order to reduce the likelihood of bias resulting from availability and representative heuristics, the following recommendations are offered:
1. Pay careful attention to the less salient details of a case and to those with which one is less familiar.
2. Individualize the approach to each patient, regardless of similarities to previous patients.
3. Refer to appropriate guidelines/criteria each time a diagnosis is made, rather than basing judgment on memory of the characteristics of various categories.
4. Consider base rates (frequency of occurrence) and multiple diagnostic possibilities (Faust, 1986). Ask, "How likely is it that a particular individual, with this set of characteristics, fits into this diagnostic category?" (Morrow & Deidan, 1992).
5. Evaluate and examine the information from different theoretical or philosophical perspectives (Arnoult & Anderson, 1988).

Fundamental Attribution Error
In the perception of responsibility for events, there often exists a discrepancy between the observers of the event and those who participated in the situation (Morrow & Deidan, 1992). Jones and Nisbett (1971) described this phenomenon as the "pervasive tendency for actors to attribute their actions to situational requirements whereas observers tend to attribute the same actions to stable personal dispositions" (p. 2). The proclivity for observers to underestimate and for actors (participants) to overestimate the degree of situational influence is known as the fundamental attribution error (Ross, 1977).

The fundamental attribution error has been demonstrated to occur within the therapy process (Batson, 1975). However, this type of bias may also cause a neuropsychologist to infer that a patient's symptoms are based on the patient's personality rather than on situational factors, such as an acquired brain injury (Batson et al., 1982). During an evaluation, the neuropsychologist would be considered the observer and the patient would be considered the actor. As a consequence of this dynamic, the actor–observer bias will make it more likely for the neuropsychologist to attribute the patient's distress or concerns to dispositional or personality factors, whereas the patient may attribute his or her problems to external variables (e.g., traumatic brain injury, spouse, stress). These attribution errors may create a situation in which the neuropsychologist and patient disagree on the etiology of the concern or complaint. Female and minority patients, who often have legitimate claims of discrimination and are subjected to significant external stressors, may be particularly at risk for this type of inferential bias. As a result of the fundamental attribution error, neuropsychologists may attempt to compensate for a patient's tendency to blame external variables by emphasizing the patient's contributions to the complaint or concern (Batson, 1975).

Many factors may contribute to a neuropsychologist's susceptibility to the fundamental attribution error. Education and training paradigms and certain philosophical positions that neuropsychologists may adopt based on experience may render them more vulnerable to the fundamental attribution error than others (Snyder, 1977). For example, some neuropsychologists that practice in the forensic arena (e.g., those retained by the defense) may have a tendency to attribute a patient's poor cognitive performance to a desire for secondary gain rather than to an injury to the brain. In contrast, neuropsychologists that practice in other settings or the other side of the legal argument (e.g., the plaintiff) may have a propensity for attributing a patient's cognitive complaints to neurophysiological factors rather than to social, situational, environmental, or motivational factors.

To avoid the fundamental attribution error, the following recommendations are offered:
1. Recognize the tendency to attribute symptoms or findings solely to either dispositional or situational factors.
2. Formulate alternative hypotheses that focus on a variety of factors that may be affecting the patient.
3. Examine the case from the position of an imagined colleague representing the opposite point of view.

Anchoring: Prior Knowledge, and Labeling

The inferential bias of anchoring occurs when initial impressions, beliefs, or preconceptions are not revised despite new, often contradictory, information. These beliefs, impressions or preconceptions are adhered to and maintained and may disproportionately influence future judgments. In the practice of neuropsychology, cognitive anchors can manifest themselves in two primary ways: (a) The formation of preconceptions or clinical impressions from the information that the neuropsychologist attains prior to meeting, interviewing, and evaluating the patient (i.e., prior knowledge), and (b) the formation of preconceptions or clinical impressions from previous conditions or diagnosis associated with the patient (i.e., labeling).

Neuropsychologists often receive referrals from professionals representing a variety of disciplines who make their impressions or beliefs of patients known to the neuropsychologist. Similarly, neuropsychologists are likely to receive medical, academic, and/or legal information prior to the first appointment with the patient. Although such procedures are thought to be time-efficient, practical, and methodical, they may not always be in the patient's best interest. Prior knowledge about a case can influence clinical judgment (e.g., Darley & Gross, 1983; Mahoney, 1977).

One of the most important and well-known studies of the effects of prior information is Temerlin's (1968) study of psychiatrists, clinical psychologists, and clinical psychology graduate students. In essence, these groups of subjects were asked to listen to a taped interview of a patient who was labeled 'healthy.' No symptomatology was found, and no diagnoses were rendered. However when a similar group of professionals was told, prior to listening to the same taped interview, that the patient was psychotic, 94% of the professionals rendered a clinical diagnosis.

Labeling and prior diagnosis also tend to persist and influence future clinical decisions and interpretations (e.g., Cantor & Mischel, 1979; Cantor et al., 1980). Once preconceptions have been formulated, it is difficult to change these beliefs as new information comes to light (Lichtenberg, 1984). The classic exemplar of the durability of prior diagnosis is the study conducted by Rosenhan (1973) in which 'normal' participants, after reporting auditory hallucinations, were given the diagnosis of schizophrenia by the medical staffs of various psychiatric facilities. The participants, subsequently, had extreme difficulty convincing the staff that they were, in fact, not schizophrenic. Anchoring would be evident in a neuropsychological context if a patient with a documented history of schizophrenia presented with new cognitive complaints and his or her symptoms were attributed to delusions rather than considered viable.

Timing of when information is obtained in the neuropsychological evaluative process may also bias a neuropsychologist's clinical impressions, with information obtained earlier seemingly having more weight than information obtained later (Friedlander & Phillips, 1984). One study was composed of five groups of psychologists, psychiatrists and social workers that were given detailed transcripts to review (Friedlander & Stockman, 1983). The transcripts presented identical information including symptomatology consistent with anorexia nervosa. The only difference between the transcripts was the timing of the presentation of the symptoms. Results indicated that the more substantial anchoring and the more pathological clinical findings were associated with transcripts presenting the symptoms of anorexia nervosa earlier in the interview.

Neuropsychologists may be influenced by these cognitive anchors when evaluating a colleague's behavior and considering whether or not it represents ethical misconduct. For example, if a neuropsychologist has knowledge that a colleague has acted unethically in the past, he or she may be more likely to perceive current behavior as unethical. If neuropsychologists are not aware of the potential for anchoring, such bias may result in the filing of frivolous complaints. Conversely, questionable behavior exhibited by a neuropsychologist that has a reputation as an ethical practitioner may go unpursued.

To counteract the anchoring effects of prior knowledge and labeling, the following recommendations are offered:

1. Delay reviewing the information from referring and collateral sources until making your own observation of the patient.
2. Keep in mind that the referral source is also susceptible to inferential bias.
3. Check with the patient to see if the first impression (anchor) is correct. If not, be open to assimilating new information that may change the initial impression.
4. Consult with colleagues and ask them to evaluate the existing information. Determine if they draw the same conclusions.
5. Challenge yourself to look for new information that may contradict preconceptions.
6. As the evaluation process unfolds, re-evaluate one's working hypothesis, the preconceived diagnosis, to determine if earlier impressions are valid.
7. Adopt a 'changing probabilities' point of view, which will allow one to examine all logical possibilities on a continuous basis.

Confirmatory Hypothesis Testing Bias

Confirmatory hypothesis testing bias occurs as a consequence of pursuing information in such a manner as to influence the type of information that one elicits from another individual. Once an initial impression has been made, it is difficult to test the accuracy of the hypothesis in an unbiased manner (Dallas & Baron, 1985; Snyder & Campbell, 1980). Thus, one is likely to make inquiries and initiate discussions that will confirm the hypotheses one has formed about the patient (Hollon & Kriss, 1984).

Some studies of confirmatory hypothesis testing bias have revealed findings that were contradictory to those of Hollon and Kriss (1984). For example, Dallas and Baron (1985) found that when participants were allowed to generate their own questions, they asked both confirmatory and nonconfirmatory questions. Other investigations have reported similar findings (Strohmer & Chiodo, 1984; Strohmer & Newman, 1983; Trope and Bassok, 1982). The results of these studies indicated that when participants were given the opportunity to behave in an unbiased manner, they did so.

Neuropsychologists that utilize the hypothesis-testing approach to neuropsychological assessment may be particularly vulnerable to this source of bias. While this approach affords the neuropsychologist the opportunity to elicit rich information relevant to the specific referral question and the unique circumstances surrounding each evaluation (Lezak, 1995), it is essential that the clinician be aware of the potential for engaging in confirmatory hypothesis testing. With an awareness of the potential for such bias and an investment in avoiding confirmatory hypothesis testing, the individualized, hypothesis-testing assessment approach retains the advantages described by Lezak (1995).

This bias, like others, becomes an ethical concern if it results in professional behavior that is incomplete or inaccurate and poses harm to the individuals served by neuropsychologists, the public at large, or the field of neuropsychology. Neuropsychologists who believe that they have observed ethical misconduct by a colleague are also susceptible to this bias if they fail to consider alternative explanations for the behavior that they have observed.

To avoid confirmatory hypothesis testing bias, the following recommendations are offered:

1. Ask questions that can both confirm and disconfirm the initial hypothesis and diagnosis (Faust, 1986).
2. Be receptive to information that appears to contradict initial impressions.
3. Generate reasons why the initial hypothesis may be incorrect (Leary & Miller, 1986).
4. In order to clarify assumptions and biases, make initial impressions explicit by writing them down (Arnoult & Anderson, 1988).

Reconstructive Memory

Reconstructive memory (Barlett, 1932) occurs when people inadvertently fill gaps in their memory or alter their memories so that they are consistent with the present experience (Loftus & Loftus, 1980; Snyder & Uranowitz, 1978; Wells, 1982). This condition is likely to occur when it seems more important to make diagnoses than to remember details of the original information. Reconstructive memory decreases the probability of recalling accurate and specific information. Individuals tend to be overconfident in the accuracy of their memories and may have the false impression that memory reconstructions represent an accurate recall of factual information (Wells, 1982).

Delays in completing clinical notes increase the probability that details of a session will be forgotten and that only information that confirms one's current hypothesis about a patient will be recalled. Thus, the use of reconstructive memory could result in inaccurate or incomplete records.

The bias inherent in reconstructive memory seems to be particularly important in the field of clinical neuropsychology due to the number of hours that are invested in a variety of professional activities often across a number of sessions. For example, behaviors observed during the initial interview or during administration of the first test may not be remembered following completion of the evaluation, particularly if the process spans a number of days and many patients are seen in the interim. Clinical case notes are vital because they are the means of documenting what transpired between the patient and the examiner (Piazza & Baruth, 1990). When providing evidence of an ethical violation perpetrated by a colleague or when defending oneself from accusations of misconduct, complete clinical notes and other documentation often provide the strongest support of one's position. The importance of maintaining current and accurate case notes has been described by Koocher and Keith-Spiegel (1998).

To avoid reconstructive memory bias, the following recommendations are offered:

1. Maintain current case notes by writing notes immediately following each session.
2 Schedule time for scoring test data, interpreting results, and writing reports immediately following completion of the evaluation.
3 Consider tape recording treatment sessions.
4. Consider videotaping cognitive remediation sessions, primarily to address the therapeutic goal of increasing a patient's awareness of his or her deficits, but also to provide documentation of a patient's performance at various points of treatment.
5. Discuss the importance of maintaining current clinical notes with colleagues and supervisors and attempt to introduce policies concerning the appropriate allotment of time for paperwork.

Addressing Ethical Misconduct of Colleagues

Neuropsychologists may, on occasion, encounter work of colleagues that raises the concern of unethical practice. Such concern may be due to disagreement with a clinical opinion in an ambiguous situation. However, the source of concern may also be due to the quality of the work and the potential for harm to patients or the reputation of neuropsychology. Determining the nature of the concern and the appropriate course of action may prove to be one of the more challenging aspects of one's role as a neuropsychologist. However, deciding whether or not to pursue a course of action may be even more challenging.

The purpose of this section of the chapter is to attempt to clarify and potentially simplify the processes involved in examining potential ethical violations of neuropsychologists, determining the best course of action, and deciding whether or not to act on the information. A recent article on this subject by Grote and colleagues (2000) provides an excellent reference. This chapter integrates the work of Grote and his colleagues with other available sources of information on this topic (e.g., ES 8, APA, 1992; Keith-Spiegel & Koocher, 1998; Minagawa, 2000; Treppa, 1998), resulting in an expanded list of recommendations. We propose the following twenty-two steps to consider when addressing potential ethical misconduct of colleagues. It is important to maintain a clear written record of the decision-making that one follows. A decision-making worksheet that was designed to facilitate this process is provided in the Appendix.

1. *Identify the problem or dilemma.* The first step in addressing potentially unethical behavior is observing that some professional behavior is inconsistent with usual and customary practices and may result in harm to an individual, an organization, or the discipline of neuropsychology.

2. *Identify the potential issues involved.* The next step is to delineate all of the relevant issues involved. The issues may be legal, professional, and moral, as well as ethical.

3. *Identify the relevant ethics codes.* In addition to the APA Ethics Code, general bioethical principles and the ethical guidelines of other organizations should be considered (American College of Physicians, 1992; Association of State and Provincial Psychology Boards, 1991; Canadian Psychological Association, 1991).

4. *Identify the relevant sections of the ethics codes.* This step is critical in that some clinical behaviors that may initially appear to be unethical may actually reflect personal philosophical differences or professional disagreement, without corresponding representation in the Ethics Code. Similarly, a given behavior may be found under the aspirational Ethical Principles rather than under the enforceable Ethical Standards.

5. *Review applicable laws and regulations.* State licensing laws provide specific requirements for the practice of psychology. State laws may mandate that a particular clinical course be followed, such as reporting child abuse. Other laws, legal decisions, and regulations may provide further guidance regarding acceptable practice parameters.

6. *Consider the context and setting.* There are situations in which unethical practice in one setting is ethical in another. For example, while it would be unethical to administer a neuropsychological screening measure to a relatively high functioning person with complaints of mild memory impairment four weeks after a sport-related concussion, administration of such a measure would represent ethical practice with many patients in acute rehabilitation settings.

7. *Consider the obligations owed.* Consider who retained the neuropsychologist and the purpose of the neuropsychological evaluation or treatment. Confidentiality issues and the nature of feedback to the patient differ in some settings and situations. For example, in military settings the results of neuropsychological evaluations may be disseminated on a "need to know" basis, without the consent of the serviceman/woman (Jaques & Folen, 1998).

8. *Identify and challenge your beliefs and values.* The field of neuropsychology is rich with controversy regarding optimal, or even acceptable, styles of practice, and those with differing points of view often feel passionately about their position and opposing positions. It is important that

one examine one's own values and beliefs and their role in creating or maintaining the dilemma. A trusted colleague may be of assistance in recognizing areas that may not be seen in oneself due to one's emotional investment in the process.

9. *Consider the significance of the violation.* Determine whether or not harm has been done or may be done in the future, either to patients or to the reputation of neuropsychology, as result of the psychologist's actions or inaction.

10. *Consider what the ethics code indicates should be done.* ES 8.04 stipulates that "When psychologists believe that there may have been an ethical violation by another psychologist, they attempt to resolve the issue by bringing it to the attention of that individual if an informal resolution appears appropriate and the intervention does not violate any confidentiality rights that may be involved." ES 8.05 further stipulates that "If an apparent ethical violation is not appropriate for informal resolution under Standard 8.04 or is not resolved properly in that fashion, psychologists take further action appropriate to the situation, unless such action conflicts with confidentiality rights in ways that cannot be resolved. Such action might include referral to state or national committees on professional ethics or to state licensing boards."
(see also, APA Standards of Practice, section H: Resolving ethical issues. Consultation, informal resolution, reporting suspected violations.)

11. *Consider the reliability and persuasiveness of the evidence of the violation.* Direct observation of objective, verifiable unethical behavior provides the strongest evidence of a violation. In contrast, evidence that is based on the report of others or that is subjective or not available for verification would carry less weight.

12. *Consider personal feelings toward the colleague.* Due to previous interactions with colleagues, personal feelings may exist toward the psychologist whose behavior is in question. The ability to remain objective toward such an individual may be limited when it is believed that that person engaged in unethical behavior, and particularly so in the adversarial context of litigation. The tendency for filing frivolous complaints intended to harm the colleague rather than minimize harm to the public may be particularly great in such situations; however, ES 8.07 specifically prohibits the filing of such complaints.

13. *Consider confidentiality issues.* APA ES 8.05 stipulates that maintaining patient confidentiality takes precedence over the responsibility to report suspected ethical violations. Obtaining informed consent from the patient prior to contacting the suspected colleague or filing a complaint would be necessary in many settings. However, in some situations, such as litigation, the patient may have waived his or her right to confidentiality as part of the proceedings. When the issue of confidentiality interferes with the ability to file a specific complaint, an anonymous complaint may be indicated in situations in which there seems to be potential for con-

siderable harm. While it may be difficult for an ethics committee to act on anonymous complaints, multiple complaints from different psychologists regarding harmful professional behavior would require action. In some situations, patients can be encouraged to file the complaints themselves.

14. *Consult written resources.* In addition to this book, a number of articles, chapters, and special volumes of journals relevant to ethical issues in neuropsychological practice have been written in the last few years (see the References sections of this book). Position papers on critical issues in neuropsychology have been written by professional organizations (e.g. the Policy and Planning Committee of the National Academy of Neuropsychology). Legal decisions and local, state, and federal laws have been established and are available for review. The numerous ethics texts that are available for general psychological practice can provide guidance for neuropsychologists as well. Also, APA has produced guidelines for general psychological practice in addition to the ethics code. Those guidelines include the following: *Guidelines for Providers of Psychological Services to Ethnic, Linguistic, and Culturally Diverse Populations* (APA, 1990), *General Guidelines for Providers of Psychological Services* (APA, 1987), *Guidelines for Ethical Conduct in the Care and Use of Animals* (APA, 1986), *Standards for Educational and Psychological Testing* (APA, 1985), and *Ethical Principles in the Conduct of Research with Human Participants* (APA, 1982).

15. *Consult others.* It is likely that few potential ethical violations will be straightforward enough and the circumstances clean enough that the best course of action will be clear. Therefore, it is important to seek the perspectives and input of knowledgeable colleagues, ethics committees, the legal department of your institution, and/or the legal department of your liability insurance carrier. Inform the colleague or legal representative that you would like to document the results of their consultation. Issues of confidentiality should be kept in mind when seeking consultation.

16. *Generate potential solutions to the problem.* In addition to identifying the problem, be prepared to suggest ways to resolve the problem. For example, if one were to contact a colleague and express concern about his or her qualifications to perform neuropsychological evaluations of individuals with multiple sclerosis, it is possible that the colleague would ask for suggestions on how to avoid making the mistakes that led to him or her being contacted. It would then be important to provide the colleague with information on how to increase their skill level with that population prior to seeing more patients with that diagnosis. Discussing the relevant heuristics involved would be of value. If the potential for harm to that individual was minimal, such an informal resolution may suffice. In addition, it is important to allow the colleague the opportunity to demonstrate that his or her behavior was ethical. Remaining open to having one's opinion changed is necessary.

17. *Consider courses of action.* ES 8.04 states that, when "appropriate", psychologists should attempt an informal resolution of the ethical violation by bringing it to the attention of the colleague. As Grote et al. (2000) suggest, "The only circumstances in which it wold be inadvisable to contact the colleague before making a report would be those rare situations in which doing so would create a risk of harm to patients or destruction of evidence" (p. 132). Initial contacts should be done in writing and delivered by registered mail.

   After attempts at informal resolution have proven unsuccessful, filing a complaint with the ethics committees of the professional organizations of which the colleague is a member or with the colleague's state regulatory board may be necessary. Complaints made to professional organizations may be sufficient to encourage the colleague to correct the unethical behavior. While some neuropsychological organizations do not have formal ethics committees, and those that do may not adjudicate cases, they will likely be able to offer advice on how to handle the situation and which organizations should be contacted. Complaints made to the state licensing board may be the most detrimental to the colleague and should be made as a last resort. Complaints should be made in writing and include copies of supporting documentation of the violation and previous attempts at resolution.

18. *Consider the potential consequences of various actions, both positive and negative.* The prospects of confronting a colleague regarding unethical behavior are daunting for a number of reasons, and one must consider those reasons when preparing for the confrontation. Potential deterrents include: (a) the possibility of facing an unpleasant interaction and creating an adversarial relationship with a colleague, (b) the fear of being counter-reported, (c) the fear of being sued for damaging the reputation or practice of the colleague, and (d) the possibility that addressing the ethical misconduct will not result in the desired changes in behavior. Nevertheless, the potential benefits of taking action to remedy unethical behavior, including minimizing harm to both patients and the public's opinion of neuropsychology, outweigh the risks. The colleague who is originally accused of unethical behavior will likely be unsuccessful with a counter-complaint unless the charges are well founded (Grote et al., 2000). Regarding litigation, while even unjustified suits can be expensive and emotionally trying, the risk of such a suit is typically minimal, and the fear of such a suit should not dissuade the neuropsychologist from reporting ethical violations (Grote et al., 2000). In addition, unless precluded by confidentiality issues, it is a violation of the ethics code if a neuropsychologist does not take appropriate action when he or she believes that another neuropsychologist has behaved unethically (Grote et al., 2000).

19. *Decide on a course of action.* Once the options for addressing the unethical behavior have been identified and discussed and the relevant issues

noted above have been considered, a decision must be made regarding which course of action to pursue. Following the steps above should provide the needed information and resources for making a sound decision; however, the ultimate responsibility for choosing a course of action or inaction falls to the observer of the ethical misconduct. Unless considerable harm is imminent, the decision should not be made quickly. The decision should also not be made in the heat of an emotional reaction to the observed unethical behavior. By considering the previous steps, the potential pitfalls of impulsive decision-making may be avoided.

20. *Implement the decision.* At this point, one should be confident that the course of action to be taken is in the best interest of the patient, other consumers of neuropsychological services, payers for neuropsychological services, the public, and/or the profession of neuropsychology.

21. *Evaluate the outcome.* Consider how the colleague responded or what steps were taken by the committee or organization that was contacted.

22. *Consider and implement alternative courses of action as needed.* Take further steps to bring the issue to a satisfactory resolution.

The following vignettes are presented to illustrate potential ethical violations that may be encountered in clinical practice. Errors in reasoning that may lead to such violations are discussed, and the process to follow to address the perceived ethical misconduct of colleagues is emphasized.

Case Illustration

Dr. A. Vail worked for a number of years on the dementia unit of a skilled nursing facility. His primary responsibilities included conducting neuropsychological screening evaluations and establishing behavior modification programs. To supplement his income, Dr. Vail decided to begin a part-time private practice. He was soon referred Mrs. Able, a 73-year-old, recently widowed, retired schoolteacher. Mrs. Able reported a recent onset of considerable cognitive difficulty. In order to examine Mrs. Able's presenting complaints, a comprehensive cognitive evaluation was performed, but no formal assessment of emotional factors was conducted. Results of the evaluation revealed moderate to severe impairment with attention, the ability to encode verbal information, word-finding ability, and speed of information processing. Dr. Vail diagnosed Mrs. Able with Dementia of the Alzheimer's Type and suggested that she move in with one of her children and begin a day treatment program for individuals with dementia.

When Mrs. Able discussed the results of her evaluation with her children, they recommended that she seek a second opinion. Dr. Leary, the second neuropsychologist, requested and reviewed the data from the cognitive testing, and conducted an assessment of Mrs. Able's mood. His findings suggested that Mrs. Able was depressed, and he recommended a combined treatment of psychotherapy and antidepressant medications. Within a few weeks, Mrs. Able reported improvement with both emotional and cognitive functioning.

Summary

Dr. Vail demonstrated bias resulting from the availability and representative heuristics, and he made a number of violations of the ethics code. Regarding the availability and representative heuristics, he relied on his primary experience with dementia patients to guide his reasoning. Since Mrs. Able met some of the criteria for dementia, Dr. Vail did not consider other diagnoses with overlapping symptoms. This reasoning may have contributed to his failure to assess Mrs. Able's mood and, thus, his diagnostic error. The significance of his error was clearly substantial. It may have resulted in increased distress for the patient, the loss of her independence, the failure to receive appropriate treatment, and possibly a hardship for her family.

Addressing the relevant heuristics

Dr. Vail would have substantially reduced his chances of making reasoning errors involving the availability and representative heuristics by considering diagnostic possibilities other than that with which he was most familiar and by considering the need to conduct a comprehensive neuropsychological examination that included measures of emotional functioning. Had he tailored his approach to this evaluation to Mrs. Able's individual needs and referred to established diagnostic guidelines, he would likely have avoided these errors in reasoning. The issue of his qualifications is discussed below.

Addressing the ethical violations

The twenty-two-step model presented above illustrates the decision-making process employed to address the ethical violations of a colleague.

The problem

Dr. Leary, having first hand knowledge of Dr. Vail's performance on this case, realized that Dr. Vail mishandled his evaluation of Mrs. Able and arrived at conclusions and recommendations that were potentially damaging to the patient and to the reputation of neuropsychology. He felt a strong responsibility to the public and to the profession to address the ethical violations of his colleague.

The potential issues involved

Dr. Leary believed that the patient was misdiagnosed, due at least in part to an incomplete evaluation. He questioned the reasoning process that led to such an evaluation. He further questioned the qualifications of a neuropsychologist that apparently did not adequately consider factors other than cognition when formulating an opinion and making recommendations.

The relevant ethics code
Dr. Leary consulted his APA membership directory and found that Dr. Vail was indeed a member of APA and, thus, subject to its ethics code. Further investigation revealed that Dr. Vail was not a member of his state psychological association nor a member of the primary neuropsychological organizations.

The relevant sections of the ethics code
In Dr. Leary's opinion, Dr. Vail violated ES 2.01(b) (Evaluation, Diagnosis, and Interventions in Professional Context), which states that "Psychologists' assessments, recommendations, reports, and psychological diagnostic or evaluative statements are based on information and techniques...sufficient to provide appropriate substantiation for their findings." In addition, it appeared that Dr. Vail violated ES 2.05 (Interpreting Assessment Results), which mandates that "When interpreting assessment results, including automated interpretations, psychologists take into account the various test factors and characteristics of the person being assessed that might affect psychologists' judgments or reduce the accuracy of their interpretations." As a result of failing to comply with ethical standards 2.01(b) and 2.05, Dr. Vail seemed to have violated EP A and ES 1.04 (Boundaries of Competence). EP A states that psychologists "recognize the boundaries of their competencies and the limits of their expertise" and "provide only those services and use only those techniques for which they are qualified by education, training, or experience." In addition, ES 1.04(b) states that "Psychologists provide services...in new areas or involving new techniques only after undertaking appropriate study, training, supervision, and/or consultation from persons who are competent in those areas or techniques."

Applicable laws and regulations
Dr. Vail was licensed for the independent practice of psychology in his state. There was no legal restriction preventing him from practicing as a neuropsychologist.

The context and setting
The context of the evaluation proved to be important. While Dr. Vail may have functioned quite efficiently in his role on the dementia unit, his ability to conduct comprehensive neuropsychological evaluations in an outpatient setting appeared to be inadequate. No special considerations, such as those involving confidentiality in some settings, were noted in the context of this case.

Obligations owed
For both clinicians involved in this case, the primary obligation was to the patient, with additional obligations to potential future patients and the reputation of neuropsychology. No special obligations were noted that would prevent pursuit of this ethical matter.

The role of one's own beliefs and values

Dr. Leary was angry about this situation for a two primary reasons. First, he was angry that Mrs. Able was misdiagnosed and would have received inappropriate treatment had her family not encouraged her to seek a second opinion. He maintains a strong belief regarding a patient's right to autonomy. He tends to be conservative regarding recommendations that would result in a reduction in a patient's autonomy and encourages aggressive treatment of factors, such as mood, that may serve to maintain one's independence. Second, he was angry that a colleague would consider himself qualified to perform such an evaluation with, at best, no recent experience working in an outpatient setting. Dr. Leary had worked hard to establish the appropriate qualifications and credentials to practice ethically as a neuropsychologist and was angry that a fellow psychologist would not see the need to do the same. In addition, he had been frustrated for years that there was no legal means of restricting the practice of neuropsychology to those demonstrating the necessary education, training, experience and, thus, skills to do so.

While considering his emotional reaction to the situation and his values and beliefs, Dr. Leary realized that Dr. Vail might have good qualifications to practice neuropsychology in some settings and with some patient populations but just not in the current context. However, he wondered about the potential for Dr. Vail to undervalue the importance of emotional factors no matter what the setting. He further realized that his longstanding frustration with the lack of licensure specific to the practice of neuropsychology was a professional issue and had little to do with Dr. Vail and the current case. Dr. Leary experienced a reduction in his anger after examining these issues, but he was no less resolved to act on the unethical behavior.

The significance of the ethical violation(s)

Dr. Leary considered the potential for harm due to continued violation of these ethical principles and standards to be substantial if not addressed. In addition, he perceived that the confidence of Mrs. Able's family in neuropsychology had been weakened as a result of Dr. Vail's work.

What the ethics code states should be done

ES 8.04 stipulates that, with consideration of the patient's confidentiality rights, Dr. Leary attempt an informal resolution of the matter by bringing his concerns to the attention of Dr. Vail. If unsatisfactorily resolved, further action, such as contacting the APA ethics committee or the state licensing board, would be indicated.

The strength of the reliability and persuasiveness of the evidence

Based on having received copies of all of the relevant records and having interviewed the patient and her family, Dr. Leary had first-hand knowledge of the situation. Thus, the evidence of ethical misconduct was reliable and persuasive.

Personal feelings toward the colleague
Dr. Leary had no prior knowledge of Dr. Vail. He remained somewhat angered that Dr. Vail had conducted such an evaluation without the appropriate skills, but he had no personal feelings toward Dr. Vail otherwise.

Confidentiality issues
Dr. Leary required Mrs. Able's consent in order to pursue the ethical misconduct with Dr. Vail. Mrs. Able gladly provided the consent.

Written resources consulted
Dr. Leary consulted the membership directories of a number of professional organizations, the APA Ethics Code (APA, 1992), and the General Guidelines for Providers of Psychological Services (APA, 1987).

Other professionals or organizations consulted
Dr. Leary contacted a local colleague who served on the ethics committee of a large teaching hospital. He then contacted the ethics committees of the APA Division of Neuropsychology (Division 40) and his state's psychological association. Dr. Leary had obtained consent from the patient to pursue this issue during their initial session. He spent a couple of days reflecting on the issues involved and consulting the written resources, mindful of the need to move quickly in order to reduce potential harm to others. His consultation with others occurred within three days of finding out about the ethical misconduct. He wrote down the names of the organizations that he contacted and individuals that he spoke with, the date and time of the contact, and their advice. All parties consulted agreed that the matter should be pursued and that an informal resolution should be attempted first.

Potential solutions to the problem
It seemed clear that Dr. Vail needed to immediately stop conducting comprehensive neuropsychological evaluations on an outpatient basis. If he wanted to pursue such work, it would be necessary for him to receive the appropriate training and supervision prior to seeing additional patients. It would be necessary for him to understand the errors in reasoning (the availability and representative heuristics) that may have contributed to his ethical misconduct. In addition, it seemed to be necessary to have him demonstrate adequate sensitivity to emotional factors in his current setting.

Possible courses of action
Dr. Leary considered attempting an informal resolution of the problem by contacting Dr. Vail directly. Due to his busy schedule and his discomfort with the prospect of confronting a colleague about ethical misconduct, he also considered filing a formal complaint with the APA ethics committee and letting them handle the matter. Although contacting the state licensing board was an option, Dr. Leary did not consider pursuing that option without filing a compliant with APA first.

Potential consequences of pursuing an informal resolution
Potential positive consequences included protecting the public and the reputation of neuropsychology and assisting a colleague with his professional development. Possible negative consequences of such action included facing a hostile response from Dr. Vail, having to file a formal complaint, receiving a counter-complaint, and facing a lawsuit.

The chosen course of action
Dr. Leary understood his responsibility to pursue a resolution of the problem. He did not believe that the matter warranted directly contacting the APA ethics committee or the state licensing board as the first step. Therefore, he chose to contact Dr. Vail directly, in writing. He believed that he could raise his concerns in a sensitive, helpful manner that would have a good chance of being accepted by an open-minded colleague.

The timing of the action
Dr. Leary chose to write the letter immediately upon making his decision.

The outcome
As it turned out, Dr. Vail was receptive to the feedback. He replied in writing that he was well trained as a neuropsychologist but that he had subsequently become specialized in working with individuals with advanced dementia in residential settings. He indicated that Mrs. Able had been the first patient that he had seen on an outpatient basis, and he acknowledged that he might have made errors in the evaluation. He agreed to follow the suggestions offered by Dr. Leary and even asked Dr. Leary if he would provide the supervision.

Alternative courses of action
The informal resolution was successful; thus, there was no need for an alternative course of action.

Vignette Summary
This vignette, while presenting an ideal resolution, illustrates ethical violations that may be encountered in the practice of clinical neuropsychology and demonstrates how the decision-making model can be applied to them. Although many situations will be more complex and more difficult to resolve, this vignette was designed to provide clarification of relevant issues, as well as guidance regarding the process to follow when addressing ethical violations of colleagues.

Summary

Deciding whether or not to confront the ethical misconduct of a colleague may be one of the most unsettling processes that a neuropsychologist can experience in professional practice. There are many reasons for that difficulty, including uncertainty about the occurrence or nature of the behavior, personal feelings toward the colleague, fear of retaliation, and uncertainty about the process involved in addressing the ethical misconduct of a colleague. The purpose of this chapter was to clarify the process through which one may go when addressing an ethical violation, thereby reducing some of the apprehension that one may experience when considering the best course of action to take when faced with concerning professional conduct by another neuropsychologist. By considering inferential biases and following the proposed decision-making model, neuropsychologists will be in a good position to determine and pursue a satisfactory course of action.

References

American College of Physicians (1992). American College of Physicians ethics manual (3rd ed.). *Annals of Internal Medicine, 117*, 947-960.

American Psychological Association (1982). *Ethical principles in the conduct of research with human participants.* Washington, DC: American Psychological Association.

American Psychological Association (1985). *Standards for educational and psychological testing.* Washington, DC: American Psychological Association.

American Psychological Association (1986). *Guidelines for ethical conduct in the care and use of animals.* Washington, DC: American Psychological Association.

American Psychological Association (1987). *General guidelines for providers of psychological services.* Washington, DC: American Psychological Association.

American Psychological Association (1990). *Guidelines for providers of psychological services to ethnic, linguistic, and culturally diverse populations.* Washington, DC: American Psychological Association.

American Psychological Association (1992). Ethical principles of psychologists and code of conduct. *American Psychologist, 47*, 1597-1611.

Arkes, H.R. (1981). Impediments to accurate clinical judgment and variable ways to minimize their impact. *Journal of Consulting and Clinical Psychology, 49*, 323-330.

Arnoult, L.H., & Anderson, C.A. (1988). Identifying and reducing causal reasoning biases in clinical practice. In M.R. Leary & R. S. Miller (Eds.), *Social psychology and dysfunctional behavior: Origins, diagnosis, and treatment* (pp. 209-232). New York: Springer-Verlag.

Association of State and Provincial Psychology Boards (1991). *ASPPB code of conduct.* Montgomery, AL: Association of State and Provincial Psychology Boards.

Barlett, F.C. (1932). *Remembering.* Cambridge, England: Cambridge University Press.

Batson, C.D. (1975). Attribution as a mediator of bias in helping. *Journal of Personality and Social Psychology, 32*, 455-466.

Batson, C.D., O'Quin, K., & Pych, V. (1982). An attribution theory analysis of trained helpers' inferences about patients' needs. In T.A. Wills (Ed.), *Basic processes in helping relationships* (pp. 59-80). New York: Academic Press.

Bishop, J.B., & Richards, T.F. (1984). Counselor theoretical orientation as related to intake judgments. *Journal of Counseling Psychology, 31*, 398-401.

Brown, B.R. (1970). Experienced and inexperienced counselor's first impressions of patient and case outcomes: Are first impressions lasting? *Journal of Counseling Psychology, 17,* 550-558.

Bush, S., & Coben, R. (1997). Optimal environmental stimulation during acute brain injury rehabilitation. *Archives of Clinical Neuropsychology, 13,* 69 [abstract].

Canadian Psychological Association (1991). *Canadian code of ethics for psychologists* (Rev. ed.). Ottawa, ON: Canadian Psychological Association.

Cantor, N., & Mischel, W. (1979). Prototypes in person perception. In L. Berkowitz (Ed.), *Advances in experimental social psychology,* Vol. 9 (pp. 4-52). New York: Academic Press.

Cantor, N., Smith, E., French, R., & Mezzich, J. (1980). Psychiatric diagnosis as prototype categorization. *Journal of Abnormal Psychology, 80,* 181-193.

Chapman, L.J., & Chapman, J.P. (1969). Illusory correlation as an obstacle to the use of valid psychodiagnostic signs. *Journal of Abnormal Psychology, 74,* 271-280.

Dallas, M.E., & Baron, R.S. (1985). Do counselors use a confirmatory strategy during interviewing? *Journal of Social and Clinical Psychology, 3,* 106-122.

Darley, J.M., & Gross, P.H. (1983). A hypothesis-confirming bias in labeling effects. *Journal of Personality and Social Psychology, 44,* 20-33.

Dawes, R.M. (1982). The value of being explicit when making clinical decisions. In T.A. Wills (Ed.), *Basic processes in helping relationships* (pp. 37-58). New York: Academic Press.

Faust, D. (1986). Research on human judgment and its application to clinical practice. *Professional Psychology: Research and Practice, 17,* 420-430.

Fischoff, B. (1982). Debiasing. In D. Kahneman, P. Slovic, & A. Tversky (Eds.). *Judgment under uncertainty: Heuristics and biases* (pp. 424-444). Cambridge, England: Cambridge University Press.

Friedlander, M.L., & Phillips, S.D. (1984). Preventing anchoring errors in clinical judgment. *Journal of Consulting and Clinical Psychology, 52,* 366-371.

Friedlander, M.L., & Stockman, S.J. (1983). Anchoring and publicity effects in clinical judgment. *Journal of Clinical Psychology, 39,* 337-371.

Grosz, H.J., & Grossman, K.G. (1964). The sources of observer variation and bias in clinical judgments: 1. The item of psychiatric history. *Journal of Nervous and Mental Disease, 138,* 105-113.

Grote, C.L., Lewin, J.L., Sweet, J.J., & van Gorp, W.G. (2000). Responses to perceived unethical practices in clinical neuropsychology: Ethical and legal considerations. *The Clinical Neuropsychologist, 14,* 119-134.

Higgins, E.T., & King, G.A. (1981). Accessibility of social constructs: Information-processing consequences of individual and contextual variability. In N. Cantor & J.F. Kihlstrom (Eds.), *Personality, cognition and social interaction* (pp. 69-121). Hillsdale, NJ: Erlbaum.

Hollon, S.D., & Kriss, M.R. (1984). Cognitive factors in clinical research and practice. *Clinical Psychology Review, 4,* 35-76.

Jaques, L.H., & Folen, R. (1998). Confidentiality and the military. In R.M. Anderson, Jr., T.L. Needles, & H.V. Hall (Eds.), *Avoiding ethical misconduct in psychology specialty areas.* Springfield, IL: Charles C. Thomas Publisher, Ltd.

Jones, E.E., & Nisbett, R.E. (1971). *The actor and the observer: Divergent perceptions of the causes of behavior.* New York: General Learning Press.

Kahneman, D., & Tversky, A. (1973). On the psychology of prediction. *Psychological Review, 80,* 237-251.

Keith-Spiegel, P., & Koocher, G.P. (1998). How to confront an unethical colleague. In G.P. Koocher, J.C. Norcross, & S.S. Hill (Eds.), *Psychologists' desk reference.* New York: Oxford University Press.

Koocher, G.P., & Keith-Spiegel, P. (1998). *Ethics in psychology: Professional standards and cases* (2nd ed.). New York: Oxford.

Kruglanski, A.W., & Ajzen, I. (1983). Bias and error in human judgment. *European Journal of Social Psychology, 19*, 448-468.

Langer, E.J., & Abelson, R.P. (1974). A patient by any other name.....: Clinician group difference in labeling bias. *Journal of Consulting and Clinical Psychology, 42*, 4-9.

Leary, M.R., & Miller, R.S. (1986). Clinical inferences. In M.R. Leary & R.S. Miller (Eds.), *Social psychology and dysfunctional behavior: Origins, diagnosis, and treatment.* New York: Springer-Verlag.

Lezak, M.D. (1995). *Neuropsychological assessment* (3rd ed.). New York: Oxford.

Lichtenberg, J.W. (1984). Believing when facts don't fit. *Journal of Counseling and Development, 63*, 10-11.

Loftus, E.F., & Loftus, G.R. (1980). On the permanence of stored information in the human brain. *American Psychologist, 35*, 409-420.

Mahoney, M. (1977). Publication prejudices: An experimental study of confirmatory bias in the peer review system. *Cognitive Therapy and Research, 1*, 161-175.

Meehl, P.E. (1954). *Clinical versus statistical prediction: A theoretical analysis and review of the evidence.* Minneapolis: University of Minnesota Press.

Minagawa, R. (2000). *Laws, ethics, and risk management.* Workshop conducted at the 20th annual conference of the National Academy of Neuropsychology, Orlando, FL.

Morrow, K.A., & Deidan, C.T. (1992). Bias in the counseling process: How to recognize and avoid it. *Journal of Counseling and Development, 70*, 571-577.

Nisbett, R.E., & Ross, L. (1980). *Human inference: Strategies and shortcomings of social judgment.* Englewood Cliffs, NJ: Prentice-Hall.

Pepinsky, H.B., & Pepinsky, P. (1954). *Counseling theory and practice.* New York: Ronald Press.

Piazza, N.J., & Baruth, N.E. (1990). Patient record guidelines. *Journal of Counseling and Development, 68*, 313-316.

Rosenhan, D.L. (1973). On being sane in insane places. *Science, 179*, 250-258.

Ross, L. (1977). The intuitive psychologist and his shortcomings: Distortions in the attribution process. In L. Berkowitz (Ed.), *Advances in Experimental Social Psychology, Vol 10.* New York: Academic Press.

Routh, D.K., & King, K.M. (1972). Social class bias in clinical judgment. *Journal of Consulting and Clinical Psychology, 38*, 202-207.

Sharf, R.R., & Bishop, J.B. (1979). Counselors' feelings toward patients as related to intake judgments and outcome variables. *Journal of Counseling Psychology, 26*, 267-269.

Snyder, C.R. (1977). "A patient by any other name" revisited: Maladjustment or attributional locus of problem? *Journal of Consulting and Clinical Psychology, 45*, 101-103.

Snyder, M., & Campbell, B.H. (1980). Testing hypotheses about people: The role of the hypothesis. *Personality and Social Psychology Bulletin, 6*, 421-426.

Snyder, M., & Uranowitz, S.W. (1978). Reconstructing the past: Some cognitive consequences of person perception. *Journal of Personality and Social Psychology, 36*, 941-950.

Strohmer, D.C., & Chiodo, A.L. (1984). Counselor hypothesis testing strategies: The role of initial impressions and self-schema. *Journal of Counseling Psychology, 31*, 510-519.

Strohmer, D.C., & Newman, L.J. (1983). Counselor hypothesis-testing strategies. *Journal of Counseling Psychology, 30*, 557-565.

Strupp, H.H. (1958). The psychotherapist's contribution to the treatment process. *Behavior Science, 3*, 34-67.

Sweet, J., & Moulthrop, M. (1999). Self-examination questions as a means of identifying bias in adversarial assessment. *Journal of Forensic Neuropsychology, 1,* 74-88.

Taylor, S.E., & Fiske, S.T. (1978). Salience, attention, and attribution: Top of the head phenomena. In L. Berkowitz (Ed.), *Advances in Experimental and Social Psychology,* Vol. 11 (pp. 249-288). New York: Academic Press.

Temerlin, M.K. (1968). Suggestion effects in psychiatric diagnosis. *Journal of Nervous and Mental Disease, 147,* 349-353.

Treppa, J.A. (1998). A practitioner's guide to ethical decision-making. In R.M. Anderson, Jr., T.L. Needles, & H.V. Hall (Eds.), *Avoiding ethical misconduct in psychology specialty areas.* Springfield, IL: Charles C. Thomas Publisher, Ltd.

Trope, Y., & Bassok, M. (1982). Confirmatory and diagnosing strategies in social information gathering. *Journal of Personality and Social Psychology, 22,* 33-40.

Turk, D.C., & Salovey, P. (1985). Cognitive structures, cognitive processes, and cognitive behavior modification: II. Judgments and inferences of the clinician. *Cognitive Therapy and Research, 9,* 19-33.

Tversky, A., & Kahneman, D. (1971). Belief in the law of small numbers. *Psychological Bulletin, 76,* 105-110.

Wells, G.L. (1982). Attribution and reconstructive memory. *Journal of Experimental Social Psychology, 18,* 447-463.

Wiggins, J.S. (1981). Clinical and statistical prediction: Where are we and where do we go from here? *Clinical Psychology Review, 1,* 3-18.

Appendix — Worksheet for Addressing the Ethical Misconduct of Colleagues

1. What is the problem or dilemma? ───────────────
───────────────────────────────────────

2. What are the potential issues involved? ───────────
───────────────────────────────────────

3. What is the relevant ethics code? ─────────────
───────────────────────────────────────

4. What are the relevant sections of the ethics code? ──────────
───────────────────────────────────────

5. What are the applicable laws and regulations and what do they indicate?
───────────────────────────────────────

6. What is the significance of the context and setting? ────────────
───────────────────────────────────────

7. What are the obligations owed? ───────────────
───────────────────────────────────────

8. What is the role of your beliefs and values? ────────────
───────────────────────────────────────

9. What is the significance of the violation? ────────────
───────────────────────────────────────

10. What does the ethics code say should be done? ──────────
───────────────────────────────────────

11. How strong is the reliability and persuasiveness of the evidence of the violation? ───────────────────────
───────────────────────────────────────

   Describe: ──────────────────────
───────────────────────────────────────

12. Have you considered your personal feelings toward the colleague? ─
───────────────────────────────────────

13. What are the confidentiality issues? ──────────────
───────────────────────────────────────

14. Which written resources have been consulted? ───────────
───────────────────────────────────────

15. Which other professionals or organizations have been consulted? When? What was suggested? ———————————————————

———————————————————————————————

16. What are potential solutions to the problem? ———————————

———————————————————————————————

17. What are possible courses of action? ———————————————

———————————————————————————————

18. What are the potential consequences of various actions?
   Positive: ——————————————————————————

———————————————————————————————

   Negative: ————————————————————————————

———————————————————————————————

19. Which course of action was chosen? ———————————————

———————————————————————————————

20. When will the decision be implemented? ————————————

———————————————————————————————

21. What was the outcome? ———————————————————

———————————————————————————————

22. Is there a need to consider and implement alternative courses of action? ————————————————————————

———————————————————————————————

   If so, describe: ——————————————————————

———————————————————————————————

Notes:

AFTERWORD

Abigail B. Sivan

Ethical Issues in Clinical Neuropsychology affords the seasoned practitioner as well as the beginner a broad sampling of research and commentary on the ethical dilemmas involved in the clinical practice of Neuropsychology. The carefully crafted vignettes allow the reader to apply these concepts to a myriad of situations confronting practicing clinical neuropsychologists. Each chapter offers a rare view into the actual practice of Neuropsychology and the examples highlight an oft-quoted observation at Ethics Committee meetings that good clinical practice is good ethical practice.

At first glance, it might appear unfortunate that this well-conceived volume predates a new Ethics Code (APA, 2001), currently being developed and scheduled to go into effect in 2003. In its current formulation, the proposed code includes a set of five general principles — Beneficence and nonmaleficence; Fidelity and responsibility; Integrity; Justice; and Respect for people's rights and dignity — that are aspirational. The enforceable part of the code consists of a set of ethical standards, organized into ten categories — Resolving ethical issues; Competence; Human relations; Privacy and confidentiality; Advertising and other public representations; Record keeping and fees; Education & training; Research and publication; Assessment; and Therapy — each of which includes enforceable rules for the conduct of the ethical psychologist.

Upon further examination, it is clear that *Ethical Issues in Clinical Neuropsychology* can easily illuminate a new code as well as the 1992 Code (APA, 1992). The discerning reader of *Ethical Issues in Clinical Neuropsychology* should have no difficulty translating between the 1992 and the proposed ethics code. Similarly, the authors will have little difficulty updating their chapters for the second edition.

References

American Psychological Association (June 24, 2001). *APA Ethics Code*, Draft 5.
American Psychological Association (1992). Ethical Principles of Psychologists and Code of Conduct. *American Psychologist,47,* 1597-1611.

AFTERWORD

ABOUT THE
EDITORS AND
CONTRIBUTORS

Shane Bush, Ph.D., ABPP-RP, ABPN, is the Director of Neuropsychological Services at the St. Johnland Head Injury Rehabilitation Center and is in private practice in Long Island, NY. He is a Clinical Assistant Professor of Pharmacy in the College of Pharmacy and Health Sciences of Long Island University. In addition, he is a neuropsychologist in the U.S. Naval Reserves. He received a master's degree from the University of Georgia and received his doctorate from the California School of Professional Psychology-Berkeley/ Alameda. He completed his internship at Yale University School of Medicine and received his postdoctoral neuropsychology fellowship training at Bacharach Institute for Rehabilitation. He is board certified in Neuropsychology by the American Board of Professional Neuropsychology and board certified in Rehabilitation Psychology by the American Board of Professional Psychology. He is a member of the Ethics Committee of the Division of Neuropsychology of the American Psychological Association and is a member of the Social and Ethical Responsibility Committee of the Division of Rehabilitation Psychology of the American Psychological Association. He is a member of New York State Psychological Association's Committee on Ethical Practice. He is a member of the Education Committee of the National Academy of Neuropsychology and is the editor of the Grand Rounds section of the NAN Bulletin. He has presented research on ethical issues in neuropsychology and rehabilitation at the Annual Conferences of the National Academy of Neuropsychology and the American Psychological Association.

Michael L. Drexler, Ph.D., was recently appointed the Director of Geropsychology at the Department of Veterans' Affairs Medical Center in San Francisco, after having been the Director of the Neuropsychology Service and Administrative Program Director of the Psychosocial Inpatient Units at Laguna Honda Hospital and Rehabilitation Center in San Francisco for more than 10 years. In addition, he is Assistant Clinical Instructor of Neurology at UCSF/Mt. Zion Campus, an Instructor in Geriatric Neuropsychology for the UC Berkeley Extension, and an Adjunct Professor of Neuropsychology and Neuropsychological Assessment at the California School of Professional Psychology, Berkeley/Alameda, and The Wright Institute in Berkeley. He is Consulting Neuropsychologist at the Morton Bakar Geropsychiatric and Neurobehavioral Center in Hayward, California, and at Geriatric Services of San Francisco. He is Past-Chair of the Education Committee and a Fellow of the National Academy of Neuropsychology.

Robert M. Anderson Jr., Ph.D., is a professor at the American School of Professional Psychology — Hawaii Campus. He holds a doctorate in philosophy from the University of Minnesota and a doctorate in psychology from the University of Hawaii. He is the author of *Practitioner's Guide to Clinical Neuropsychology* and coeditor of *Avoiding Ethical Misconduct in Psychology Specialty Areas*.

Jeffrey T. Barth, Ph.D., ABPP-CN, presently holds the position of professor and chief of the Division of Medical Psychology and of the Neuropsychology Center in the Department of Psychiatric Medicine, with a joint appointment in the Department of Neurological Surgery at the University of Virginia Medical School. Dr. Barth received his Bachelor's degree from Vanderbilt University in 1971 and his doctoral degree in psychology in 1976 from the George Peabody College of Vanderbilt University. He completed his internship in 1977 at the Ft. Logan Mental Health Center in Denver, Colorado and was awarded a two year post doctoral fellowship in clinical neuropsychology at the University of Virginia Medical School. He holds the diplomate certification in Clinical Neuropsychology from the American Board of Professional Psychology and is board certified at the diplomate level in medical psychotherapy, behavioral medicine, and disability analyses. He is a fellow of the American Psychological Association and the National Academy of Neuropsychology and has received several distinguished teaching awards. Dr. Barth is past president of the National Academy of Neuropsychology, past president of the Virginia Psychological Association and holds the emeritus distinction of the Virginia Psychological Foundation. He is on the editorial board of seven scientific journals, co-chief editor of *Advances in Medical Psychotherapy and Psychodiagnosis*, and has co-authored two books (including *The Halstead–Reitan Neuropsychological Battery: Guide to Interpretation and Clinical Application*) and over one hundred scholarly articles and book chapters. He is recognized nationally and internationally for his research on the neuropsychological sequelae of mild head trauma and he has been involved as a co-investigator and consultant on 22 funded research grants. In 1992 he was awarded the John Edward Fowler Professorship in Clinical Psychology, an endowed chair in the Eminent Scholars Program.

Bruce Becker, Ph.D., ABPP-CN, CL, is in private practice. He earned a Ph.D. in Clinical Psychology at Loyola University, Chicago, and moved almost immediately into neuropsychology, spending three years in a neurology hospital, seeing neurology patients exclusively and absorbing training in neuropsychology, neuroanatomy, neuropathology, and EEG, as well as clinical neurology. After being awarded board certification in clinical psychology by ABPP he became Director of Clinical Psychology Training for the U.S. Navy, also maintaining an active neuropsychology laboratory at the Bethesda Naval hospital, holding adjunct/clinical faculty positions at three medical schools and five graduate schools and publishing more than a dozen articles or book chapters. He was awarded board certification in clinical neuropsychology in 1984 by ABPP (ABCN). He was an invited delegate to the Houston Conference, served six years on the Division 40 Ethics Committee, three as chair, and four years on the Maryland Psychological Association Ethics Committee, two as chair. He is a fellow of the American Psychological Association.

Cecilia Theresa Deidan, Ph.D., has a practice in Pembroke Pines, Fl, dealing with the assessment, intervention and treatment of various psychological and organic concerns affecting younger and older adults ranging from adjustment disorders to memory concerns, anxiety, depression, and brain injury. She received a B.A. in Psychology, a B.A. in Biology, and a B.A. Spanish from St. Louis University in 1985. In 1997 she earned her Masters in Counseling Psychology from the University of Missouri-Columbia, Missouri, and in 1992 she received her Ph.D. in Counseling Psychology. In 1993, she completed a postdoctoral fellowship in Adult and Geriatric Neuropsychology at the University of Miami School of Medicine and Mount Sinai Medical Center in Miami Beach, Florida.

Eileen B. Fennell, Ph.D., ABPP-CN, is a Professor in the Departments of Clinical and Health Psychology and Neurology of the University of Florida, Gainesville. She also serves as the Co-Director of the University of Florida Center for Neuropsychological Studies and is a faculty member of the University of Florida Brain Institute. She has authored or co-authored over 50 refereed articles, 10 book chapters and one book, *Pediatric Neuropsychology in a Medical Setting*. Dr. Fennell has served on a number of Boards and Committees of professional organizations in the field of clinical neuropsychology including Division 40 of APA, the National Academy of Neuropsychology, the American Board of Clinical Neuropsychology and the Board of Trustees of the American Board of Professional Psychology. She was elected President of Division 40 for 1996–1997. She is Board Certified in Clinical Neuropsychology by the American Board of Professional Psychology and continues to teach, see patients and supervise graduate students at the University of Florida where she is Director of the Specialty Track in Clinical Neuropsychology in the Department.

Jerid M. Fisher, Ph.D., ABPN, has been a private consultant in the field of neuropsychology since 1993. He received his bachelor's degree from Duke University in 1975 and his doctoral degree in clinical psychology in 1981 from The University of Rochester. He completed postdoctoral fellowships in the Departments of Psychiatry (Psychology) and Neurology at the University of Rochester's Strong Memorial Hospital. After receiving his Ph.D., Dr. Fisher served on the faculty of Psychiatry (Psychology) and Neurology at Strong Hospital for several years before becoming a Program Director and Developer of inpatient brain injury rehabilitation programs for New Medico Associates. In 1986 he founded Neurorehab Associates, Inc., and developed outpatient and inpatient brain injury rehabilitation centers in freestanding and hospital settings. He holds Diplomate certification from the American Board of Professional Neuropsychology and is a fellow of The National Academy of Neuropsycholgy. Dr. Fisher coauthored *The Practice of Forensic Neuropsychology*. He has also authored or coauthored scholarly articles and book chapters.

Chris Grote, Ph.D., ABPP-CN, is a neuropsychologist at Rush-Presbyterian-St. Luke's Medical Center and is the executive director of the Midwest Neuropsychology Group. He received his doctorate from the University of Louisville. He is board certified in neuropsychology through ABPP/ABCN. He has published on ethics and other topics. He is currently chair of the Division 40 Practice Advisory Committee.

Ruben C. Gur, Ph.D., ABPP-CN, is a Professor of Psychology in Psychiatry, Neurology and Radiology at the University of Pennsylvania. He is the Director of the Brain Behavior Laboratory in the Department of Psychiatry at the Hospital of the University of Pennsylvania. Dr. Gur received his B.A. from Hebrew University in Jerusalem and his M.A. and Ph.D. from Michigan State University. He completed a postdoctoral fellowship at Stanford University. He is board certified in Clinical Neuropsychology by the American Board of Professional Psychology. He is a fellow of the National Academy of Neuropsychology, the American Psychological Association (Divisions 6 and 30), and the American Psychological Society. Dr. Gur is a member of the Ethics Committee of the American College of Neuropsychopharmacology. He has published numerous articles in the areas of neurology, psychiatry, and neuropsychology.

Josette G. Harris, Ph.D., is an Assistant Professor in the Departments of Psychiatry and Neurology at the University of Colorado School of Medicine and is the Executive Director of National Academy of Neuropsychology. She is also Post-Doctoral Training Faculty with the Developmental Psychobiology Research Group at the University of Colorado School of Medicine. She received her B.A. in Psychology from Texas Tech University and both her M.A. and Ph.D. in Psychology from the University of Denver. She completed internships at Denver General Hospital and Denver Veterans Administration Hospital. She completed a postdoctoral fellowship in Neuropsychology (Center for Neuroscience and Schizophrenia; Developmental Psychobiology Research Group; Neuropsychology Laboratory) at the University of Colorado School of Medicine. She has numerous awards, presentations, publications, and research grants based on her work with cross-cultural factors in neuropsychology.

Doug Johnson-Greene, Ph.D., ABPP-CL, RP, is Director of Neuropsychological Services and Assistant Professor of Physical Medicine and Rehabilitation at the Johns Hopkins University School of Medicine. He is a 1993 graduate of the University of Mississippi. He completed his internship at the Portland VA & Oregon Health Sciences University and his residency in neuropsychology and neuroimaging at the University of Michigan. He is a Diplomate of the American Board of Professional Psychology in the areas of Clinical and Rehabilitation psychology. In addition to being an active investigator, teacher, and clinician in the areas of clinical, rehabilitation, and neuropsychology, he has served on numerous editorial boards and committees for professional societies such as the International Neuropsychological Society and American Psychological Association, including an appointment as a Board Member of the Division 40 (neuropsychology) Ethics Committee. Among his accolades is a recent appointment to the Board of Psychologists in Maryland by the Governor. An author of over 60 articles, book chapters, reviews, and abstracts, Dr. Johnson-Greene continues to conduct research and obtain grant funding to examine ethics in medical settings, effects of alcohol abuse, cerebrovascular disease, and assessment of premorbid abilities.

A. John McSweeny, Ph.D., ABPP-CN, is Professor of Psychiatry and Neurology, and Director of the Neuropsychology Laboratory, at the Medical College of Ohio (MCO). He received his Ph.D. in clinical psychology from Northern Illinois University in 1975. He completed his clinical psychology internship at Baylor College of Medicine in Houston, Texas and a post-doctoral fellowship in methodology and evaluation research at Northwestern University in Evanston, Illinois. He was a member of the faculties at Northwestern University and West Virginia University before coming to MCO. Dr. McSweeny is a Diplomate in Clinical Neuropsychology of the American Board of Professional Psychology and a Fellow of the American Psychological Association and the National Academy of Neuropsychology. He served on the APA Division 40 Ethics Committee from 1992 to 2000 and chaired the Committee from 1993–1996. Dr. McSweeny has conducted research on several topics in neuropsychology for 25 years and is the author of multiple research articles and the co-editor of two books.

Paul Moberg, Ph.D., ABPP-CN, is an Associate Professor of Neuropsychology in the Departments of Psychiatry and Otorhinolaryngology: Head and Neck Surgery at the University of Pennsylvania School of Medicine. He is the Director of Clinical Services for the Brain-Behavior Laboratory. He received his B.A. in Psychology from Augsburg College in Minneapolis, Minnesota in 1982 and his M.A. in Clinical Psychology from Loyola College in Baltimore, Maryland in 1985. He received his initial training in Neuropsychology at the Johns Hopkins University School of Medicine in Baltimore and subsequently obtained his Ph.D. in Clinical Psychology (1990) from the University of Health Sciences/The Chicago Medical School in North Chicago, Illinois. Dr. Moberg completed his Predoctoral internship at the University of Florida in Gainesville with an emphasis in Neuropsychology. He subsequently completed Postdoctoral training in Neuropsychology at the same institution. Dr. Moberg is board certified in Clinical Neuropsychology by the American Board of Professional Psychology.

Joel E. Morgan, Ph.D., ABPP-CN, practices clinical neuropsychology in New Jersey and is an Assistant Professor in the Department of Neurosciences at UMDNJ-New Jersey Medical School. For nearly 20 years he was Director of

Neuropsychology and Director of Training at the Department of Veterans Affairs Medical Center in East Orange, New Jersey. Dr. Morgan recently retired from the VA system to devote full time to private practice, supervision and teaching, and myriad professional activities in clinical neuropsychology. Dr. Morgan is board certified in clinical neuropsychology by the American Board of Clinical Neuropsychology/American Board of Professional Psychology. He is a Fellow of the National Academy of Neuropsychology (NAN) and an Accreditation Site Visitor for the Committee on Accreditation of the American Psychological Association (APA). Dr. Morgan devotes a good deal of time to APA, and serves as the Editor of Division 40's Newsletter, *Newsletter40,* as well as many committee assignments, including the Division 40 Program Committee for the APA Annual Convention. He is also the President of the Association for Internship Training in Clinical Neuropsychology (AITCN), which represents neuropsychology specialty track internships at the division level of APA. Dr. Morgan recently completed NAN's *DistanCE* Program on *Ethics in Neuropsychology.* Dr. Morgan does a good deal of forensic neuropsychology in his private practice.

Ann Mary Palozzi, Psy.D., works with the Craine Institute of Neuropsychology and Rehabilitation and with the State of Hawaii Department of Education. She received her B.S. and M.Ed. from the University of Maine, Orono and her doctorate from the American School of Professional Psychology— Hawaii Campus. She was formerly a special education teacher who specialized in learning disabilities.

Albert 'Skip' Rizzo, Ph.D., has joint faculty appointments with the University of Southern California Integrated Media Systems Center (IMSC) and the USC School of Gerontology. Skip is also the director of the IMSC Virtual Environments Lab, which designs, develops and evaluates the usefulness/feasibility/ efficacy of Virtual Reality systems targeting the assessment and rehabilitation of spatial abilities, attention, and other cognitive functions. Additionally, he is conducting research on computerized facial recognition, facial avatar animation, VR applications that use 360 Degree Panoramic video for exposure therapy (social phobia) and role playing applications (anger management), and is involved in designing better human-computer interface systems for the elderly and persons with disabilities. He has recently been funded to direct the testing and evaluation research component at the USC Institute of Creative Technology on VR applications that will incorporate artificially intelligent agents (virtual human representations) that will serve as characters within U.S. Army peacekeeping mission rehearsal training scenarios. His interest in Virtual Reality and cognitive processes stems from his previous clinical work in neuropsychological assessment and rehabilitation with clients having acquired brain injuries. He feels that an ideally suited match exists for VR applications in the neuropsychological assessment and rehabilitation areas, and has presented and published numerous papers in these areas. He is the associate editor of the journal, *CyberPsychology and Behavior*; and is also on the editorial boards of *Presence: Teleoperators and Virtual Environments*, *The International Journal of Virtual Reality*, and *Cognitive Technology*, and is the creator of the Virtual Reality Mental Health Email Listserver (VRPSYCH). He has also recently guest-edited a theme issue of the MIT journal *Presence: Teleoperators and Virtual Environments* on 'Virtual Reality and Neuropsychology' to appear in August 2001. He received his Ph.D. in Clinical Psychology from the State University of New York at Binghamton.

Barbara Olasov Rothbaum, Ph.D., is a tenured associate professor in psychiatry at the Emory School of Medicine in the Department of Psychiatry and Behavioral Sciences and director of the Trauma and Anxiety Recovery Program at Emory. She received her Ph.D. in clinical psychology in 1986. Dr. Rothbaum specializes in research on the treatment of individuals with anxiety disorders, particularly focusing on exposure therapy. She has won both state and national awards for her research, is an invited speaker internationally, authors scientific papers and chapters, has published 2 books, and received the Diplomate in Behavioral Psychology from the American Board of Professional Psychology. She is currently Associate Editor of *Journal of Traumatic Stress* and on the Editorial Board for the journal *CyberPsychology and Behavior*. Dr. Rothbaum is co-founder with Dr. Larry Hodges, a Georgia Tech computer scientist, of Virtually Better, Inc., and together they have pioneered the application of virtual reality to the treatment of psychological disorders. Two patents have been granted, and they have received approximately $1,000,000 in research funding for this application of virtual reality.

Maria T. Schultheis, Ph.D., is a Clinical Research Scientist in the Neuropsychology and Neuroscience Laboratory at KMRREC and an Assistant Professor in the Department of Physical Medicine and Rehabilitation at the University of Medicine and Dentistry of New Jersey-New Jersey Medical School. She received her B.S. in Biological Sciences from Rutgers, The State University of New Jersey; received her M.A. in Biological Sciences, with a specialization in Neurobiology, from Temple University; and completed her Ph.D. in Clinical Psychology, with a specialization in Neuropsychology, from Drexel University. During her graduate training her work was recognized by awards from the National Academy of Neuropsychology and the Philadelphia Neuropsychological Society. She was a National Institutes of Health Postdoctoral Fellow at Kessler Medical Rehabilitation Research and Education Corporation (KMRREC), West Orange, NJ. Her clinical and research experiences have focused on the rehabilitation of cognitively impaired populations, with primary emphasis on studying driving capacity following neurological injury and developing new driving assessment protocols. Her research has focused on the application of new technologies, such as Virtual Reality, to neuropsychological assessment and treatment and has been funded by such organizations as the National Institutes of Health, the National Multiple Sclerosis Society, and the National

Institute on Disability and Rehabilitation Research. She has published and presented in the area of neuropsychological assessment and rehabilitation. Dr. Schultheis is active in several professional organizations related to neuropsychology and rehabilitation and serves on the Transportation Research Board of the National Research Council. She also serves as an Editorial Consultant to the *Journal of Head Trauma Rehabilitation*, *Rehabilitation Psychology*, and *Archives of Physical Medicine and Rehabilitation*.

Abigail Sivan, Ph.D., is in independent practice in Chicago, IL. She received her AB degree from Oberlin College, and her M.A. and Ph.D. from New York University where she specialized in Educational Research and worked with Leonard Diller at Rusk Rehabilitation Institute on her dissertation research. While teaching at Michigan State University, she continued her education in Clinical Psychology. From 1975–1981, Dr. Sivan lived in Israel where she worked with Y. Ben-Yishay at the Rehabilitation Division of the IDF, directed the Kibbutz Child Development Center, taught at several medical schools, and did research with A. Carmon at the Brain Behavior Research Unit at Hadassah/Hebrew University Hospital. After returning to the U.S. in 1981, Dr. Sivan completed her internship with Nils Varney at the VAMC in Iowa City where she also researched the applicability of adult neuropsychological measures to normal and special children. Between 1983 and 1987, she was the staff psychologist on a multidisciplinary team at the Child Development Clinic at the Division of Developmental Disabilities at the University of Iowa. Between 1988 and 1999, Dr. Sivan worked as a pediatric neuropsychologist in the Section of Child Psychiatry at Rush Presbyterian St. Luke's Medical Center, Chicago. After two years at Evanston Northwestern Healthcare in January, 2001, she entered private practice in Chicago where she maintains an appointment as a Clinical Associate Professor at Northwestern University Department of Psychiatry. Her research has focused on neuropsychological test development for children and adults. Dr. Sivan served on the Iowa Board of Psychology Examiners (1985–1987) and most recently on the APA Ethics Committee (1999–2001) and the APA Ethics Code Task Force (2000–2001). In 1994, she consulted with the U.N. Commission on War Crimes in the former Yugoslavia.

Jerry J. Sweet, Ph.D., ABPP-CN, CL, is Director of the Neuropsychology Service at Evanston Northwestern Healthcare, Evanston, IL. He is Professor of Psychiatry and Behavioral Sciences at Northwestern University Medical School, and is board certified in clinical neuropsychology and clinical psychology by the American Board of Professional Psychology. He is presently on the Board of Directors of the American Academy of Clinical Neuropsychology. He is a Fellow of the Division of Clinical Neuropsychology (Division 40) and the Division of Clinical Psychology (Division 12) of the American Psychological Association and is also a Fellow of the National Academy of Neuropsychology. He served on the Ethics Committee of the Illinois Psychological Association for four years. Dr. Sweet edited the textbook *Forensic Neuropsychology: Fundamentals and Practice*, co-authored *Psychological Assessment in Medical Settings* and co-edited *Handbook of Clinical Psychology in Medical Settings*. He has authored and co-authored numerous book chapters and peer-reviewed research studies. He is founding Associate Editor of *Journal of Clinical Psychology in Medical Settings*, and presently serves on the editorial boards of *The Clinical Neuropsychologist, Archives of Clinical Neuropsychology, Journal of Forensic Neuropsychology, and Journal of Clinical Psychology*.

Dennis P. Swiercinsky, Ph.D., ABPN, created Brain Training, a treatment program for persons with traumatic brain injury in Kansas City in 1983. Brain Training offers a range of basic cognitive remediation, vocational retraining, and family educational and support components. He conducted that program until 1997 when he relocated to San Francisco to direct a neurobehavioral treatment program in a long-term care facility for persons with severe impairments. Prior to entering private practice in Kansas City in 1981 he served for five years as a merit reviewed researcher–practitioner for the Veterans Administration Medical Center in Topeka, Kansas. Dr. Swiercinsky received his doctorate in rehabilitation psychology from the University of Kansas in 1974. He is a diplomate of the American Board of Professional Neuropsychology. He now resides in Portland, Oregon, and is completing a book on brain injury rehabilitation for patients and families and continues an active consultant role with Bay Area Psychological Testing Associates for neuropsychological assessment development.

Laetitia L. Thompson, Ph.D., ABPP-CN, is an associate professor in the departments of psychiatry and neurology and she is the Director of the UCHSC Neuropsychology Laboratory. She obtained her Ph.D. in clinical psychology from the University of Kansas in 1980. Her postdoctoral fellowship in clinical neuropsychology was completed at the University of Oklahoma Health Sciences Center in 1983. She then joined the faculty at the University of Colorado School of Medicine and has remained there since. She is board certified in Clinical Neuropsychology by the American Board of Professional Psychology. She is a Fellow of the National Academy of Neuropsychology and was Treasurer of NAN from 1998 to 2000. She has had an interest in ethical issues for a number of years. She co-authored with Dr. Laurence Binder one of the first articles relating the 1992 APA Ethics Code to neuropsychological assessment, published in the *Archives of Clinical Neuropsychology* in 1995. She also served on the APA Division 40 Ethics Committee from 1995 to 1999.

Wilfred G. van Gorp, Ph.D., ABPP-CN, is Associate Professor of Psychology in Psychiatry at the Weill Medical College of Cornell University and Associate Attending Psychologist at the Memorial Sloan Kettering Cancer

Center. He currently serves as Director of the Neuropsychology Program in the Department of Psychiatry of Cornell University. Dr. van Gorp is a Fellow of the American Psychological Association (Division 40) and a diplomate in Clinical Neuropsychology from the American Board of Professional Psychology. He has served on the Executive Committee of Division 40 of the American Psychological Association for the past 6 years. Dr. van Gorp is currently President of the American Academy of Clinical Neuropsychology and is a member of the Board of Governors of the International Neuropsychological Society. He is Editor of the *Journal of Clinical and Experimental Neuropsychology*, and sits on the editorial boards of the *Journal of the International Neuropsychological Society* and *The Clinical Neuropsychologist*. Dr. van Gorp also serves as Chair of the Committee on Psychological Tests and Assessment of the American Psychological Association. He has authored over 120 peer-reviewed research papers, book chapters, and books.

Elisabeth Wilde, Ph.D., received her doctorate in clinical psychology with a focus in neuropsychology from Brigham Young University. She completed an internship in neuropsychology at the Ann Arbor VA Medical Center and is completing her postdoctoral fellowship in neuropsychology at the University of Michigan. She is a member of NAN, INS, and APA division 40. She has previously published on competency issues in older, cognitively-impaired patients. Her current research interests include functional neuroimaging, dementia, and cognitive changes in normal aging.

Paul Root Wolpe, Ph.D., is a Senior Fellow of the Center of Bioethics at the University of Pennsylvania, where he holds appointments in the Department of Psychiatry and the Department of Sociology. He is the Director of the Program in Psychiatry and Ethics at Penn, and is also a Senior Fellow of the Leonard Davis Institute for Health Economics. Dr. Wolpe also serves as the first Chief of Bioethics (Care and Protection of Research Subjects and Patients) for the National Aeronautics and Space Administration (NASA). The office is responsible for safeguarding the protections of research subjects and astronauts both within NASA and among our international space partners. Dr. Wolpe received his Ph.D. from Yale University in 1987 in Medical Sociology, funded by an NIMH traineeship in Mental Health Services Research and Evaluation. He has served as the Director of the Project of Informed Consent at the Center for Bioethics, and is Principle Investigator of a project exploring the ethical issues of psychiatric research, as well as an ongoing project exploring the emerging ethical issues in Neuroimaging and Cognitive Neuroscience. He has published numerous articles/chapters on ethics and psychology.

Penelope Zeifert, Ph.D., is a Clinical Assistant Professor in the Department of Neurology and Neurological Sciences at Stanford University Medical Center. She serves as Director of the Neuropsychology Service, and Co-Director of the Stanford Memory Clinic. She is also Chief Psychologist on the Behavioral Medicine Units at Stanford. Dr. Zeifert currently serves as the Education Chair of the National Academy of Neuropsychology. Areas of specialization include post-encephalitic cognitive sequelae, epilepsy, dementia, mood disorders, and the evaluation and management of complex neuropsychiatric conditions.

CONTRIBUTORS
ADDRESS LIST

Robert M. Anderson, Jr., Ph.D.
PO Box 61446
Honolulu, HI 96839-1446
(808) 595-4964
rma@pixi.com

Jeffery T. Barth, Ph.D.
John Edward Fowler Professor
Chief, Medical Psychology/
Neuropsychology
University of Virginia, School of
Medicine
Psychiatric Medicine
Box 203, HSC
Charlottesville, VA 22908-0002
(804) 924-2718
jtb4y@virginia.edu

Bruce Becker, Ph.D.
9508 Newbold Place
Bethesda, MD 20817
(301) 365-9109
neuropsybb@aol.com

Shane S. Bush, Ph.D.
26 Pembrook Drive
Stony Brook, NY 11790
(631) 334-7884
sbushphdnp@medscape.com

Cecilia T. Deidan, Ph.D.
18459 Pines Blvd. #324
Pembroke Pines, FL 33029
(954) 430-7772 ctdphd@aol.com

Michael L. Drexler, Ph.D.
1705 11th Avenue
San Francisco, CA 94122
(415) 759-6158
michaeldrexler@netscape.net

Eileen B. Fennell, Ph.D.
Professor
Department of Clinical & Health
Psychology
Box 100165 HSC
Gainesville, FL 32610
(352) 395-0680 x. 46893
efennell@hp.ufl.edu

Jerid M. Fisher, Ph.D.
12 Brigden Lane
Pittsford, NY 14534
(716) 425-4771
beaucoup93@aol.com

Doug Johnson-Greene, Ph.D.
Assistant Prof. & Director of Neu-
ropsychological Services
Dept. Physical Medicine and
Rehabilitation
Johns Hopkins University School of
Medicine
Good Samaritan, POB Suite 406
5601 Lock Raven Blvd.
Baltimore, MD 21239
(410) 532-4700
FAX: (410) 532-4770
johnsong@jhmi.edu

Christopher Grote, Ph.D.
Rush Presbyterian – St. Luke's Medical Center
Department of Psychology
1653 W. Congress Parkway
Chicago, IL 60612
(312) 942-5932
cgrote@rush.edu

Ruben C. Gur, Ph.D.
University of Pennsylvania / Psychology
36th & Spruce St.
10th Floor, Gates Pavillion
Philadelphia, PA 19104-4283
(215) 662-2915
gur@bblmail.psycha.upenn.edu

Josette G. Harris, Ph.D.
University of Colorado School of
Medicine

4200 E. 9th Avenue
Denver, CO 80220-3706
(303) 315-4610
josette.harris@uchsc.edu

A. John McSweeny, Ph.D.
Medical College of Ohio
Department of Psychiatry
3120 Glendale Avenue
Toledo, OH 43614-5809
(419) 383-5695
jmcsweeny@mco.edu

Paul J. Moberg, Ph.D.
Hospital of the University of Pennsylvania
Brain-Behavior Lab., Dept. of Psychiatry
10th Floor Gates Bldg.
3400 Spruce St.
Philadelphia, PA 19104
(215) 615-3608
moberg@bbl.med.upenn.edu

Joel E. Morgan, Ph.D.
Assistant Professor of Neurosciences
UMDNJ-New Jersey Medical School
49 Greenwood Drive
Millburn, NJ 07041
(973)-921-2889
joelmor@comcast.net

Richard I. Naugle, Ph.D.
Department of Psychology and Psychiatry
Cleveland Clinic Foundation
9500 Euclid Avenue (P57)
Cleveland, OH 44195-0001
(216) 444-7748
naugler@ccf.org

Ann Mary Palozzi, Psy.D.
Kailua Medical Arts Building
407 Uluniu Street, Suite 112

Kailua, Hawaii
(808) 261-1624
annpalozzi@att.net

Albert 'Skip' Rizzo, Ph.D.
Research Assistant Professor Integrated Media Systems Center and School of Gerontology
University of Southern California
3715 McClintock Ave. MC-0191
Los Angeles, CA 90089-0191
(213) 740-9819
arizzo@usc.edu

Barbara O. Rothbaum, Ph.D.
Associate Professor in Psychiatry
Director, Trauma and Anxiety Recovery Program
Emory University School of Medicine
1365 Clifton Rd., NE
Atlanta, GA 30322
(404) 778-3875
brothba@emory.edu

Maria T. Schultheis, Ph.D.
Kessler Medical Rehabilitation Research & Education Corporation
1199 Pleasant Valley Way
W. Orange, NJ 07052
(973) 731-3600 x. 2270
mschultheis@kmrrec.org

Abigail B. Sivan, Ph.D.
P.O. Box 605
Glenview, IL 60025-0605
(847) 730-3100
a-sivan@nwu.edu

Jerry J. Sweet, Ph.D.
Evanston Northwestern Healthcare
500 Davis St., 8th floor
Evanston, IL 60201
(847) 425-6445
j-sweet@northwestern.edu

Dennis P. Swiercinsky, Ph.D.
PO Box 1726
Portland, OR 97207-1726
(503) 450-0599
FAX: (413) 228-5950
denswier@earthlink.net

Laetitia L. Thompson, Ph.D.
University of Colorado Health
Sciences Center Neuropsychology
Lab
4200 E. 9th Avenue, #C268-29
Denver, CO 80220
(303) 315-2511
FAX: (303) 315-2527
laetitia.thompson@uchsc.edu

Wilfred G. van Gorp, Ph.D.
NY Hospital Cornell Medical
Center
Psychiatry Department
525 East 68th Street
Box 140
New York, NY 10021
(212) 821-0596
wvangorp@mail.med.cornell.edu

Elisabeth A. Wilde, Ph.D.
University of Michigan
Division of Neuropsychology
C-480 Med Inn Bldg., Box 0840
1500 E. Medical Center Drive
Ann Arbor, MI 48109
(734) 936-9277
ewilde@med.umich.edu

Paul Root Wolpe, Ph.D.
University of Pennsylvania
Center for Bioethics
3401 Market St., Suite 320
Philadelphia PA 19104
(215) 898-7136
wolpep@mail.med.upenn.edu

Penelope Zeifert, Ph.D.
Stanford University School of Medicine
Neurology Department, Room
A343
300 Pasteur Drive
Stanford, CA 94305-5235
Penelope.zeifert@stanford.medcenter
.edu

SUBJECT INDEX

AUTHOR INDEX